Challenging Neuropathic Pain Syndromes

Challenging Neuropathic Pain Syndromes

Evaluation and Evidence-Based Treatment

MITCHELL K. FREEDMAN, DO
Associate Professor
Physical Medicine and Rehabilitation
Thomas Jefferson University Hospital;
Director
Physical Medicine and Rehabilitation
Rothman Institute
Philadelphia, PA, United States

JEFFREY A. GEHRET, DO
Attending Physician
Rehabilitation Medicine
Rothman Institute;
Clinical Assistant Professor of Rehabilitation
Medicine
Sidney Kimmel Medical College
Philadelphia, PA, United States

GEORGE W. YOUNG, DO
Attending Physician
Physical Medicine and Rehabilitation
Rothman Institute;
Clinical Instructor
Sydney Kimmel Medical College at
Thomas Jefferson University
Department of Rehabilitation Medicine
Philadelphia, PA, United States

LEONARD B. KAMEN, DO
Clinical Director
MossRehab Outpatient Center
Einstein Hospital;
Clinical Associate Professor
Physical Medicine and Rehabilitation
Temple University Hospital
Philadelphia, PA, United States

ELSEVIER

ELSEVIER

3251 Riverport Lane
St. Louis, Missouri 63043

Content Strategist: Kayla Wolfe
Content Development Manager: Taylor Ball
Project Manager: Deepthi Unni
Designer: Gopalakrishnan Venkatraman

Printed in United States of America

Last digit is the print number: 9 8 7 6 5 4 3 2 1

Working together
to grow libraries in
developing countries

www.elsevier.com • www.bookaid.org

This book is dedicated to the memory of Dr Lisa Marino, who led her life as a courageous and exemplary physician and associate. Those of us who have had the privilege of knowing Lisa, strive to emulate her intelligent and caring approach to treating patients with painful syndromes. You will be remembered by us all Lisa.

Contributors

Nazish Ahmad, MD
Endocrinology Fellow
Department of Endocrinology
Thomas Jefferson University Hospital
Philadelphia, PA, United states

John M. Barbis, MA, PT
Clinical Assistant Professor
Physical Therapy
Thomas Jefferson University
Philadelphia, PA, United States

Mitchell J. Cohen, MD
Professor of Psychiatry Human Behavior
Vice Chair for Education
Director
Pain Medicine Program
Department of Psychiatry and Human Behavior
Sidney Kimmel Medical College at Thomas Jefferson
    University
Philadelphia, PA, United States

Houman Danesh, MD
Director of Integrative Pain Management
Department of Anesthesiology, Perioperative and Pain
    Medicine
Icahn School of Medicine at Mount Sinai Hospital
New York, NY, United States

Madhuri Dholakia, MD
Clinical Assistant Professor of Rehabilitation Medicine
Sidney Kimmel Medical College at Thomas Jefferson
    University
Philadelphia, PA, United States

Natacha Falcon, DO
The Rothman Institute
Thomas Jefferson University
Philadelphia, PA, United States

Renae Fisher, MD
Sidney Kimmel Medical College at Thomas Jefferson
    University
Philadelphia, PA, United States
PGY-1 Transitional Year Resident
Mercy Catholic Medical Center
Darby, PA, United States

Mitchell K. Freedman, DO
Associate Professor
Physical Medicine and Rehabilitation
Thomas Jefferson University Hospital;
Director
Physical Medicine and Rehabilitation
Rothman Institute
Philadelphia, PA, United States

Jeffrey A. Gehret, DO
Attending Physician
Rehabilitation Medicine
Rothman Institute;
Clinical Assistant Professor of Rehabilitation Medicine
Rehabilitation Medicine
Sidney Kimmel Medical College
Philadelphia, PA, United States

Ari C. Greis, DO
Clinical Assistant Professor
Department of Rehabilitation Medicine
Sydney Kimmel Medical College at Thomas Jefferson
    University
Clinical Assitant Professor
Department of Physical Medicine and Rehabilitation
Rothman Institute
Thomas Jefferson University
Philadelphia, PA, United States

Tulasi Gude, MD
Clinical Instructor
Department of Physical Medicine and Rehabilitation
Sidney Kimmel Medical College at Thomas Jefferson
    University
Philadelphia, PA, United States

Shivani Gupta, DO
Department of Rehabilitation Medicine
Sydney Kimmel Medical College at Thomas Jefferson
    University
Philadelphia, PA, United States

Kimberly Heckert, MD
Assistant Professor
Department of Physical Medicine and Rehabilitation
Sidney Kimmel Medical College at Thomas Jefferson
    University
Philadelphia, PA, United States

Victor Hsu, MD
Professor of Medicine
Department of Medicine
Harvard Medical School
Brigham and Women's Hospital
Boston, MA, United States

William C. Jangro, DO
Assistant Professor of Psychiatry and Human Behavior
Associate Director
Adult Residency Training Program
Department of Psychiatry and Human Behavior
Sidney Kimmel Medical College at Thomas Jefferson
    University
Philadelphia, PA, United States

Leonard B. Kamen, DO
Clinical Director
MossRehab Outpatient Center
Einstein Hospital;
Clinical Associate Professor
Physical Medicine and Rehabilitation
Temple University Hospital
Philadelphia, PA, United States

Mary S. Keszler, MD
Fellow
Physical Medicine and Rehabilitation
Amputation Rehabilitation
University of Washington
Seattle, WA, United States

Yury Khelemsky, MD
Program Director
Pain Medicine Fellowship
Department of Anesthesiology, Perioperative and Pain
    Medicine
Icahn School of Medicine at Mount Sinai Hospital
New York, NY, United States

Brian T. Kucer, MD
Assistant Professor of Rehabilitation Medicine
Sidney Kimmel Medical School at Thomas Jefferson
    University
Magee Rehabilitation Hospital
Philadelphia, PA, United States

Mendel Kupfer, MD
Assistant Professor Sidney Kimmel Medical College at
    Thomas Jefferson University
Magee Rehabilitation Hospital
Philadelphia, PA, United States

Priyanca B. Magdalia, DO
Sydney Kimmel Medical College at Thomas Jefferson
    University
Department of Physical Medicine and Rehabilitation
Philadelphia, PA, United States

Santiago M. Mazuera-Mejia, MD
Neurologist
Clinical Appointment in Headache Medicine at
    The Sandra and Malcolm Berman Brain & Spine
    Institute;
Clinical Appointment in Department of Neurology
Sinai Hospital
Baltimore, MD, Unites States

Michael J. Mehnert, MD
Attending Physician
Physical Medicine and Rehabilitation
Rothman Institute;
Clinical Instructor
Department of Rehabilitation Medicine
Sydney Kimmel Medical College of Thomas Jefferson
    University
Philadelphia, PA, United States

David Neckman, MD
Resident
Anesthesiology
Department of Anesthesiology, Perioperative and Pain
    Medicine
Icahn School of Medicine at Mount Sinai Hospital
New York, NY, United States

Daniel Neff, MD
PGY-3 Psychiatry Resident
Department of Psychiatry and Human Behavior
Thomas Jefferson University Hospital
Philadelphia, PA, United States

Harla O'Donnell, DO
Department of Rehabilitation Medicine
Thomas Jefferson University
Philadelphia, PA, United States

Jason Pan, MD
Resident Physician
Physical Medicine & Rehabilitation
University of Pennsylvania
Philadelphia, PA, United States

Ziva Petrin, MD
Resident, Physical Medicine and Rehabilitation
Sidney Kimmel Medical College at Thomas Jefferson
    University
Philadelphia, PA, United States

Michael Saulino, MD, PhD
Physiatrist
PMR
MossRehab
Elkins Park, PA, United States
Assistant Professor
Rehabilitation Medicine
Thomas Jefferson University
Philadelphia, PA, United States

Saloni Sharma, MD
Attending Physician
Rothman Institute;
Clinical Assistant Professor of Rehabilitation
    Medicine
Sidney Kimmel Medical College, Thomas Jefferson
    University Hospital
Philadelphia, PA

Eric Shiffrin, MD
Endocrinology Fellow
Department of Endocrinology
Thomas Jefferson University Hospital
Philadelphia, PA, United States

Jeremy Simon, MD
Division Chief
Department of Physical Medicine and Rehabilitation
Rothman Institute;
Assistant Professor of Rehabilitation Medicine
Sidney Kimmel Medical College at Thomas Jefferson
    University
Philadelphia, PA, United States

Anupam Sinha, DO
Department of Rehabilitation Medicine
Clinical Assistant Professor, Thomas Jefferson
    University
Associate Physician, Rothman Institute
Philadelphia, PA, United States

Nicole M. Spare, DO
Clinical Assistant Professor
Clinical Appointment in the Department of Neurology;
Academic Appointment in the Department of
    Rehabilitation Medicine
Thomas Jefferson University
Jefferson Headache Center
Philadelphia, PA, United States

Dave Stolzenberg, DO
Attending Physician
Physical Medicine and Rehabilitation
Rothman Institute Orthopaedics;
Clinical Assistant Professor
Rehabilitation Medicine
Sidney Kimmel Medical College
Thomas Jefferson University
Philadelphia, PA, United States

Fatima Z. Syed, MD
Chair, ACP CRFM
Fellow
Thomas Jefferson University Hospital
Philadelphia, PA, United States

Sanya Thobani, MD
Endocrinology Fellow
Department of Endocrinology
Thomas Jefferson University Hospital
Philadelphia, PA, United States

John M. Vasudevan, MD
Assistant Professor
Physical Medicine & Rehabilitation
University of Pennsylvania
Philadelphia, PA, United States

Stanley Yoo, MD
Attending Physician
Physical Medicine and Rehabilitation
Moss Rehab
Elkins Park, PA, United States

George W. Young, DO
Attending Physician
Physical Medicine and Rehabilitation
Rothman Institute;
Clinical Instructor
Department of Rehabilitation Medicine
Sydney Kimmel Medical College at Thomas Jefferson
    University
Philadelphia, PA, United States

Elina Zakin, MD
Chief Resident
Department of Neurology
Icahn School of Medicine at Mount Sinai Hospital
New York, NY, United States

Allison Zibelli, MD
Division Director
Regional Cancer Care
Jefferson Kimmel Cancer Center
Philadelphia, PA, United States

Contents

CHAPTER 1

Pathophysiology of Pain

MITCHELL J. COHEN, MD • WILLIAM C. JANGRO, DO • DANIEL NEFF, MD

INTRODUCTION

Pain is defined by the International Association for the Study of Pain as "an unpleasant sensory and emotional experience associated with actual or potential tissue damage, or described in terms of such damage."[1] It is a complex multidimensional concept that includes a sensory component, assessment of that sensory component, and perception and cognitive appraisal to determine whether or not the sensation is associated with suffering, and pain behaviors initiated in response to the unpleasant sensation. Pain serves a protective function in alerting a person to tissue damage or threats to bodily integrity and survival. However, the pathways that convey pain from body surface and organs to brain are subject to modulation at multiple levels, which can alter sensitivity and reactivity of the pain pathways over time. Genetics, internal metabolic factors, emotional states, and ambient variables, such as temperature and barometric pressure, all impact these built-in modulatory mechanisms. As a result of this wired-in capacity for modulation, also called *plasticity*, of the peripheral and central pain pathways, these mechanisms are acted upon by factors internal and external to individuals. Plasticity can dampen or intensify pain across time. Therefore, pain intensity experienced by a particular individual suffering from disease or injury, can vary greatly over time. Plasticity also leads to significant differences in pain intensity experienced across individuals suffering similar illness or injury and between experimental subjects exposed to the same standardized pressure, chemical, heat, or cold stimuli. In certain unfortunate patients, somatosensory signaling can be modulated at the spinal and supraspinal levels to create chronic pain states with much more intense pain levels and suffering than usually seen in association with similar injuries or diseases.

NOCICEPTION VERSUS PAIN

Somatosensation is the physiologic result of transduction of a physical stimulus into a neural signal that activates afferent pathways resulting in the sensations of touch (mechanoreception), temperature (thermosensation), and pain (nociception). Noxious stimuli activate neural pathways that convey signals that ultimately lead to pain perception. Nociception refers to the neural processes *associated* with pain, as distinguished from the unpleasant sensory and emotional experience that *is* pain. *Nociceptors* are primary afferent neurons activated by noxious stimuli. Nociceptors have free nerve endings in the periphery, cell bodies located in the dorsal root ganglia, and axons that make first-order synapses with spinal cord cells. Conversion of noxious peripheral stimuli (physical or chemical) into electrical energy (action potential) is called *transduction*. Transduction occurs in the free nerve endings of nociceptors and makes possible communication of peripheral noxious stimulation to the central nervous system. *Transmission* is the receipt (from nociceptors) and communication through spinal cord cells to higher brain centers. Communication to supraspinal centers starts when the primary (first-order) afferents or nociceptors synapse with second-order central transmission cells in the dorsal horn of the spinal cord. These second-order cells are part of ascending pathways that convey stimuli transduced by nociceptors to the brainstem, thalamus, limbic structures, and finally to neocortex. Psychological, metabolic, and ambient factors can trigger *modulation* of aspects of nociception from spinal through cortical levels. The end result of pain transmission is conscious *experience* of pain as a multidimensional experience involving emotional, sensory-discriminative, and behavioral components.[2]

In the sections that follow, we describe each of the aforementioned aspects of ascending pain signaling from periphery to brain pain processing, including afferent mechanisms such as transduction, central transmission through spinal pathways, and brain areas activated by these pathways. The discussion of ascending pathways is followed by a description of the top-down or descending modulation of pain signals from brain to periphery.

Aβ fibers
- Fastest, large diameter, and heavily myelinated
- Usually transmit sensations of light touch, pressure, or hair movement
- Conduction velocity: 35–90 m/s
- Diameter 6–12 μm

C-fibers
- Nociceptive
- Predominant type of afferent fibers in peripheral nerves
- Associated with delayed, prolonged burning sensation
- Unmyelinated
- Smallest fibers, diameter 0.2–1.5
- Conduction less than 2 m/s

Aδ fibers
- Nociceptive
- Thinly myelinated
- Activation evokes sharp, intense, or tingling sensation
- Smallest fibers, diameter 1–5 μm
- Conduction velocity: 5–40 m/s

PERIPHERAL MECHANISMS

Nociception, somatosensation involving noxious stimuli, begins with transduction at free nerve endings and activation of primary peripheral afferent fibers. Cell bodies of these peripheral afferents as mentioned are located in the dorsal root ganglia. These fibers can be grouped into three classes with distinct behaviors and conduction velocities (see Box 1.1).[3] Nociceptors include the smallest fibers Aδ- and C-fibers. Their stimulation can cause a dual pain sensation as that seen with an intense brief heat stimulus.[4] Aδ-fibers, which conduct faster than C fibers, transmit the first pain sensation, which is felt as a prickling pain of rapid onset. The second pain sensation, transmitted by slower C-fibers, is a delayed aching or burning sensation. In addition to being classified based on conduction velocity, nociceptors can be further subclassified based on molecules expressed on their cell surface, molecules they store and release, and enzymes they contain. Noxious stimuli must be converted to chemical and electrical signals, however, before they can be propagated along Aδ- and C-fibers.

For noxious stimuli to travel from the periphery to the brain, it first has to be encoded into signals appropriate for the architecture of the nervous system. Transduction is this process of encoding touch, temperature, pressure, and other stimuli in the periphery into electrochemical signals. The free nerve endings of primary afferent fibers directly carry out this transduction function, with multiple factors functioning to modulate pain transduction.

One of the most important modulators of pain transduction is the microenvironment and chemical milieu in which it occurs. In the setting of tissue injury, inflammation contributes many potent modulators. Factors such as bradykinin, serotonin, and histamine all have dual roles in initiating the inflammatory response to tissue injury as well as mediating pain.[5–8] Other cell-derived factors such as eicosanoids (arachidonic acid derivatives, including prostaglandins, thromboxanes, and leukotrienes) also act directly on nociceptors in potentiating pain.[9] Further inflammatory contributors to peripheral modulation include cytokines such as tumor necrosis factor α that act to sensitize nociceptors. Compensatory mechanisms balance these factors and dampen pain transduction and nociceptor sensitization. Afferent fibers upregulate opioid receptors in the setting of inflammation.[10] γ-Amino-butyric acid (GABA) may affect transduction differently depending on local factors, increasing or decreasing transduction.[11] Somatostatin also helps counteract excessive cytokine activity. Acetylcholine acting at muscarinic receptors can desensitize C-fibers.[12] After stimulus transduction, primary nociceptive afferents from the body surface synapse with spinal cord transmission cells in the dorsal horn while those from the face make their first synapse in the spinal trigeminal nucleus.

SPINAL MECHANISMS: THE DORSAL HORN

Primary somatosensory afferent fibers, whether conveying painful or nonpainful stimuli, terminate in the spinal cord dorsal horn on the same side of the body as their origin. The dorsal horn is anatomically organized in the form of layers of laminae (Rexed laminae).[13] Afferent C-fibers terminate primarily in the most superficial laminae (I and II), Aδ-fibers terminate in laminae I and III-V, and nonpain larger Aβ-fibers terminate in laminae III-V.

Second-order nociceptive spinal and spinal trigeminal projection neurons include *wide-dynamic-range* (WDR) neurons and *nociceptive-specific* (NS) neurons.[14] WDR cells are concentrated in deeper laminae (III-IV) and receive somatosensory input from Aβ-, Aδ-, and C-fibers and are activated by both noxious and innocuous stimuli. WDR cells produce a graded response from mild nonpainful sensation at low stimulation of

Aβ-fibers to intense pain at high levels of stimulation. NS neurons are located in the more superficial laminae I and II and do not exhibit such graded activation. NS cells fire only after noxious stimuli exceed a high threshold. Axons of WDR and NS second-order neurons cross the midline close to the spinal level where primary afferents synapse with spinal cord transmission cells. They gather into bundles in the contralateral, anterolateral quadrant of the spinal cord and then ascend as the spinothalamic tract (STT) toward targets in the brainstem, diencephalon, and cortex.

Noxious input at the spinal level can be modulated by neurotransmitters released in the spinal cord as well as descending inputs to the dorsal horn from the brainstem. Central sensitization is a special type of spinal modulation that is involved in the development and maintenance of chronic pain states.[15] It occurs when a noxious stimuli of sufficient intensity and duration increases the firing frequency and intensity of spinal neurons for a given stimulus. An example of this is the phenomenon of *wind-up*, caused by persistent nociceptive signals from C-fibers into the dorsal horn spinal transmission cells. The barrage of C-fiber transmission to WDR cord cells provokes central sensitization, characterized by an increased WDR firing, allodynia (experience of pain from typically innocuous stimuli), and hyperalgesia (painful stimulus perceived as more painful than in it would be in healthy states).

ASCENDING PAIN TRANSMISSION: SPINAL PATHWAYS AND SUPRASPINAL MECHANISMS

The STT is the major ascending pain pathway in the spinal cord conveying noxious, painful information to higher centers. The STT is located in the anterolateral region of the spinal cord. The STT has two components, a lateral and medial pathway. The lateral pathway encodes for the sensory-discriminative aspect of pain perception (see Box 1.2), that is, the nature and bodily location of the noxious stimulus. The medial pathway conveys no spatial information or features of the noxious stimulus. It encodes for the motivational-affective component of pain perception; that is, it creates the conscious emotional urgency to focus on and contain the pain.[16]

Some nonpainful sensory information travels with the STT in the anterolateral quadrant of the spinal cord, but most nonpainful stimuli are transmitted through the dorsal columns and ultimately activate the dorsomedial nucleus gracilis, for information from the upper extremities, and the dorsolateral nucleus cuneatus, for

---

BOX 1.2
Multidimensional Systems Related to Processing Nociceptive Stimuli

Sensory-discriminative
- Sense of the intensity, location, quality, and duration of the pain

Motivational-affective
- Unpleasantness and urge to escape the unpleasantness

Cognitive-evaluative
- Cognitions such as appraisal, cultural values, distraction, and hypnotic suggestion

---

the lower extremities. The dorsal column pathways do not cross sides at the level of the first-order synapse in the dorsal horn as opposed to the STT fibers. The dorsal columns, instead, carry nonpainful sensory input up to the brainstem and nucleus cuneatus and nucleus gracilis where they cross the midline to form the medial lemniscus.

The STT ascends to the brainstem, the diencephalon, and various cortical sites that are involved with somatosensory processing at the supraspinal level.[17] Some fibers from the STT and parallel pathways in the anterolateral cord activate spinal projection neurons that terminate in brainstem and midbrain nuclei. Brainstem sites include those that regulate autonomic functions (cardiovascular and respiratory) and contribute to autonomic changes in respiratory rate, pulse, and blood pressure seen in individuals in pain. Midbrain sites include those that affect descending and ascending modulation of painful and nonpainful transmission. The midbrain parabrachial nucleus projects to the amygdaloid nucleus in the temporal lobes, contributing to fear and emotional arousal associated with pain. The output from the brainstem reticular activating system projects diffusely to the cortex and increases general alertness and attentional focus on pain. Other STT fibers pass through the brainstem and midbrain to terminate in diencephalic structures including the hypothalamus. Hypothalamic activation leads to neuroendocrine changes associated with pain, such as the increased release of corticotropin-releasing hormone and increased blood levels of cortisol, the last a biological marker of physical and emotional stress.

At the level of the thalamus, STT fibers terminate in the *ventral posterior lateral nucleus* (VPL) and *ventral posterior medial nucleus* (VPM). The VPL primarily receives input from the body surface, whereas the VPM receives major input from the face. Third-order projections from the VPL and VPM project to the limbic lobe, neocortex, and prefrontal cortex. Some of these projections are highly organized and specific, whereas others are diffuse. Neurons from the core of the VPL project to somatosensory cortical areas SI and SII and the insular cortex. Medial thalamic nuclei project to the anterior cingulate cortex. These cortical areas, primary and secondary somatosensory cortices (areas SI and SII), insular cortex, anterior cingulate cortex, and medial prefrontal cortex have been shown to be activated in a wide range of human pain states.[18] These areas play roles in different aspects of pain. For example, activation of the cingulate cortex and medial prefrontal cortex contributes to the emotional dimension of pain, whereas the insular cortex may help focus cognitive-analytic processes on pain.[19] At the same time, these brain regions are robustly and reciprocally interconnected. Together they integrate and regulate pain intensity, affective reactions, and cognitive appraisal of the seriousness of pain.[20] Dynamic brain imaging techniques, including positron emission tomography, magnetoencephalography, and functional magnetic resonance imaging, have revealed this interconnectedness and clear sequential activation of these brain regions during human pain.[21] As such, these areas are among the most prominent components of the brain's "pain matrix." Human pain, like human consciousness, is not associated with a single brain region but relies upon connectivity and activation of multiple cortical and subcortical structures.

DESCENDING MODULATION: SPINAL PATHWAYS AND SUPRASPINAL PERIAQUEDUCTAL GRAY

Supraspinal descending modulation of nociception can have inhibitory and facilitatory effects on primary afferent neurons in the dorsal horn. Descending modulation can have varied effects on pain transmission, from attenuation of acute pain to the development of chronic pain states (i.e., central sensitization). The *periaqueductal gray* (PAG) and *rostral ventromedial medullary* (RVM) pathways are well-characterized supraspinal components of descending modulation.[22] They receive descending projections from cortical and limbic regions of the brain's pain matrix. The PAG projects to the RVM, which sends either inhibitory or excitatory impulses to spinal NS and WDR neurons in the dorsal horn. The RVM facilitates inhibitory or excitatory effects in the dorsal horn via "ON" and "OFF" cells.[23] "OFF" cells are tonically active except during nociceptive input and are required for descending inhibition and are activated by analgesics like morphine. "ON" cells become more active during nociceptive input, tending

to enhance pain signaling. The activation of "ON" cells and inhibition of "OFF" cells has been implicated in chronic pain states.

Various neurotransmitters are involved in descending modulation. Glycine is the predominant inhibitory neurotransmitter in the spinal cord, whereas GABA predominates at higher central nervous system levels. GABA neurotransmission is a target for clinical intervention at the $GABA_A$ ionotropic and $GABA_B$ metabotropic receptors. Note that the same neurotransmitter can have different effects in the periphery versus central pathways. As mentioned earlier, GABA can have inhibitory or facilitating effects at the site of trauma and transduction while it suppresses pain centrally through descending pathways. Norepinephrine activates interneurons in the spinal cord through the dorsolateral funiculus to decrease pain transmission.[24] Serotonin functions in a similar descending modulatory fashion. In conditions associated with abnormal peripheral afferent activation, such as peripheral neuropathies, trigeminal neuralgia, and postherpetic neuralgia, drugs that inhibit the reuptake of serotonin and norepinephrine are important therapeutic tools.

SUMMARY

This chapter defined pain as a sensory and emotional mental experience and nociception as the neural processes underlying that experience. We examined nociception from transduction in the periphery, to the first-order synapse in the spinal cord dorsal horn, to spinal transmission pathways in the anterolateral cord, to the supraspinal targets they activate. We discussed emerging cortical components of the brain's pain network. Finally, we described descending supraspinal and spinal mechanisms that modulate the pain experience and permit significant differences in pain experienced by individuals subjected to the same noxious stimulus. Excessive excitation by persistent noxious stimuli can lead to sensitization of peripheral and central afferents, overwhelm descending modulatory pathways, and ultimately lead to development of difficult chronic pain conditions.

REFERENCES

1. International Association for the Study of Pain: http://www.iasp-pain.org/Taxonomy.
2. Melzack R, Casey KL. Sensory motivational and central control determinants of pain: a new conceptual model. In: Kenshalo D, ed. *The Skin Senses*. Springfield, IL: Charles C. Thomas; 1968:423–443.
3. Besson JM, Chaouch A. Peripheral and spinal mechanisms of nociception. *Physiol Rev.* 1987;67(1):67–186.

4. Meyer RA, Campbell JN. Myelinated nociceptive afferents account for the hyperalgesia that follows a burn to the hand. *Science*. 1981;213(4515):1527–1529.

5. Dray A. Kinins and their receptors in hyperalgesia. *Can J Physiol Pharmacol*. 1997;75(6):704–712.

6. Couture R, Harrisson M, Vianna RM, Cloutier F. Kinin receptors in pain and inflammation. *Eur J Pharmacol*. 2001;429(1–3):161–176. pii:S0014299901013188.

7. Beck PW, Handwerker HO. Bradykinin and serotonin effects on various types of cutaneous nerve fibers. *Pflugers Arch*. 1974;347(3):209–222.

8. Mizumura K, Minagawa M, Koda H, Kumazawa T. Influence of histamine on the bradykinin response of canine testicular polymodal receptors in vitro. *Inflamm Res*. 1995;44(9):376–378.

9. Cunha FQ, Ferreira SH. Peripheral hyperalgesic cytokines. *Adv Exp Med Biol*. 2003;521:22–39.

10. Machelska H, Stein C. Pain control by immune-derived opioids. *Clin Exp Pharmacol Physiol*. 2000;27(7):533–536.

11. Carlton SM, Zhou S, Coggeshall RE. Peripheral GABA(A) receptors: evidence for peripheral primary afferent depolarization. *Neuroscience*. 1999;93(2):713–722. pii:S0306-4522(99)00101-3.

12. Wess J. Novel insights into muscarinic acetylcholine receptor function using gene targeting technology. *Trends Pharmacol Sci*. 2003;24(8):414–420. pii:S0165-6147(03)00195-0.

13. Rexed B. The cytoarchitectonic organization of the spinal cord in the cat. *J Comp Neurol*. 1952;96(3):414–495.

14. Willis Jr WD. The pain system. The neural basis of nociceptive transmission in the mammalian nervous system. *Pain Headache*. 1985;8:1–346.

15. Woolf CJ. Evidence for a central component of post-injury pain hypersensitivity. *Nature*. 1983;306(5944):686–688.

16. Melzack R. From the gate to the neuromatrix. *Pain*. 1999;(suppl 6):S121–S126.

17. Albe-Fessard D, Berkley KJ, Kruger L, Ralston 3rd HJ, Willis Jr WD. Diencephalic mechanisms of pain sensation. *Brain Res*. 1985;356(3):217–296.

18. Rapps N, van Oudenhove L, Enck P, Aziz Q. Brain imaging of visceral functions in healthy volunteers and IBS patients. *J Psychosom Res*. 2008;64(6):599–604. http://dx.doi.org/10.1016/j.jpsychores.2008.02.018.

19. Villemure C, Bushnell MC. Mood influences supraspinal pain processing separately from attention. *J Neurosci*. 2009;29(3):705–715. http://dx.doi.org/10.1523/JNEUROSCI.3822-08.2009.

20. Apkarian AV, Bushnell MC, Treede RD, Zubieta JK. Human brain mechanisms of pain perception and regulation in health and disease. *Eur J Pain*. 2005;9(4):463–484. pii:S1090-3801(04)00148-X.

21. Fomberstein K, Qadri S, Ramani R. Functional MRI and pain. *Curr Opin Anaesthesiol*. 2013;26(5):588–593. http://dx.doi.org/10.1097/01.aco.0000433060.59939.fe.

22. Helmstetter FJ, Tershner SA, Poore LH, Bellgowan PS. Antinociception following opioid stimulation of the basolateral amygdala is expressed through the periaqueductal gray and rostral ventromedial medulla. *Brain Res*. 1998;779(1–2):104–118. pii:S0006-8993(97)01104-9.

23. Fields HL, Malick A, Burstein R. Dorsal horn projection targets of ON and OFF cells in the rostral ventromedial medulla. *J Neurophysiol*. 1995;74(4):1742–1759.

24. Basbaum AI, Fields HL. Endogenous pain control mechanisms: review and hypothesis. *Ann Neurol*. 1978;4(5):451–462. http://dx.doi.org/10.1002/ana.410040511.

CHAPTER 2

Central Sensitization, Central Sensitization Syndromes, and Chronic Neuropathic Pain

LEONARD B. KAMEN, DO

BACKGROUND AND DEMOGRAPHICS OF CHRONIC PAIN AND CENTRAL SENSITIZATION

In the 2010 Web-based survey of 35,718 US adults, 30.7% of responders identified themselves to meet criteria for chronic pain defined as "chronic, recurrent, or long-lasting pain lasting for at least 3–6 months."[1] That a near third of our adult population identifies themselves as afflicted with this sensory experience should not be a surprise. Pain is an interpretation of collective signals from our central nervous system monitoring systems that there are measured consequences to physical or emotional real or perceived threats.[2] Central sensitization (CS) is a key concept to comprehend in developing an essential foundation of knowledge of how sensory communication can misfire and lead to chronic pain encompassing a host of central sensitization syndromes (CSSs) that are discussed in this chapter (Fig. 2.1). Identification of a physically altering or damaging life event as chronic pain implies a real or anticipated threat to homeostasis (maintenance of a constant internal environment) or allostasis (neuroendocrine adaption to stress). Pain and suffering are an experiential reality of our cognitive-emotional species. In an imperfect world where humankind is assaulted with an uneven or seemingly unfair advantage and disadvantage, it is no wonder that 30% of US adults relate their life experience as being in a state of chronic pain, physical, psychological, or metaphysical, with a heightened state of perceived threat.

Those 70% of us with a baseline absent awareness of somatic pain symptoms have a privileged vantage point. Neuropathic pain (NP) symptoms in particular present a heuristic challenge to track down the generator or source of what appears to be a referred symptom or cluster of symptoms. Clinicians are frequently consulted by individuals with very different daily reference points of wellness, obscured by chronic pain, and they offer them only temporizing treatments. Connecting the somatic signals or semiotics of the sensory experience within the realm of chronic neuropathic pain (CNP) requires a working knowledge of how the central nervous system (CNS) processes and defuses or amplifies mechanical, thermal, or chemically mediated peripheral stimuli to be interpreted as central CNP. This chapter aims to provide a working scheme for clinicians seeking to interpret and modulate the signs and symptoms of chronic pain that has become centralized then sensitized or found to be primarily generated and perpetuated within the CNS itself.

What Is Central Sensitization?

CS of pain as described by Woolf in a seminal article in 2011 refers to an amplification of neural signaling within the CNS eliciting pain hypersensitivity.[3] An enhanced pain response to noxious stimulus occurs in somatosensory pathways attributed to bidirectional (i.e., afferent or efferent) increases in synaptic efficacy and reductions in inhibition. Amplification of the nociceptive signal is attributed to an augmented amplitude, duration, and spatial extension of pain in the somatosensory cortex. Temporal summation, a repetitive, consistent level of noxious stimulus to peripheral C-fibers, has been shown to create a progressive increase in the perceived intensity of the stimulus. A decreased sensory threshold required for pain perception is produced. Additional strengthening of normally ineffective synapses recruits subliminal inputs such that inputs in low threshold sensory inputs can now activate the pain circuit. The two parallel sensory pathways, i.e., strengthened stimuli and low thresholds, converge to augment pain perception.[4,5] Terms frequently referred to in this chapter are summarized briefly in Box 2.1.

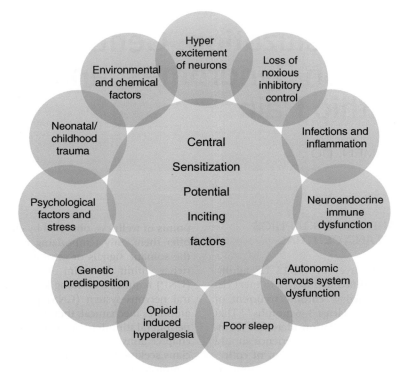

FIG. 2.1 Central sensitization syndromes characterized by amplified sensory, motor, or autonomic responses often interfacing with emotional and/or neuroendocrine-immune amplified responses.[26] (From Yunus MB. Central sensitivity syndromes: a new paradigm and group nosology for fibromyalgia and overlapping conditions, and the related issue of disease versus illness. *Semin Arthritis Rheum*. 2008;37(6):339–352; with permission.)

BOX 2.1
Terms and Brief Definitions of Key Elements of Central Sensitization

CENTRAL SENSITIZATION
- Increase responsiveness (amplification) of nociceptive neurons in the central nervous system to normal or subthreshold afferent input

PERIPHERAL SENSITIZATION
- Increase responsiveness and reduce threshold of nociceptive neurons in the periphery to the stimulation of their receptive fields

NEUROPATHIC PAIN
- Pain caused by a lesion or disease of the somatosensory nervous system

CENTRAL SENSITIZATION SYNDROMES
- Syndromes with features of amplification of nociceptive or neuroendocrine-immune stress

NOCICEPTION
- Neural process of encoding noxious stimuli

WINDUP
- Repeated stimulation of C-fibers increasing the intensity of pain

KINDLING
- Causation model whereby small stimuli induce an enhanced pain response

Why Is Central Sensitization an Important Topic to Pain Clinicians?

Irrespective of the source, pain remains a subjective end point of a host of sensory, electrochemical impulses, physical and emotional, pathologically perceived aspects of the human environment. The qualia or sensory experience of one individual may be starkly different from that of another person, which speaks to the very fabric of what makes humans unique. Sensory associations are collected and interpreted throughout our lives. Sensitization is a reflection of multiple processes that go awry in the process of encoding the sensory experiences of our physical and emotional environment. A better understanding of the factors that contribute to the sensation of pain allows pain clinicians to untangle this web and address what is correctable or develop adaptations to what cannot be "fixed."

Pain Syndromes Associated With Central Sensitization

Disease states that amplify pain associated with CSS are often those conditions that defy imaging or straightforward laboratory analysis. Fibromyalgia syndrome (FMS) and complex regional pain syndrome (CRPS) are common conditions seen in our pain clinics. Additional medical diagnoses associated with the CSS (Fig. 2.1) include chronic mechanical low back pain, chronic whiplash-associated disorders, temporomandibular joint disorders, myofascial pain syndrome, pelvic pain disorders, osteoarthritis and rheumatoid arthritis, chronic fatigue syndrome (CF), chronic headache, and irritable bowel syndrome. Symptoms associated with these conditions may include hypersensitivity to bright light, touch, noise, chemical pesticides and herbicides, mechanical pressure, and extremes of temperature and intolerance to multiple medications. Additional symptoms (Fig. 2.2) associated with CS may be difficult to differentiate from other commonly seen chronic pain settings, which include unrefreshed sleep, concentration difficulties, a sense of swelling in the limbs, tingling, and numbness.[6]

PERIPHERAL TO CENTRAL SENSITIZATION

Organisms require a pain defense mechanism to survive. The early warning system of our human peripheral nervous system (PNS) comprises specialized mechanical, thermal, and/or chemical peripheral receptors or

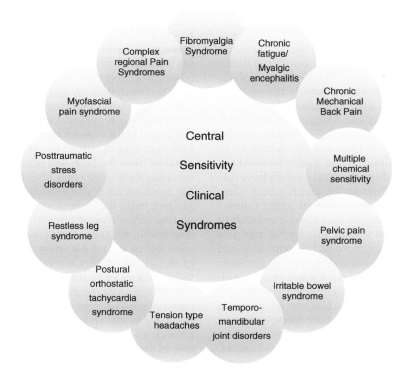

FIG. 2.2 Potential inciting factors in common among central sensitivity syndromes.

nociceptors. These nociceptors are unusually simplistic and respond uniquely only to mechanical, thermal, or chemical established threshold stimuli to initiate transduction or the process of electrochemical transformation of a noxious signal into a transmissible neural signal. The transduced signal is then transmitted by high-threshold primary sensory neurons. During inflammation, cutaneous and deeper mechanosensitized nociceptors in joints and muscle are recruited from a resting, silent state to barrage the dorsal horn of the spinal cord. Wide dynamic range neurons first described by Mendell in 1966 identified in the dorsal horn receive peripheral nociceptive signals from mechanical, thermal, and chemical activity within a broad range of intensities.[7] Interneurons within the gray matter of the spinal cord relay afferent signals and then perpetuate a nociceptive action potential in the ascending tracts of the cord. Ectopic discharges from inflamed and impaired nerve fibers may occur in rhythmic to intermittent bursts along the low-threshold $A\beta$- and higher threshold $A\partial$- and C-fibers. Additional theory holds that the contiguous uninjured nerve fibers may be responsible for nociceptive transmission. For example, damage to the L5 nerve root was found to propagate spontaneous action potentials in C fibers of the unaffected L4 dorsal root.[8]

Clinical Manifestations of Central Sensitization

On a clinical level, CS manifested by myofascial trigger points has been demonstrated to represent histologic changes that differ from normal muscle tissue. Using microanalytic methods and equipment, Shah et al.[9] have measured by lower pH levels, increased levels of substance P (SP), calcitonin gene-related peptide, tumor necrosis factor (TNF) α, and interleukin 1β in muscles with active and/or latent trigger points. Each of these inflammatory histochemical markers has a role in increasing pain and sensitivity and has been identified as elevated in or near myofascial trigger points.[9] Sensitized muscle nociceptors have lower thresholds to weak and/or innocuous stimuli and are hallmarks of CS-related muscle pain symptoms.[9] Latremoliere and Woolf have extensively illustrated that neuroplastic changes in the properties of neurons and neural transduction and transmission best represent the underpinnings of CS.[6] Complex CNS mechanisms are daunting to explain or demonstrate. With this collected research, CS has become a scientific challenge to the medical community to explore, better characterize, understand, explain, and develop equally sophisticated systems of assessment and management. All told, peripheral

sensitivity is a veritable soup of chemosensitizing mediators and pop-up expressed receptors navigating through channels by various means. The end game is transduction of noxious mechanical, thermal, or chemical stimuli. This is manifested clinically by the sensitization or amplification of nociception at available specialized peripheral neural terminals. What clinicians detect may be the trigger points of myofascial pain or tender points of fibromyalgia. What imaging and standard electrophysiologic testing detect at this point is not perceptible or practically reproducible at this time.

ANATOMY OF CENTRAL SENSITIZATION IN THE BRAIN: THE PAIN NEUROMATRIX

To paraphrase Moseley, "pain detectors are the eyes of the brain, one mechanism by which the body is protected."[10] Extending that logic to a view of persistent pain, sensitization represents the "amplitude knob" of these sensors becoming out of control in chronic pain. Touch or mechanoreception is the only primary sensory experience that cannot be turned on or off. Taste, smell, sight, and hearing can be voluntarily suppressed or completely averted. The capacity of being aware of oneself physically (kinesthesia) is attributed to the neuromatrix of mesolimbic structures and the somatosensory cortex that provide feedback as to spatial awareness, magnitude and localization of touch, pressure, and painful threats to existence. Differentiating pleasant from painful touch is meaning or context related; thus, cognitive and complex mechanoreception is transmitted through similar Aδ- and C-fiber pathways to the dorsal root ganglion and then through to the spinothalamic-cortical system. The pain neuromatrix of the brain's neural network receives an aberrant neurosignature described by Melzack as a "continuous out-flow from the body-self neuromatrix." The neurosignature forms after cyclic CNS processing and creates the synthesis of a characteristic "signature" on what Melzack terms the "neural sentient hub."[11]

Four major cortical areas of the brain are felt to be responsible for the neurosignature of pain. The area identified as the primary pain neuromatrix is inclusive of the somatosensory cortex (SI), secondary somatosensory cortex (SII), the anterior insula cortex, and the anterior cingulate cortex (ACC). Registration of pain or threat of pain requires interoception or the capacity of the brain to incorporate the self-perceptive subjective physical and emotional sense of the physiologic condition of the individual.[12]

Contrasting views of the neuromatrix have been disseminated. Canavero finds the pain matrix to be a multimodal network related to the detection of and reaction to salient sensory inputs regardless of a nociceptive pathway but more likely to involve nonnociceptive cognitive processes.[13] Apkarian likewise states that there is no unitary set of brain areas imaged precisely, especially for chronic pain conditions.[14] Physical versus social pain may differ in selective brain imaging studies. Anticipation of pain lights up affective areas of the prefrontal cortex and motor areas of the cerebellum.[15] Ghosts of the CP neurosignature stem from a systemic failure to protect the homeostasis of the person perceiving the tissue damage or threat of injury. Changes in the way these structures connect or communicate (connectomies) within the neuromatrix are more likely to be at fault in CP.[16]

Regional areas of the brain involved in sensory, affective, and cognitive aspects of pain have been demonstrated by functional magnetic resonance imagery (fMRI).[17] Increased fMRI activity in patients with identified acute pain sensation and emotional representations overlap in the forebrain area.[18] This includes the ACC in the prefrontal cortex and insula. The overactive pain neural matrix in CSS enhances brain activity in these regions not involved in acute pain sensations, including the brainstem, the dorsolateral frontal cortex, and the parietal associated cortex. The brainstem may specifically play a role in the maintenance of CS. Long-term potentiation (LTP) is a key neuroplastic capacity of the CNS that facilitates chemical synapses to change their strength. LTP is one of the essential elements in the neural mechanism of memory and learning initially derived from neuroscience experiments by Lomo in 1966.[19] Long-term potentiation of synapses in the ACC, nucleus accumbens, insula, and sensorimotor cortex embeds this disproportionate nociceptive neuromatrix response.

Neuroendocrine Immune System Function in Central Sensitization Syndromes

CSSs, with limited objective markers, have long been burdened with an onus of proving their legitimacy. These conditions are often considered among syndromes labeled with the terminology of medically unexplained symptoms. Common to each of these constellations of conditions, such as FMS, CF, CRPS, and IBS, is the theme of "stress-related illness." Tremendous strides have been made since the 1970s in the understanding of the role of the hypothalamic-pituitary-adrenal axis (HPAA) in the perpetuation and formation of stress-related disease conditions. CSSs are now better recognized but are still defined primarily by clinical diagnosis. CSS-related brain pathology may now be objectively demonstrated by fMRI and MR spectroscopy as other well-recognized and studied neuroendocrine immune–related conditions.

Communication between the immune system and the brain is mediated by proinflammatory cytokines, including TNF, interleukin-1 (IL-1), and IL-6. These cytokines are responsible for the early immune response to stressful challenge by attracting and activating immune cells. Blocking the action of these cytokines can prevent the generation of sickness responses normally elicited by peripheral immune challenges. Proinflammatory cytokines within the CNS are instrumental in creating sickness responses. These responses include fever, myalgias, arthralgias, neuralgias, decreased activity, and changes in sleep, along with decreased social and sexual behavior.

Glial cells (or microglia) in the spinal cord or astrocytes are the predominant sources of cytokines. Blockade of their actions in the CNS prevents simulated sickness responses, and cytokines introduced to the CNS induce expression of sickness. Proteins from cytokines have two key sites of action, at the site of peripheral immune challenge and within the CNS sites that create this sickness sequela.[20] Microglia express proinflammatory cytokines that exert indirect effects on neuronal nociception, including potentiating N-methyl-D-aspartic acid (NMDA) channel openings and glutamate transport.[20,21] When sufficient amounts of SP and glutamate are released in the dorsal horn, Mg^{2+} is detached or unplugged from the NMDA channels, allowing Ca^{2+} to flow into these ion-gated channels activating nitric oxide and prostaglandins. An exaggerated release of these transmitters results in the amplification of nociceptive messages relayed to higher brain thalamic and the brain's pain neuromatrix areas.[21]

Opioids and Glial Activity

Exposure to chronic opioids for the management of pain has paradoxically been demonstrated to stimulate glial activation and thus thwart pain control. Opioid treatment failure is mediated through a class of pattern recognition immune receptors termed toll-like receptors (TLRs).[22] Enantiomers of various opioid analgesics (morphine, fentanyl, methadone) as well as their metabolites (morphine3-glucoronide) act as agonists to TLR4, promoting a constant low-level release of cytokines, chronic fatigue-fibromyalgia syndrome and IL-1 β. Consequent loss of opioid efficacy, tolerance, dependence, and potential allodynia and hyperalgesia are thus promulgated.[23] Antagonists to TLRs and attenuation of glial activity suppress pain and present a promising pharmacologic target for nonopioid treatment of

NP. The role of TLRs is felt to be pivotal to perpetuating NP. Glial-modulating drugs (methotrexate, low-dose naltrexone) may calm the activated glia, causing them to revert to their quiescent resting state.

Biopsychosocial Aspects of Central Sensitization Syndromes

It is critical to the management of any chronic pain disorder that practitioners take into account where and in whom the pain exists. The meaning of pain to each individual patient is embodied in the environment in which that individual lives and functions. The capacity to interpret CS symptoms as a threat or perceived threat is an instinctive, emotional, and cognitive function filtered through a fine mesh of memories and learned behaviors. Whether the noxious stimuli lead to habituation or sensitization is determined by multiple neural exchanges and relays, in part biology and in part psychology, and finally is culturally or socially influenced (Fig. 2.3).

Psychosocial stressors are commonly seen in CSS along with sleep disorders, cognitive-memory disturbances, and fixation on symptoms that may not be demonstrable. Failure to mount an adequate psychological adjustment to stress has been shown to be associated with low cortisol levels.[24] This challenge in the HPAA is a measurable index of susceptibility to chronic widespread pain. Psychosocial maladaptations may occur in greater frequency with CS but cannot be seen without careful consideration as the singular source of these complex symptoms.

Clinicians responding to the lack of consistently objective signs and diagnostic analysis often consider individuals with CS symptoms with the differential diagnosis of somatization disorder. Somatization in the International Classification of Disease, sixth edition, of the World Health Organization (ICD 10) is defined as "a pattern of recurrent poly symptomatic somatic complaints resulting in medical treatment or impaired daily function. Symptoms usually begin before age 30 and

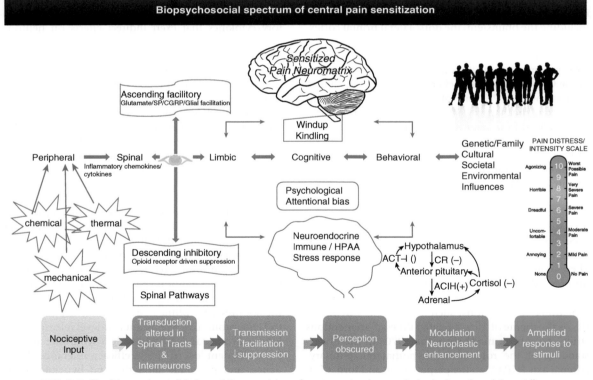

FIG. 2.3 The biopsychosocial view of the spectrum of neuroanatomic, psychological, and social contributors to the process of pain amplification seen in central sensitization. *ACTH*, adrenocorticotropic hormone; *CGRP*, calcitonin gene related protein; *CRF*, corticotropin-releasing factor; *HPAA*, hypothalamic pituitary adrenal axis; *SP*, substance P.

extend over a period of years."[25] The ambiguity of this diagnostic category is purposeful, as it allows a billing code to be entered in electronic medical records and payments to be collected despite an otherwise unexplained symptom. The term somatization does not account for individual differences in tolerance and acceptance of the biology of nociception. Many studies have refuted the concept of subjectivity in CSS.[26] Trigger points in FMS (also known as chronic widespread pain) demonstrate objectively consistent interrater reliability.[27] Quantitative thermal sensitivity testing and additional psychometric methods of detecting CNS hypersensitivity have been employed with objective significance, although these are not commonly employed on a clinical basis because of the lack of specificity, reimbursement concerns, or neglected need to demonstrate CS for treatment purposes.[28]

Sensitization of the interplay between the mind and body is described best by the concept of kindling. This term was first applied to neuroscience by Goddard in 1949 who used repeated subthreshold electric stimulation of the amygdala to induce seizures in rats.[29,30] Kindling in the corticolimbic system as influenced by emotions, memory, and cognitive and behavioral background represents a change in "gain" or intensity of a noxious experience into a neuroplastic engram of heightened sensitization. This convergence of sensory, affective, and cognitive processes is referred to as a limbically augmented pain syndrome (LAPS) by Rome et al., with a behavioral or illness response to persistent nociceptive input in a subset of predisposed individuals.[31] By modeling this convergence of spinal and cortical levels of nociception, we may eventually determine the best psychological, pharmacologic, and physical interventions. Depression and the behaviors associated with CSS may be better understood and addressed clinically within the conceptual framework of the kindling phenomena exacerbated by LAPS.

CENTRAL SENSITIZATION SYNDROMES

Central sensitization (occasionally referred to as central sensitivity) syndromes are characterized by a cluster of symptoms reflecting enhanced pain reception in a regional or targeted systemic distribution (see Fig. 2.1). As noted earlier, this terminology encompasses conditions that fall into the caldron of "medically unexplained symptoms" or "idiopathic pain disorders." Yunus in his article on the nosology of CSS calls for acceptance of the biopsychosocial nature of CSS.[26] This requires a conceptual bridge between the physical evidence that has been collected in great detail regarding pathologic relay systems from the PNS to the CNS and

the psychological interpretation of these electrochemical signals. Clinical symptoms are grouped by the organ system in which the symptoms predominate.

FMS connotes a widespread muscle pain syndrome. Chronic low back pain (CLBP) refers to nonradicular or otherwise nonclassified lower back pain that meets the model of amplification of signal beyond recognition of anatomic pathology. CRPS by definition is at least initially a localized limb or anatomically confined sensitivity syndrome that is beyond a simple peripheral nociceptive phenomenon. Interstitial cystitis is confined to the pelvic organ system. CF now identified as myalgic encephalomyelitis (CF/MES) is characterized by chronic debilitating fatigue; sleep; cognitive, immune, and autonomic dysfunctions; postexertional malaise, and myalgic pain.[32] CF/MES represents multisystem oversensitivity without a unifying trigger. CSS terminology has been applied to additional nonanatomic immune system and HPAA-related stress or neuroendocrine physiologic function disorders, including posttraumatic stress disorder. The Venn diagram illustrating the overlap of these sensitivity-related syndromes has expanded dramatically over the last 30 years (Figs. 2.1 and 2.2).

The principle criterion for establishing a CSS is, like many clinical conditions, to exclude a known pathologic state of the PNS or CNS (Table 2.1). The definition of NP has been accepted as "pain arising as a direct consequence of a lesion or disease affecting the somatosensory system."[33] Once a nonneuropathic explanation has been demonstrated, the criterion of disproportionate pain and/or physical impairment to the extent of known injury or pathology is applicable. If there is a plausible nociceptive generating condition, i.e., underlying osteoarthritis, but disproportionate pain and suffering, CS may remain as a component of the disorder. In addition, the second criterion involves self-reports of pain distribution that is atypical for the specific condition as well. Pain diagrams may be diffuse, bilateral, and caudal to rostral out of the lines of known local or regional syndromes. Finally, hypersensitivity of senses unrelated to the musculoskeletal system has been identified as a third cardinal criterion for CSS. This may be inclusive of expressions of hypersensitivity to environmental elements not otherwise recognized as noxious, i.e., bright lights, food, chemical smells, weather, and situational stress. These responses should represent a change to the individual and not a baseline state.[34]

The Central Sensitivity Inventory: Assessment Tool

Efforts to further the objective analysis of CS have been increasingly appearing in the pain literature.

TABLE 2.1
Clinical Criteria for the Classification of Central Sensitization Syndromes[33]

Elemental Assessment	Descriptors	Confirmatory Process
Exclude neuropathic pain (NP)	"Pain arising as a direct consequence of lesion or disease affecting the somatosensory system"	NP is neuroanatomic and logical. Diagnostic studies demonstrate neuropathology. Descriptors of NP are frequently used
Central sensitization pain (CSP) experience is disproportionate to the identified nature and extent of injury/pathology	Objective and subjective assessment are not otherwise classifiable	CSP represents an impairment beyond that which is commonly expected for disease state, i.e., osteoarthritis, Chronic mechanical low back pain, traumatic tendinitis
Diffuse pain distribution with allodynia/hyperalgesia	Pain drawings out of perspective of usual anatomic distribution, widespread, spreading out of usual pathways	Self-reported pain may be beyond outlines of pain drawings
Hypersensitivity of senses unrelated to the musculoskeletal system	Central sensitization represents increased responsiveness to a variety of stimuli	Mechanical, chemical, and thermal responses are elicited at low thresholds. Central Sensitivity Inventory >40

From Treede RD, Jensen TS, Campbell JN, et al. Neuropathic pain: redefinition and a grading system for clinical and research purposes. *Neurology*. 2008;70(18):1630–1635; with permission.

Consensus has not been definitively established, but proposals for acceptance of a straightforward schema to identify CSS have evolved using validated methods.[35] The Central Sensitization Inventory (CSI) (Fig. 2.4) was designed to provide a clinical tool using a symptom-based questionnaire to help qualify a cluster of symptoms as belonging to this class.[36] Applying a scale with both sensitivity and specificity criteria to CSS offers a framework for better recognition of the complexities of CS and a brighter future for better treatment. Using a validated instrument for identification of CSS is a critical step toward engaging the neuroscience and clinical community in acceptance of these conditions. The CSI was developed by a consortium of researchers. Scores greater than 40/100 are identified as showing a strong correlation with central sensitivity.[36] The CSI was applied to a psychiatric practice setting dealing with chronic pain. It was felt to be valid and sensitive in 82.8% (n = 82) of patients with CSS and 54.8% of non-CSS patients using the 40/100 cutoff. False positives were noted among those patients with comorbid psychiatric disease, severe pain, abuse history, and low function.[37] With this reproducible and validated recognition tool, rehabilitative interventions should evolve that can treat central sensitivity and hyperexcitable CNS pathways with greater accuracy. Neuroplastic change in a positive inhibitory biased fashion is more likely when the proper diagnosis and tools for treatment are assembled.

PHARMACEUTICAL MANAGEMENT OF CENTRAL SENSITIZATION PAIN

Medical management of CSS is in its infancy. Clinicians have been prescribing medications for somatosensory pain and hypersensitivity over many centuries. No profoundly sensitive or specific class of medication has excelled in anything much more than placation of this condition. The current principal pharmacopeia for chronic pain has been limited to agents that have been on the market for over 100 years (morphine was isolated in 1803; oxycodone emerged in 1913). Opioids have assumed a large share of the burden in the treatment of chronic pain without a coincident universal satisfaction of an increase in quality of life or function by prescribers or consumers. The role of glial cell activity in the undermining of opioid effects has been advanced as described.[22,38] Antiinflammatory drugs, antiepileptic agents, and antidepressants have varied efficacy and are not all specifically targeted to the spectrum of electrophysiologic, chemical, and somatosensory dysfunction seen in CSS. Meta-analyses of the efficacy and safety of these widely used classes of drugs for the treatment of FMS as a useful prototype for all the CSSs have been published and updated recently.[39,40]

Prescribing currently available medication for CS entails understanding of the mechanisms of these drugs as well as of the ascending and descending pathways and intraspinal, cortical, cognitive, and psychosocial aspects of nociceptive transmission and perception.

CENTRAL SENSITIZATION INVENTORY: PART A

Name: _____   Date: _____

Please circle the best response to the right of each statement.

1	I feel tired and unrefreshed when I wake from sleeping.	Never	Rarely	Sometimes	Often	Always
2	My muscles feel stiff and achy.	Never	Rarely	Sometimes	Often	Always
3	I have anxiety attacks.	Never	Rarely	Sometimes	Often	Always
4	I grind or clench my teeth.	Never	Rarely	Sometimes	Often	Always
5	I have problems with diarrhea and/or constipation.	Never	Rarely	Sometimes	Often	Always
6	I need help in performing my daily activities.	Never	Rarely	Sometimes	Often	Always
7	I am sensitive to bright lights.	Never	Rarely	Sometimes	Often	Always
8	I get tired very easily when I am physically active.	Never	Rarely	Sometimes	Often	Always
9	I feel pain all over my body.	Never	Rarely	Sometimes	Often	Always
10	I have headaches.	Never	Rarely	Sometimes	Often	Always
11	I feel discomfort in my bladder and/or burning when I urinate.	Never	Rarely	Sometimes	Often	Always
12	I do not sleep well.	Never	Rarely	Sometimes	Often	Always
13	I have difficulty concentrating.	Never	Rarely	Sometimes	Often	Always
14	I have skin problems such as dryness, itchiness, or rashes.	Never	Rarely	Sometimes	Often	Always
15	Stress makes my physical symptoms get worse.	Never	Rarely	Sometimes	Often	Always
16	I feel sad or depressed.	Never	Rarely	Sometimes	Often	Always
17	I have low energy.	Never	Rarely	Sometimes	Often	Always
18	I have muscle tension in my neck and shoulders.	Never	Rarely	Sometimes	Often	Always
19	I have pain in my jaw.	Never	Rarely	Sometimes	Often	Always
20	Certain smells, such as perfumes, make me feel dizzy and nauseated.	Never	Rarely	Sometimes	Often	Always
21	I have to urinate frequently.	Never	Rarely	Sometimes	Often	Always
22	My legs feel uncomfortable and restless when I am trying to go to sleep at night.	Never	Rarely	Sometimes	Often	Always
23	I have difficulty remembering things.	Never	Rarely	Sometimes	Often	Always
24	I suffered trauma as a child.	Never	Rarely	Sometimes	Often	Always
25	I have pain in my pelvic area.	Never	Rarely	Sometimes	Often	Always

Total=

FIG. 2.4 Central Sensitivity Inventory developed at PRIDE in Dallas, Texas, parts A & B. Scoring 0–4 (part A only). Severity ranges have been recommended: Subclinical=0–29; Mild=30–39; Moderate=40–49; Severe=50–59; and Extreme=60–100. >40=high index of symptoms being consistent with a CSS.[36] (From Neblett R, Cohen H, Choi Y, et al. The central sensitization inventory (CSI): establishing clinically significant values for identifying central sensitivity syndromes in an outpatient chronic pain sample. *J Pain*. 2013;14(5):438–445; with permission.)

CENTRAL SENSITIZATION INVENTORY: PART B

Name: _____

Date: _____

Have you been diagnosed by a doctor with any of the following disorders?

Please check the box to the right for each diagnosis and write the year of the diagnosis.

		NO	YES	Year Diagnosed
1	Restless Leg Syndrome			
2	Chronic Fatigue Syndrome			
3	Fibromyalgia			
4	Temporomandibular Joint Disorder (TMJ)			
5	Migraine or tension headaches			
6	Irritable Bowel Syndrome			
7	Multiple Chemical Sensitivities			
8	Neck Injury (including whiplash)			
9	Anxiety or Panic Attacks			
10	Depression			

FIG. 2.4, cont'd.

There have only been three medications approved in the United States for FMS. Pregabalin, an antiepileptic, was approved in 2007; duloxetine and milnacipran, both selective serotonin and norepinephrine reuptake inhibitors, were approved in 2008 and 2009, respectively. The treatment of NP is likewise confined to a limited number of agents, each with a narrow band of US Food and Drug Administration–approved indications as to the specific disease state allowable by these standards. In light of the intricate mechanisms of NP and especially when this is amplified as in CSS, this constrictive construct for prescribing makes little sense. Consequently, there has been a robust utilization of the available pharmaceutical options, including oral, transdermal, parenteral, epidural, and intrathecal delivery of off-label chemotherapy for these "difficult-to-treat" and nonobjectively demonstrated painful conditions.

In a brief review of the available desensitizing pharmaceuticals, mixed serotonin and norepinephrine reuptake (SNRI) drug(s) have a proposed mechanism of action on the descending inhibitory pathway of spinal transmission and the cognitive-behavioral aspects of pain-related anxiety and depression, sleep disruption, catastrophic thinking, and improved coping abilities are clinically addressed. Tricyclic antidepressants alone have played a role in similar ways, but a balanced norepinephrine (NE) and serotonin (5-HT) approach has been proved to be more effective. There is some evidence of recruitment of opioid receptors in the spinal interneurons with selective serotonin-biased reuptake inhibitors, but clinical practice has focused on the SNRIs for pain.[41] Second-generation analgesics have emerged in the US market that combine modulating effects on both descending and ascending spinal nociceptive transmission. Tapentadol and to a lesser degree tramadol represent single-molecule synthetic opioids that combine NE reuptake with a more moderate μ opioid receptor (MOR) agonism.[42] No active metabolic activation is necessary for tapentadol activation, and there are no active metabolites. Less nausea and gastrointestinal-related adverse effects are reported. Tapentadol extended release was approved for treating chronic diabetic NP in the United States in 2012.

Opioid agonists and partial agonists are perhaps used more predominantly in the US medical system for the management of CSS. The partial MOR agonist and k opioid receptor antagonist buprenorphine is approved in selective low-dose slow-release delivery systems in the United States for chronic pain. Buprenorphine is selectively antihyperalgesic and differs from other opioids.[43] This molecule has a broader mechanism of action for pain, with a high affinity to MOR, less euphoria, and a ceiling on respiratory depression. Buprenorphine transdermal or transbuccal delivery systems in low-dose delivery systems are approved to treat chronic pain in the United States and may exhibit less tendency to tolerance and dose creep because of the high affinity and partial agonism to receptors. Owing to lower dose levels employed in these pain-related buprenorphine preparations, there is no conflict in the concomitant use of low-dose pure agonist shorter acting opioids for breakthrough pain.

Levorphanol is an older, more potent opioid agent. Levorphanol is a multitasking MOR, delta, kappa1-3 agonist, and NE and 5-HT reuptake inhibitor, with NMDA antagonism in the spectrum of nociceptive transmission.[44] It may prove useful in the setting of CSS resistant to traditional opioids.

Opioid therapy for CSS, however, is fraught with precautions regarding the medical and psychosocial consequences of employing this class of drug. The most significant caveat to the use of opioids in CSS is the distinct possibility of initiating a long-term dependence on an agent for a disease state with no end in sight. Opioid-induced hyperalgesia, glial cell induction of spinal cord changes, increasing tolerance and neuroplastic behavioral shifts with drug craving, and

entrenched belief systems by the consumer are factors that make withdrawing these agents daunting, to say the least.

Nonpharmacologic Management of CSS

Pain neuroscience education has come to the forefront of nonpharmacologic intervention for chronic pain and centralization symptoms. Evidence-based reviews (Table 2.2) and grading studies with low- to high-quality and weak to strong recommendations showed compelling results of educational strategies employing neuroscience foundations. End points of these interventions, including positive impacts on outcomes including pain, disability, catastrophic thinking, and physical performance, have been validated.[45] Engagement of patients in techniques of narrative medicine, reflective listening, motivational interviewing, and cognitive behavioral therapy for desensitization is an additional validated approach. Randomized controlled studies have demonstrated that individuals with CF and other musculoskeletal pain syndromes respond to pain physiology education during the course of care.[46] Hypnosis, relaxation training, mindfulness meditation, and variations on cognitive behavior acceptance therapies have proven efficacy in chronic pain conditions in those patients with the financial resources to pursue these strategies.[47] Reconceptualizing pain and the meaning of pain to entrenched individuals requires technical skills acquired through approaches such as motivational interviewing with theatrical-like training seminars.[47] Carefully crafting a challenge to old thinking, creating a cultured and controlled cognitive dissonance provides a seedbed for novel and constructive problem solving. Studies have shown that changing maladaptive pain beliefs leads to changes in brain activation in pain areas and positive changes in descending nociceptive facilitation.[48]

Therapeutic Exercise for Central Sensitization

In the 2007 Cochrane study review of "Exercise for treating fibromyalgia syndrome," results of up to 34 studies with 2276 subjects were presented.[49] The ultimate conclusion was that there was significant evidence of the beneficial effects of aerobic exercise on physical capacity and fibromyalgia symptoms. Additional studies were suggested for the determination of the benefits of exercise and muscle strengthening and flexibility. Moderate-intensity aerobic exercise for 12 weeks improved overall well-being and physical function but showed little to no difference in pain or tender points. Strength training at a similar intensity reduced pain tender points and

TABLE 2.2
Complementary and Alternative Therapies Frequently Used in the Treatment of Fibromyalgia and Central Sensitization Syndromes

Complementary Therapy	Characteristics/Assets of Treatment	Comments—Adverse Events (AEs)
Acupuncture	Drug free, techniques are variable	AE minor with limited duration
Biofeedback	Noninvasive, multiple feedback targets, i.e., heart rate variability, thermal skin sensor, electromyogram biofeedback	Studies varied in frequency and intensity
Manipulative/manual Medicine	Includes spinal manipulation, massage, stretching, resistance training	Mild-moderate transient adverse effects of spinal manipulation
Cognitive behavioral therapy	Median duration 10 weeks, 10 sessions = 18 h. Median follow-up 6 months	AE—worsening comorbid mental health disorders
Exercise	Aerobics > 20 min (or 2 × 10 min), 2–3 days/week. Strength training > 8 reps/exercise, 2–3 days/week	Initial deterioration in symptoms. Generally considered safe
Hydrotherapy/spa treatments	Water or mud baths at temperatures 36–45°C; median treatment 240 min over several weeks	Little to no AE, expect slight flashes, chlorine sensitivity
Hypnotherapy	Variations between trials regarding time and days or weeks duration	No AE reported
Massage	Therapy time variable	No AE reported
Meditative moment	Variations in trials, Yoga, Tai chi. Qigong or body awareness therapy. Median duration 16 h (6–24 h) over 4–12 weeks	AE minor—with pain, muscle inflammation. Safety overall high for meditative movement therapies
Mindfulness	2- to 3.5-h sessions/week, programs include daily home practice (30–45 min)	No AE reported
Guided imagery	Audiotape, individual 30 min/day × 6 weeks	No AE reported

Adapted from Macfarlane GJ, Kronisch C, Dean LE, et al. EULAR revised recommendations for the management of fibromyalgia. *Ann Rheum Dis*. 2016; with permission.
Comments and adverse events associated with therapies as per multiple observational reports.[40]

depression with overall well-being but no difference in physical function. The assessment of practicality and continuity of the benefits were limited to 12 weeks.[49] These findings do not address the totality of a physical approach to CSS. Multiple modalities may be considered, although there is little to no collective evidence specific to the symptoms of amplified pain sensitivity common to these conditions. Transcutaneous electric stimulation for desensitization of muscular pain in other somatic conditions has been applied generously over the years with little long-term benefit even in trials showing short-term efficacy.[50] Exercise therapies for CLBP are strongly promoted with only moderate evidence of efficacy along with spinal manipulation, cognitive behavioral therapies (CBT), and interdisciplinary rehabilitation.[51] Functional restoration programs likewise showed fair evidence of efficacy in this full analysis. As noted in Fig. 2.4, there are multiple modalities

explored for the treatment of chronic amplified pain symptoms applicable to CSS with limited quality of studies demonstrating strong preferences.

SUMMARY

Recognition of chronic pain and especially chronic NP as a complex neuroscience and social science challenge has evolved over the last several decades. Identification of a large cohort of the US population with some form of chronic pain will likely drive additional scientific as well as nonscientific interventions in the current healthcare environment. CS of chronic pain is best viewed through the prism of the well-documented neuroscience of pain with biological complexity and multisystem complicity (Fig. 2.3). It is clear that the human nervous system may adapt negatively to noxious stimulation in our challenging physical and psychosocial environment. When biological systems become challenged, they attempt to engage compensatory and collateral pathways (ascending and descending suppression or facilitation) to achieve homeostasis. When these homeostatic systems fail or become hyperexcitable, the organism perceives and suffers pain. By attaining insight in regards to the peripheral to central and central to peripheral transmission of nociception, we do understand the response of the whole organism to a real or perceived threat. Understanding the impact of amplified nociception in CS and how the organism responds biologically and psychosocially is critical to the holistic management of the multiple central sensitivity syndromes identified in this chapter. Modulation of chronic NP employing multiple pathways from bottom-up to top-down in a bidirectional fashion (i.e., peripheral to central reciprocally) seems to be our best defense against this crescendo effect of nociception. Employment of cognitive-behavioral interventions along with physical, biological, and pharmaceutical science may help mitigate the maladjustment of these profound neurosensory disturbances within the "body-self." Fine-tuning of the neuroendocrine-immune system, judicious utilization of the available and evolving CNS pathway facilitatory and/or inhibiting medications, and novel engaging cognitive-behavioral strategies are critical elements to employ in this common clinical challenge. Dependence on imperfect single-entity medical treatments without promoting self-efficacy or incorporating quality-of-life enhancement (bio-psycho-social) techniques is likely to result in disappointing outcomes. Acceptance of this model of hypersensitized nociceptive signal transmission influenced by stress and by a disrupted CNS homeostatic balance is critical to evolving effective future management strategies for CS and chronic NP.

REFERENCES

1. Johannes CB, Le TK, Zhou X, Johnston JA, Dworkin RH. The prevalence of chronic pain in United States adults: results of an internet-based survey. *J Pain.* 2010;11(11): 1230–1239.
2. Merksey H, Bogduk N. *Classification of Chronic Pain. Descriptions of Chronic Pain Syndromes and Definitions of Pain Term;* 1994:59–71.
3. Woolf CJ. Central sensitization: implications for the diagnosis and treatment of pain. *Pain.* 2011;152(3):S2–S15.
4. Ossipov MH, Dussor GO, Porreca F. Central modulation of pain. *J Clin Invest.* 2010;120(11):3779–3787.
5. Ossipov M, Morimura K, Porreca F. Descending pain modulation and chronification of pain. *Curr Opin Support Palliat Care.* 2014;8(2):143–151.
6. Latremoliere A, Woolf CJ. Central sensitization: a generator of pain hypersensitivity by central neural plasticity. *J Pain.* 2009;10(9):895–926.
7. Mendell LM. Physiological properties of unmyelinated fiber projection to the spinal cord. *Exp Neurol.* 1966;16(3): 316–332.
8. Canavero S. Central pain and Parkinson disease. *Arch Neurol.* 2009;66(2):282–283.
9. Shah JP, Gilliams EA. Uncovering the biochemical milieu of myofascial trigger points using in vivo microdialysis: an application of muscle pain concepts to myofascial pain syndrome. *J Bodyw Mov Ther.* 2008;12(4):371–384.
10. Moseley GL. *Pain Is One Mechanism by Which the Body Is Protected… Pain Sensors Are the "Eyes of the Brain".* BodyinMind. org: Research into the Role of the Brain and Mind in Chronic Pain; 2016. Web site: www.BodyinMind.org/what-is-pain.
11. Melzack R. Pain and the neuromatrix in the brain. *J Dent Educ.* 2001;65(12):1378–1382.
12. Melzack R. From the gate to the neuromatrix. *Pain.* 1999;82:S121–S126.
13. Canavero S, Bonicalzi V. Pain myths and the genesis of central pain. *Pain Med.* 2015;16(2):240–248.
14. Apkarian AV, Hashmi JA, Baliki MN. Pain and the brain: specificity and plasticity of the brain in clinical chronic pain. *Pain.* 2011;152(3 suppl):S49–S64.
15. Vincent K, Warnaby C, Stagg CJ, Moore J, Kennedy S, Tracey I. Brain imaging reveals that engagement of descending inhibitory pain pathways in healthy women in a low endogenous estradiol state varies with testosterone. *Pain.* 2013;154(4): 515–524.
16. Denk F, McMahon SB, Tracey I. Pain vulnerability: a neurobiological perspective. *Nat Neurosci.* 2014;17(2):192–200.
17. Borsook D, Moulton EA, Schmidt KF, Becerra LR. Neuroimaging revolutionizes therapeutic approaches to chronic pain. *Mol Pain.* 2007;3(1):1.
18. Vogt BA. Pain and emotion interactions in subregions of the cingulate gyrus. *Nat Rev Neurosci.* 2005;6(7):533–544.
19. Lomo T. The discovery of long-term potentiation. *Philos Trans R Soc Lond B Biol Sci.* 2003;358(1432):617–620.
20. Watkins L, Maier S. Immune regulation of central nervous system functions: from sickness responses to pathological pain. *J Intern Med.* 2005;257(2):139–155.
21. Milligan ED, Watkins LR. Pathological and protective roles of glia in chronic pain. *Nat Rev Neurosci.* 2009;10(1):23–36.
22. Hutchinson MR, Bland ST, Johnson KW, Rice KC, Maier SF, Watkins LR. Opioid-induced glial activation: mechanisms of activation and implications for opioid analgesia, dependence, and reward. *Sci World J.* 2007;7:98–111.
23. Hutchinson MR, Lewis SS, Coats BD, et al. Possible involvement of toll-like receptor 4/myeloid differentiation factor-2 activity of opioid inactive isomers causes spinal proinflammation and related behavioral consequences. *Neuroscience.* 2010;167(3):880–893.
24. McBeth J, Chiu YH, Silman AJ, et al. Hypothalamic-pituitary-adrenal stress axis function and the relationship with chronic widespread pain and its antecedents. *Arthritis Res Ther.* 2005; 7(5):1.

25. World Health Organization. *The ICD-10 Classification of Mental and Behavioural Disorders: Clinical Descriptions and Diagnostic Guidelines.* Geneva: World Health Organization; 1992.

26. Yunus MB. Central sensitivity syndromes: a new paradigm and group nosology for fibromyalgia and overlapping conditions, and the related issue of disease versus illness. *Semin Arthritis Rheum.* 2008;37(6):339–352.

27. Tunks E, McCain G, Hart L, et al. The reliability of examination for tenderness in patients with myofascial pain, chronic fibromyalgia and controls. *J Rheumatol.* 1995;22:5.

28. Desmeules J, Cedraschi C, Rapiti E, et al. Neurophysiologic evidence for a central sensitization in patients with fibromyalgia. *Arthritis Rheum.* 2003;48(5):1420–1429.

29. Goddard GV, McIntyre DC, Leech CK. A permanent change in brain function resulting from daily electrical stimulation. *Exp Neurol.* 1969;25(3):295–330.

30. Goddard MJ, Dean BZ, King JC. Pain rehabilitation. 1. Basic science, acute pain, and neuropathic pain. *Arch Phys Med Rehabil.* 1994;75(5):S4–S8.

31. Rome HP, Rome JD. Limbically augmented pain syndrome (LAPS): kindling, corticolimbic sensitization, and the convergence of affective and sensory symptoms in chronic pain disorders. *Pain Med.* 2000;1(1):7–23.

32. Smith MB, Haney E, McDonagh M, et al. Treatment of myalgic encephalomyelitis/chronic fatigue syndrome: a systematic review for a National Institutes of Health pathways to prevention workshop. *Ann Intern Med.* 2015;162(12):841–850.

33. Treede RD, Jensen TS, Campbell JN, et al. Neuropathic pain: redefinition and a grading system for clinical and research purposes. *Neurology.* 2008;70(18):1630–1635.

34. Nijs J, Torres-Cueco R, van Wilgen P, et al. Applying modern pain neuroscience in clinical practice: criteria for the classification of central sensitization pain. *Pain Physician.* 2014;17(5):447–457.

35. Mayer TG, Neblett R, Cohen H, et al. The development and psychometric validation of the central sensitization inventory. *Pain Pract.* 2012;12(4):276–285.

36. Neblett R, Cohen H, Choi Y, et al. The central sensitization inventory (CSI): establishing clinically significant values for identifying central sensitivity syndromes in an outpatient chronic pain sample. *J Pain.* 2013;14(5):438–445.

37. Neblett R, Hartzell MM, Cohen H, et al. Ability of the central sensitization inventory to identify central sensitivity syndromes in an outpatient chronic pain sample. *Clin J Pain.* 2015;31(4):323–332.

38. Watkins LR, Hutchinson MR, Rice KC, Maier SF. The "toll" of opioid-induced glial activation: improving the clinical efficacy of opioids by targeting glia. *Trends Pharmacol Sci.* 2009;30(11):581–591.

39. Hauser W, Petzke F, Uceyler N, Sommer C. Comparative efficacy and acceptability of amitriptyline, duloxetine and milnacipran in fibromyalgia syndrome: a systematic review with meta-analysis. *Rheumatology (Oxford).* 2011;50(3):532–543.

40. Macfarlane GJ, Kronisch C, Dean LE, et al. EULAR revised recommendations for the management of fibromyalgia. *Ann Rheum Dis.* 2016;0:1–11. http://dx.doi.org/10.1136/annrheumdis-2016-209724.

41. Basbaum AI, Fields HL. Endogenous pain control systems: brainstem spinal pathways and endorphin circuitry. *Annu Rev Neurosci.* 1984;7(1):309–338.

42. Tzschentke TM, Christoph T, Kogel B, et al. (-)-(1R,2R)-3-(3-dimethylamino-1-ethyl-2-methyl-propyl)-phenol hydrochloride (tapentadol HCl): a novel mu-opioid receptor agonist/norepinephrine reuptake inhibitor with broad-spectrum analgesic properties. *J Pharmacol Exp Ther.* 2007;323(1):265–276.

43. Koppert W, Ihmsen H, Körber N, et al. Different profiles of buprenorphine-induced analgesia and antihyperalgesia in a human pain model. *Pain.* 2005;118(1):15–22.

44. Gudin J, Fudin J, Nalamachu S. Levorphanol use: past, present and future. *Postgrad Med.* 2016;128(1):46–53.

45. Louw A, Diener I, Butler DS, Puentedura EJ. The effect of neuroscience education on pain, disability, anxiety, and stress in chronic musculoskeletal pain. *Arch Phys Med Rehabil.* 2011;92(12):2041–2056.

46. Nijs J, Malfliet A, Ickmans K, Baert I, Meeus M. Treatment of central sensitization in patients with 'unexplained' chronic pain: an update. *Expert Opin Pharmacother.* 2014;15(12):1671–1683.

47. Jensen MP. Psychosocial approaches to pain management: an organizational framework. *Pain.* 2011;152(4):717–725.

48. Gracely RH, Geisser ME, Giesecke T, et al. Pain catastrophizing and neural responses to pain among persons with fibromyalgia. *Brain.* 2004;127(Pt 4):835–843.

49. Busch AJ, Barber KA, Overend TJ, Peloso PMJ, Schachter CL. *Exercise for Treating Fibromyalgia Syndrome.* The Cochrane Library; 2007.

50. Deyo RA, Walsh NE, Martin DC, Schoenfeld LS, Ramamurthy S. A controlled trial of transcutaneous electrical nerve stimulation (TENS) and exercise for chronic low back pain. *N Engl J Med.* 1990;322(23):1627–1634.

51. Chou R, Huffman LH. Nonpharmacologic therapies for acute and chronic low back pain: a review of the evidence for an American Pain Society/American College of Physicians clinical practice guideline. *Ann Intern Med.* 2007;147(7):492–504.

CHAPTER 3

A Physiatric Approach to the Treatment of Complex Regional Pain Syndrome

MITCHELL FREEDMAN, DO • JEFFREY GEHRET, DO

INTRODUCTION

This chapter is meant to complement the other chapters in this book on complex regional pain syndrome (CRPS). Its goal is not to review all of the treatments that are available. Rather, it is an attempt to create a progressive treatment approach to what is often an arduous and potentially chronic problem. There is also a discussion of evidence base surrounding rehabilitative approaches to treatment.

A syndrome is defined as "a group of signs and symptoms that occur together and characterize a particular abnormality or condition or a set of concurrent things (as emotions or actions) that usually form an identifiable pattern."[1] CRPS is a syndrome that can present in a variety of ways. It is characterized by varying degrees by pain and vasomotor, sudomotor, and motor changes. It is not only painful but also threatening to both quality of life and function. Patients are frequently depressed and anxious as a result of the severity of the impact of this disease on their lives. Further complexity is added to the diagnosis and treatment by the fact that it can be a complication of nociceptive and/or neuropathic injuries.

With all of these variables, coupled with the fact that it is a relatively infrequent syndrome (see introductory chapter on CRPS), it becomes challenging to objectively evaluate treatments. Diagnostic criteria have also changed over the years, and outcome measures vary between studies. Thus, there is a dearth of evidence base surrounding its treatments. Recent treatment guidelines depend on systemic reviews, randomized and controlled studies, retrospective studies, open-label trials, pilot studies and anecdotes, case reports, and clinical experience to arrive at recommendations.[2–5]

Furthermore, there is a paucity in disease-specific outcome measures that are designed to specifically evaluate CRPS. The Radboud skills questionnaire was constructed to analyze disability in patients with upper extremity reflex sympathetic dystrophy.[6] A multitude of scales and questionnaires have been used in studies on CRPS. The neuropathic pain scale is designed to assess specific pain qualities associated with neuropathic pain.[7] Nonspecific unidimensional scales, such as the visual analogue scale, numeric rating scale, and verbal rating scale, have been used to evaluate pain intensity.[8] The McGill Pain is a general questionnaire that evaluates pain intensity as well as the sensory, affective, and evaluative dimensions of pain.[9] Other examples of common questionnaires used in the assessment of depression include the Minnesota Multiphasic Personality Inventory[10] and the Beck Depression Inventory.[11] The State Trait Anxiety Inventory is a questionnaire that evaluates anxiety.[12] Further work needs to be done to create questionnaires that specifically evaluate function, pain, quality of life, depression, anxiety, and costs associated with treatment so that we are better able to evaluate treatment interventions.

Although there is a suboptimal literature that supports many of our proven treatments, it is incumbent on the practitioner to formulate a logical approach to address the many facets of treatment that must be utilized to treat the physiologic and functional challenges that beset the patient. Pain, swelling, range-of-motion deficits, weakness and dystonias, functional deficits, depression and anxiety, and social and financial problems must all be addressed in the treatment plan. The initial treatment plan must be continually reassessed and updated based on the progress or lack thereof in the individual case in light of new and changing signs and symptoms that may develop as the syndrome passes from an acute injury to a potential chronic life-altering disease.

INTERDISCIPLINARY TREATMENT

There are many specialties of healthcare practitioners who treat pain. Physicians specializing in surgery (neurosurgery, orthopedics, vascular, general), anesthesia, neurology, psychiatry, family medicine, and rehabilitative medicine may have special interest in pain management. Other healthcare professionals, such as physical therapists, occupational therapists, psychologists, social workers, nurses, recreational therapists, and vocational therapists, may play a part in treatment. These practitioners may treat patients as individuals or as part of a multidisciplinary or interdisciplinary team of professionals.

An interdisciplinary team is a group of healthcare professionals from complementary fields who work in tandem to treat a patient. The core team frequently consists of a physician (often a physiatrist), physical therapist, occupational therapist, and psychologist. Social work, nursing, recreational therapist, and vocational therapist may be involved. The team meets on a regular basis to discuss progress and treatment adjustments. The team leader is often the physician or psychologist. Although these are practitioners with different backgrounds and expertise, they have the individual and complementary skills and the team approach helps to foster communication.

Perhaps the most important part of the team is the patient. The patient meets with these various team members to establish goals, including pain management and relief, function (activities of daily living [ADLs], ambulation, recreation, vocation, childcare, sexuality, etc.), mood, and anxiety. The patient must be motivated to achieve these goals, or the program cannot succeed.

Harden and Cole suggested that interdisciplinary treatment "always be considered early in every complicated case" with a neuropathic pain syndrome.[13] Interdisciplinary pain treatment has long been a standard of care for treatment of chronic nonmalignant pain. Peters et al. reported that 68% of inpatients and 61% of outpatients who received multidisciplinary treatment had improvements in pain rating, analgesic use, and activity levels.[14] A meta-analysis of 65 studies evaluating multidisciplinary treatments for chronic back pain tended to support the improvement of pain, mood, return to work, and use of the healthcare system in a stable fashion. Caution was urged because of limitations in the quality of the studies.[15] Guzman et al. also reviewed multidisciplinary treatment of back pain and concluded that there was moderate evidence that intensive biopsychosocial rehabilitation with functional restoration improves function relative to nonmultidisciplinary rehabilitation. Contradictory evidence existed regarding vocational outcomes with these programs.[16]

Singh et al.[17] treated a group of 12 patients with CRPS type I for 4 weeks with physical therapy, occupational therapy, water therapy, psychotherapy, stellate ganglion blocks, and drug therapy. Anxiety levels remained stable and function improved. At 2-year follow-up, 75%

of patients were working. Daly et al. rated this study as good-quality evidence that an outpatient treatment program is effective for CRPS.[18]

The concept behind treating patients with complicated biopsychological syndromes in a multidisciplinary way is to reset the altered central processing and normalize the distal environmental level.[5,16] There have been three consensus meetings that have gradually molded a therapeutic approach to the treatment of CRPS.[2,3,19] Treatment addresses function immediately. ADLs and mobility issues should be addressed. Medication, procedural treatment, and psychological treatments are gradually worked into the treatment as the clinical course unfolds.

The initial step in treating the patient involves a comprehensive evaluation. A thorough history and physical examination may lead to an underlying problem that can be treated effectively, such as an unstable fracture or a compressed nerve. The patient's concurrent medical problems must be understood, because these other diagnoses may have an impact on pain or on the potential treatments that may be considered for pain. Underlying psychological issues and the presence of depression or anxiety must be addressed. Inability to perform simple tasks, such as washing and dressing, homemaking, toiletry, childcare, vocational activities, and recreational activities, must be a part of the history. The functional requirements of the patient must also be understood, and goals should be created to address those specific activities whenever feasible. Strife in relationships with a spouse, parent, child, or coworker or boss may be factors in care.

THERAPEUTIC TREATMENT

The initial therapeutic treatment begins with the activation of presensorimotor cortices via motor imagery, visual and tactile discrimination, and desensitization. Treatment guidelines have been created, but these are conceptual and flexible and should flow in the context of the individual's specific needs (see Fig. 3.1). It progresses to edema control, range of motion, and isometric strengthening. Treatment of posture and secondary positional deviations ensues. As the patient tolerates more, isotonic and isokinetic strengthening can be added in combination with stress loading. Aerobic conditioning and postural strategies are utilized. More advanced strategies are added as the patient makes progress, including ergonomics, movement strategies, and normalization of use, and vocational and functional rehabilitation progresses to hierarchical goals as the syndrome improves.[5] The progression of the treatment should not be based on

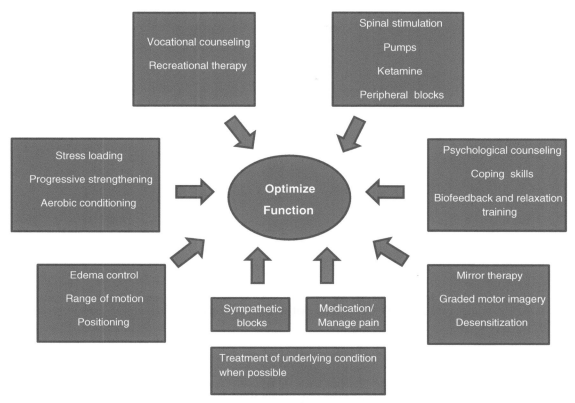

FIG. 3.1 Approach to the treatment of complex regional pain syndrome.

a time sequence because of the variability in the course of the syndrome. When there is lack of progress, medication and psychological treatment and procedural interventions may be considered if appropriate.

Physical therapy and occupational therapy often form a complementary team with separate but potentially overlapping roles. It has been stated that "physical therapy is the cornerstone and first line treatment for CRPS."[20] In addition to mobilization, the physical therapist addresses functional activities, including transfers and ambulation on levels, steps, and uneven surfaces. The occupational therapist may help with some of the transfer activities but concentrates more on upper extremity mobilization and strengthening as well as functional activities such as ADLs, homemaking, childcare, vocational activities, and any other functional goals that are important to the individual patient. "Functional restoration" is at the core of treatment of CRPS.[2,3,5] Several studies have supported the benefits of these disciplines in CRPS.[18,21–28]

Mirror Visual Feedback and Graded Motor Imagery

Mirror visual feedback (MVF) was first used by Ramachandran and Roger-Ramachandran in amputees to lessen phantom pain[29–31] It has also subsequently been used to treat phantom limb pain, stroke, CRPS, and persistent pain following wrist fracture and hand surgery. In 2003, McCabe et al. performed a pilot study with MVF in eight patients with CRPS type 1. After 6 weeks, patients with disease that was present for less than 1 year had normalization of pain and improved thermal changes. No improvements were found in patients with chronic CRPS.[30,31]

Mechanism of action for MVF is unclear, but proposed mechanisms revolve around correcting or improving the mismatch between the motor and sensory systems in CRPS, improving attention to the painful limb, lessening kinesiophobia, and improving body perception disturbance. Moseley et al.[32] demonstrated that a limb could be cooler if that limb was perceived as less important than the contralateral limb. Moseley also

Treatment 1 Treatment 2

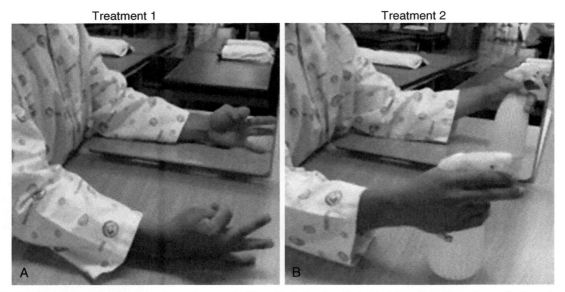

FIG. 3.2 Mirror visual feedback involves placement of the affected extremity behind the mirror. The mirror reflects an image of the healthy limb so that it appears that there are two intact hands. Goals are to improve perception of the affected limb and lessen kinesiophobia.

demonstrated that imagined movements can also cause pain and swelling in a patient with CRPS.[33] Patients with CRPS have a distorted body image.[34] Patients with chronic pain develop shrunken or enlarged changes in the primary motor and sensory maps with representations of the affected body part, as seen on functional MRI. Changes are also seen in the thalamus, visual cortex, and brainstem.[31,35,36] Pain reduction may cause reversal of these changes.[37,38]

McCabe emphasizes that MVF "is not a stand-alone therapy[31] but should be used within a multidisciplinary rehabilitation program and may instead of pay be a useful adjunct to desensitization therapy." As in most treatments in CRPS (not unlike many other pain syndromes) there is a limited evidence base supporting MVF use and even less information supporting any specific protocol. O'Connell et al. concluded that there was low-quality evidence that mirror therapy reduced pain and improved upper limb function in poststroke CRPS compared with covered mirror therapy and the effect may have moderate clinical significance.[39]

The patient is generally introduced to the idea of mirror therapy by having them create an awareness of the limbs in their body and trying to help them to understand the difference in how their brain perceives the affected limb versus the contralateral unaffected limb. The concept may be explained to the patient as an attempt to "trick" the brain into improving the image

of the damaged extremity. Imagined movements may be rehearsed before the initiation of MVF. McCabe suggests the "Bath MVF Treatment Protocol."[31] The affected limb is placed on the nonreflective side of the mirror, whereas the unaffected limb is seen in the reflective surface of the mirror (Fig. 3.2). The patient is asked to gradually begin movements bilaterally and synchronously. The patient is asked to perform this technique "little, but often" up to five or six times per day for no more than 5 min. Treatment should be discontinued if pain levels increase, if tremor and/or dystonia worsens significantly, and if the patient cannot understand the treatment. Some patients may not be able to move the hidden affected extremity when it is hidden from their vision, even though the limb is capable of movement when it is not hidden; this is called motor extinction. It may be related to deficits in attention in patients with impaired sensory feedback, leading to difficulty with motor function. This represents a severe disturbance in body image. MVF should not be used in these patients, as it may increase pain and motor deficits.

Moseley[40] hypothesized that activating the premotor cortex might be improved by starting out with a treatment that does not initially involve movement through the use of motor imagery. Part of the theory was that pain would be less likely to occur with imagined movements and that pain and motor function are so closely related that movement execution commands may induce pain. In 2004 a standardized motor imagery plan was evaluated in 26 patients with chronic upper extremity CRPS I over 6 weeks. Patients were treated with three stages, each of 2 weeks' duration. Thirteen of the patients received the motor imagery program and were compared with 13 patients who received normal management; the control group then crossed over to the motor imagery program.

Stage one consisted of identification of hand laterality. Forty-two pictures of the right and left hand (total of 82 pictures) in various postures were presented in a random order on a monitor in front of a seated patient. The patient pressed a button as rapidly as possible to identify which hand was on the screen. This activity was performed on a computer and was to be performed three times per each waking hour. It took approximately 10 min.

In stage two the patient performs imagined hand movements with the affected hand that were similar to 28 pictures of the same hand in various postures randomly selected from a picture bank. Patients performed the task three times per hour for the entire time that they were awake. Emphasis was on accuracy and not on speed.

Stage three involves mirror therapy; the patient simulates postures similar to 20 pictures of the unaffected hand that were seen on paper copies. They were told to perform this activity with both hands with the use of mirror therapy 10 times each waking hour with the affected hand concealed behind the nonreflective part of the mirror while they watched the unaffected hand perform these movements in the mirror.

Treatment resulted in significant decrease in the pain intensity and finger circumference, which was maintained for 12 weeks. The control group achieved similar gains after it crossed over to the motor imagery program. At 12 weeks after the program, a total of six patients (four in the initial motor imagery program and two from the control group after it crossed over) no longer fulfilled the criteria for CRPS I.[40] Moseley performed a larger randomized controlled study with 51 patients with CRPS or phantom pain; gains in pain and function were made in the group that was treated with graded motor imagery (GMI).[41]

Moseley confirmed that the sequence of preceding mirror therapy with imagined movement before mirror imagery was critical for successful treatment in 2005 when he randomized the order of treatment. Hand laterality recognition/imagined movements/mirror movements were compared with imagined movements/hand laterality recognition/imagined movements and hand laterality recognition/mirror group/hand laterality recognition. The group of hand laterality recognition/imagined movements/mirror movements made the greatest gains in pain and disability. The hand laterality recognition diminished pain and disability in all groups to a lesser degree, and imagined movements lessened pain and disability only when they followed hand laterality recognition. The mirror therapy reduced pain and disability only when it followed imagined movements. The conclusion was that it is important to sequentially activate the premotor and motor networks before mirror therapy to achieve the best outcome.[42]

Bowering et al. performed a literature review and concluded that GMI and mirror therapy alone may be effective, but there is limited evidence. It was concluded that rigorous studies are needed in a wider population with pain.[43] In a separate review of interventions of CRPS, O'Connell et al. opined that there is low-quality evidence that GMI and medical management are more effective at reducing pain and improving function than medical management alone and that ordered GMI is more effective than unordered GMI in reducing pain in patients with CRPS I.[39]

Desensitization

Desensitization is critical early in CRPS to allow the patient to begin to mobilize the injured limb. Pleger et al. demonstrated that intractable pain in CRPS resulted in shrinkage in cortical maps on the contralateral primary (SI) and secondary somatosensory cortex as demonstrated on functional MRI. Behavioral treatment over 1–6 months with sensorimotor retuning (desensitization and graded sensory and motor tasks) resulted in decreased pain, improved tactile discrimination, and improvement in the map size in the primary and secondary somatosensory cortex.[38] Proprioceptive feedback enhancement via vibratory stimulation also led to less pain and improved proprioception.[44]

Edema Control

Swelling and range of motion of the upper extremity must be addressed in tandem with desensitization. Edema control may be accomplished with training the patient to position the affected limb in an attitude that allows fluid to drain from the swollen extremity. Centripetal massage, Coban wrapping (when tolerated), and pressure garments may also be utilized to combat swelling. Contrast baths improve circulation by alternating vasodilation (heat) with vasoconstriction (cold). The heat and cold are also beneficial in desensitization. Splinting, when tolerated, may be employed to maintain or increase motion but has a limited role, and active motion is encouraged.

Mobilization and Strengthening

The clinician who is attempting to mobilize the affected limb or joint must overcome the patient's fear of movement (kinesiophobia). This fear is based both on fear of nociception and the actual degree of pain that may be encountered with mobilization. Learned behaviors may result in less activity and secondary weakness and functional deficits as well. In back pain, lowering fear may reduce avoidance of motion and improve function.[45] In an attempt to reduce pain-fears and subsequent functional deficit, de Jong et al. utilized graded exposure in vivo (GEXP) as a treatment modality in CRPS I. Eight patients were taught about the vicious cycle posed by pain, catastrophic thought, fear, and avoidance and lessening function with subsequent worsening of pain. They then were placed into a program in which they were gradually exposed to situations that patients thought were dangerous or threatening to their painful extremity. Patients were initially encouraged to perform these activities while in treatment and then, eventually, on their own. The therapist was gradually withdrawn. Pain-related fear, pain intensity, disability, and physiologic signs and symptoms all improved.[46]

A balance in intervention must be achieved that allows the patient to progress in range of motion and strength, which are the predicates of function. Peripheral nociceptive stimulation, which is a part of CRPS, sustains central sensitization. Overaggressive mobilization may exacerbate this process. By normalizing motion and activity, the idea is to normalize the afferent input and lessen the central nervous system hypersensitivity. Improving motion and activity in a given extremity lessens pain, range of motion, osteoporosis, swelling, and autonomic disturbance.[47]

Pain exposure physical therapy (PEPT) directly exposes patients to painful stimuli. Patients are advised to return to activity without medication; they are advised to ignore the pain. Patients and their involved family members are educated about the condition and the program; the patient's partner is directed to abandon nurturing behavior and is instructed to motivate the patient to be active. The therapists and the patient's partner are to ignore verbal and nonverbal expressions of pain. Self-massage, range of motion, and progressive-loading exercises are instituted. Positive reinforcement is given for progression of movement and activity. Assistive devices such as crutches or canes are discouraged. The goal is to restore function, with the secondary effect being decrease in pain and secondary consequences of immobilization and inactivity.

PEPT has been studied in CRPS several times with mixed results. Ek and van Gijn retrospectively evaluated 106 patients with chronic CRPS treated with PEPT. Functional improvement was seen in 95 patients and full functional recovery was seen in 49 patients, although 23 of those patients had increased pain.[48] van de Meent et al. studied 20 patients with CRPS treated with PEPT and improvements were noted in pain intensity, muscle strength, upper extremity function, walking speed, and kinesiophobia.[49] On the other hand, Barnhoom et al. found more equivocal results with PEPT. Conventional treatment was compared with PEPT in a randomized controlled study of 56 patients with CRPS I. Patients in both groups made significant gains, but there was no significant difference in gains between the two groups other than greater improvement in active range of motion in the PEPT patients.[50]

As patients improve, more advanced mobilization treatments may be employed. Carlson and Watson describe a stress-loading program that utilizes active exercises that minimize joint motion while placing stress through the upper extremity. The patient utilizes a scrub brush to scrub a plywood board with gradual increase in time and pressure. They also carry a weighted briefcase or bag in the affected hand when the patient stands or walks throughout the day. They studied 41 patients over 2 years and patients reported improvements in pain, range of motion, and grip strength. Of 31 patients who worked, 26 people returned to their normal job and 95% of patients returned to full duty, although 50% of them still had difficulty with heavy lifting, buttons, and handling change.[22,23] As the patient makes progress, stress loading with ambulation and functional activities important to their everyday function (vocational and recreational activities) can be introduced.

Other options to mobilize patients who have difficulty with weight bearing and pain may include aquatic therapy. In general, water must be warm. The buoyancy of the water allows for lesser forces with weight bearing while the water provides some resistance. It has been used with some success in children.[51] As the patient tolerates more weight bearing in the water, weight bearing on land can gradually be introduced and progressed as tolerated.

Recreational therapy can be utilized to help motivate patients to incorporate their personal interests with their exercise routine. Having patients participate in an activity that they perceive as pleasurable may help them to overcome the pain and fear associated with movement of the injured extremity. Socialization with other patients may also be fostered through recreational activities. One of the goals of the good practitioner is to help patients begin to take responsibility for their own care. Having patients enjoy their movement therapy can certainly provide a bridge to independence with exercise.

Group therapies with other patients with disabilities or similar injuries can often provide a great support system. Patients may be willing to try to perform activities that they were loath to perform on their own, with the support of a group that is experiencing similar physical problems. Feldenkrais, yoga, and tai chi are other "mind-body strategies" that can be options for the patient.

Vocational therapy can help to create a program that allows the patient to get back to work. Work conditioning/hardening can be an option for the more advanced patient. The patient may need to regain strength, endurance, and agility to return to their previous job. Vocational counseling can help patients to decide whether or not they can return to their previous job. Patient can be helped to create a new vocational plan that is feasible for the individual with a significant impairment or disability.

PSYCHOLOGICAL ASSESSMENT AND TREATMENT

It is critical to initially assess and continually monitor the psychological state of patients who have CRPS, just as this is important in any severe pain syndrome. Anxiety and depression are frequently encountered in most patients who suffer from chronic pain of any etiology and may be exacerbated in patients with premorbid history of psychiatric pathology. Prevalence of anxiety and depression is present in 24%–46% of patients with CRPS.[52,53] Initial psychological evaluation should include screen for comorbid axis one disorders. Evaluation of the patient and possibly the family's cognitive, behavioral, and emotional responses to CRPS, as well as concurrent life stressors, should be undertaken.[5]

It is unclear as to whether or not patients with a certain psychological profile are more likely to develop CRPS. High-quality studies are lacking. Harden et al. demonstrated that preoperative anxiety and severity of pain were associated with a significant increase in the development of CRPS 1 month after total knee arthroplasty.[54] An increase in depression and anxiety from baseline presurgical levels at 4 weeks post surgery predicted greater CRPS symptoms at 6 months after surgery.[55] In contrast, no significant differences in personality or depression scales were seen in patients with distal radius fractures who developed CRPS relative to those patients who did not develop CRPS.[56] In a study comparing patients with chronic back pain with CRPS I patients, similar findings of major depressive and personality disorders were seen.[52] In a systematic review of the literature since 1980, Beerthuizen et al. concluded that there was no relationship between psychological factors and CRPS other than

being associated with life events such as divorce or death of a spouse.[57] Geertzen et al. also reported that a difficult time in life or a painful affective loss was more common during the onset of CRPS by comparing a group of patients with CRPS with a group of patients preparing for hand surgery over the next 24 h.[58]

Psychological treatment options include cognitive strategies to help convert the patient with an external locus of control to having an internal locus of control. Cognitive pain coping strategies, relaxation strategies, and thermal and superficial electromyographic biofeedback can be useful interventions. Psychologic counseling for anxiety and depression for both the patients and their family members is often critical. Group therapies that involve not only the psychologist but also potentially other therapeutic team members (physical therapy, occupational therapy, social service, etc.) may be useful in fostering peer support and potentially pressure toward improving pain management and function. Education regarding CRPS is critical because there is a great deal of misinformation available to patients that may contribute to fear, anxiety, and depression.

"Pain is an unpleasant sensory and emotional experience associated with actual or potential tissue damage, or described in terms of such damage."[59] As such pain is an individual experience that leads to unique responses on the part of each patient. The behaviors that develop as a result of pain is influenced not only by the nociceptor, but also the meaning of the disease to the individual, as well as the responses of other people and friends and family members that they encounter. Patients may develop anxiety in anticipation of movement or activity. They may lessen their activity to avoid pain and develop weakness and range of motion deficits, which exacerbate the underlying problem. A cycle of disuse and pain can lead to worsening pain, mood, and anxiety even if the underlying nociceptor has improved or resolved. Family members who mean well may inadvertently nurture these behaviors.[60]

Behavioral treatment programs have been utilized to treat excessive disability and expressions of suffering, not necessarily to treat pain. However, frequently pain does improve. These are functionally driven programs in which patients focus on activity, not pain relief. Education, fear reduction, stress management, and pain management strategies are provided as well. Certainly, the patient with CRPS must be monitored carefully for objective signs of tissue injury. Operant methods such as positive reinforcement, extinction, shaping, and modeling may be employed. These are generally multidisciplinary programs. Behavioral and cognitive-behavioral treatment has been used with success in chronic pain. Improvements may be seen in pain, distress, pain behavior, and function. It has not been well studied in CRPS so much as in patients with chronic back pain.[60-62]

ALTERNATIVE TREATMENTS

In general, these studies are not high quality and have low numbers of patients. They do show promise, and further research is required.

Acupuncture

There is low-quality evidence that acupuncture is not superior to sham acupuncture for short-term pain relief in patients with CRPS.[63] There is also low-quality evidence that acupuncture combined with rehabilitation might be effective with short-term pain relief in patients with shoulder hand syndrome post stroke compared with rehabilitation therapy alone, and electroacupuncture and rehabilitation may be better than triamcinolone acetonide and vitamin B12.[39,64]

Qigong

Wu et al. compared Qigong exercises while patients listened to music and were shown visual images of abstract art with sham Qigong therapy whereby patients were shown similar visual images and listened to similar music without exercise. There was a 91% decrease in pain intensity in the patients who had Qigong treatment compared with the sham group. Both groups had improvement in anxiety, although anxiety improved to a greater degree in the sham group. O'Connell et al. concluded that there is very low evidence that Qigong is superior to sham therapy in reducing CRPS-related pain.[39,65]

Hyperbaric Oxygen

Hyperbaric oxygen therapy has been utilized in patients with CRPS with some success in case reports as well as a double-blinded placebo-controlled randomized study. Kiralp et al. evaluated 71 patients with CRPS, and 37 received hyperbaric oxygen, whereas 34 had placebo treatment with room air. At day 45, there was a clear reduction in pain intensity and edema as well as improvement in range of motion.[66,67]

CONCLUSION

CRPS is a potentially devastating problem that can destroy lives. A team effort generally leads to the best outcomes with both pain and function. Furthermore, because these cases can be emotionally and physically draining, a multidisciplinary team provides support for the treating practitioners as well as the patient. Mirror therapy and GMI, desensitization, edema control, mobilization and strengthening, and psychological support are keystones to treatment. Medication, injection procedures, surgery, and spinal stimulation are adjunctive options that may be helpful. Evidence base behind treatment is lacking and further research is critical.

REFERENCES

1. www.merriam-webster.com/dictionary/syndrome/04/01/2017.
2. Stanton-Hicks MD, et al. Complex regional pain syndromes: a guidelines for therapy. *Clin J Pain*. 1998;14(2):155–166.
3. Stanton-Hicks MD, et al. An updated interdisciplinary clinical pathway for CRPS: report of an expert panel. *Pain Pract*. 2002;2(1):1–16.
4. Peres RS, et al. Evidence based guidelines for complex regional pain syndrome type 1. *BMC Neurol*. 2010;10:20.
5. Harden RN, et al. Complex regional pain syndromes practical diagnostic and treatment guidelines, 4th edition. *Pain Med*. 2013;14:180–229.
6. Oerlemans HM, Cup EHC, et al. The Radboud skills questionnaire: construction and reliability in patients with reflex sympathetic dystrophy of one upper extremity. *Disabil Rehabil*. 2000;22(5):233–245.
7. Galer BS, Jensen MP. Development and preliminary validation of a pain measure specific to neuropathic pain: the neuropathic pain scale. *Neurology*. 1997;48:332–338.
8. Ferreira-Valente MA, Pais-Ribeiro JC, Jensen MP. Validity of four pain intensity rating scales. *Pain*. 2011;152:2399–2404.
9. Melzack R. The McGill pain questionnaire major properties and scoring methods. *Pain*. 1975;1:275–299.
10. Leavitt F, Garron DC. Validity of a back pain classification scale for detecting psychological disturbance as measured by the MMPI. *J Clin Psychol*. 1980;39(1):186–189.
11. Beck ET, et al. An inventory for measuring depression. *Arch Gen Psychiatry*. 1961;4:561–571.
12. Spielberger CD, Gorsuch RL, Lushene RE. *Manual for the State-Trait Anxiety Inventory*. Palo Alto, CA: Consulting Psychologists Press; 1970.
13. Harden RN, Cole PA. New developments in rehabilitation of neuropathic pain syndromes. Interdisciplinary team approach. *Neurol Clin*. 1998;16(4):937–950.
14. Peters J, Large RG, Elkind G. Follow up results from a randomized controlled trial evaluating in and outpatient pain management programs. *Pain*. 1992;50:41–50.
15. Flor H, Fydrich T, Turk DC. Efficacy of multidisciplinary pain treatment centers: a meta-analytic review. *Pain*. 1992;49:221–230.
16. Guzman J, et al. Multidisciplinary rehabilitation for chronic low back pain: systematic review. *BMJ*. 2001;322:1511–1516.

17. Singh G, Willen SN, et al. The value of interdisciplinary pain management in complex regional pain syndrome type I: a prospective outcome study. *Pain Physician*. 2004;7(2):203–209.
18. Daly AE, Bialocerkowski AE. Does evidence support physiotherapy management of adult complex regional pain syndrome type one? A systemic review. *Eur J Pain*. 2009;13:339–353.
19. Harden RN. The rationale for integrated functional restoration. In: Wilson PR, Stanton-Hicks M, Harden RN, eds. *CRPS: Current Diagnosis and Therapy*. Seattle, WA: IASP Press; 2006:163–171.
20. Rho RH, Brewer RP, et al. Complex regional pain syndrome. *Mayo Clin Proc*. 2002;77:174–180.
21. Birklein F, Riedl B, et al. Neurological findings in complex regional pain syndromes - analysis of 145 cases. *Acta Neurol Scand*. 2000;101:262–269.
22. Carlson LK, Watson HK. Treatment of reflex sympathetic dystrophy using the stress loading program. *J Hand Ther*. 1988;1:149–154.
23. Watson HK, Carlson L. Treatment of reflex sympathetic dystrophy of the hand with an active "stress loading" program. *J Hand Surg Am*. 1987;12:779–785.
24. Oerlemans HM, Oostendorp RA, et al. Pain and reduced mobility in complex regional pain syndrome I: outcome of a prospective randomized controlled clinical trial of adjuvant physical therapy versus occupational therapy. *Pain*. 1999;83:77–83.
25. Oerlemans HM, Goris J, et al. Do physical therapy and occupational therapy reduce the impairment percentage in reflex sympathetic dystrophy? *Am J Phys Med Rehabil*. 1999;78:533–539.
26. Severens JL, Oerlemans HM, et al. Cost-effectiveness analysis of adjuvant physical therapy or occupational therapy for adults with reflex sympathetic dystrophy. *Arch Phys Med Rehabil*. 1999;80:1038–1043.
27. Lee BH, Scharff L, et al. Physical therapy and cognitive-behavioral treatment for complex regional pain syndromes. *J Pediatr*. 2002;141:135–140.
28. Phillips ME, Katz JA, Harden RN. The use of nerve blocks in conjunction with occupational therapy for complex regional pain syndrome type I. *Am J Occup Ther*. 2000;54(5):544–549.
29. Ramachandran VS, Roger- Ramachandran D. Synaesthesia in phantom limbs induced with mirrors. *Proc R Soc Lond B Biol Sci*. 1996;263:377–386.
30. McCabe CS, Haigh RC, et al. A controlled pilot study of the utility of mirror visual feedback in the treatment of complex regional pain syndrome (type I). *Rheumatology*. 2003;42:97–101.
31. McCabe C. Mirror visual feedback therapy. A practical approach. *J Hand Ther*. 2011;24:170–179.
32. Moseley GL, Olthof N, et al. Psychologically inducing cooling of a specific body part caused by the illusory ownership of an artificial counterpart. *Proc Natl Acad Sci USA*. 2008;105:13169–13173.
33. Moseley GL. Imagined movements cause pain and swelling in a patient with complex regional pain syndrome. *Neurology*. 2004;62:1644.
34. Moseley GL. Distorted body image in complex regional pain syndrome. *Neurology*. 2005;65:773.
35. Flor H, Elbert T, et al. Phantom-limb pain as a perceptual correlate of cortical reorganization following arm amputation. *Nature*. 1995;375:482–484.
36. Maihofner C, Baron C, et al. The motor system shows adaptive changes in complex regional pain syndrome. *Brain*. 2007;130:2671–2687.
37. Maihofner C, Handwerker H, et al. Patterns of reorganization in complex regional pain syndrome. *Neurology*. 2003;61:1707–1715.
38. Pleger B, Tegenthoff M, et al. Sensorimotor retuning in complex regional pain syndrome parallels pain reduction. *Ann Neurol*. 2005;57:425–429.
39. O'Connell NE, Wand BM, et al. Interventions for treating pain and disability in adults with complex regional pain syndrome - an overview of systemic reviews (review). *Cochrane Database Syst Rev*. 2013;(4). Art. No: CD009416. http://dx.doi.org/10.1002/14651858.CD009416.pub2.
40. Moseley GL. Graded motor imagery is effective for longstanding complex regional pain syndrome: a randomized controlled trial. *Pain*. 2004;108:192–198.
41. Moseley GL. Graded motor imagery for pathologic pain. A randomized controlled trial. *Neurology*. 2006;67:2129–2134.
42. Moseley GL. Is successful rehabilitation of complex regional pain syndrome due to sustained attention to the affected limb? A randomized clinical trial. *Pain*. 2005;114:54–61.
43. Bowering KJ, O'Connell NE, et al. The effects of graded motor imagery and its components on chronic pain: a systemic review and meta-analysis. *J Pain*. 2013;14(1):3–13.
44. Gay A, Parratte S, Salazard B, et al. Proprioceptive feedback enhancement induced by vibratory stimulation in complex regional pain syndrome type I: an open comparative pilot study in 11 patients. *Joint Bone Spine*. 2007;74:461–466.
45. Boersma K, Linton S, et al. Lowering fear-avoidance and enhancing function through exposure in vivo: a multiple baseline study across six patients with back pain. *Pain*. 2004;108:8–16.
46. de Jong J, Vlaeyen J, Onghena P, et al. Reduction of pain related fear in complex regional pain syndrome type one: the application of graded exposure in vivo. *Pain*. 2005;116:241–248.
47. Guo TZ, Offley SC, et al. Substance P signaling contributes to the vascular and nociceptive abnormalities observed in a tibial fracture rat model of complex regional pain syndrome type I. *Pain*. 2004;108:95–107.
48. Ek JW, van Gijn JC. Pain exposure physical therapy may be a safe and effective treatment for longstanding complex regional pain syndrome type I: a case series. *Clin Rehabil*. 2009;23:1059–1066.
49. van de Meent H, Oerlemans M, et al. Safety of "pain exposure" physical therapy in patients with complex regional pain syndrome type I. *Pain*. 2011;152:1431–1438.

50. Barnhoom KJ, van de Meent H, et al. Pain exposure physical therapy (PEPT) compared to conventional treatment in complex regional pain syndrome type I: a randomized controlled trial. *BMJ Open.* 2015;5:e008282. http://dx.doi.org/10.1136/bmjopen-2015-008283.

51. Sherry DD, Wallace CA, et al. Short and long-term outcomes of children with complex regional pain syndrome type I treated with exercise therapy. *Clin J Pain.* 1999;15(3):218–223.

52. Monti DA, Herring CL, et al. Personality assessment of patients with complex regional pain syndrome type I. *Clin J Pain.* 1998;14(4):295–302.

53. Rommel O, Malin JP, et al. Quantitative sensory testing, neurophysiological and psychological examination in patients with complex regional pain syndrome and hemisensory deficits. *Pain.* 2001;93:279–293.

54. Harden RN, Bruehl S, et al. Prospective examination of pain-related and psychological predictors of CRPS-like phenomena following total knee arthroplasty: a preliminary study. *Pain.* 2003;106(3):393–400.

55. Harden RN, Bruehl S, et al. Development of a severity score for CRPS. *Pain.* 2010;151:870–876.

56. Puchalski P, Zyluk A. Complex regional pain syndrome type 1 after fractures of the distal radius: a prospective study of the role of psychological factors. *J Hand Surg Br.* 2005;30(6):574–580.

57. Beerthuizen A, van't Spijker A, et al. Is there an association between psychological factors and the complex regional pain syndrome type I (CRPS I) in adults? A systematic review. *Pain.* 2009;145(1–2):52–59.

58. Geertzen JH, de Bruijn-Kofman AT, et al. Stressful life events and psychological dysfunction in complex regional pain syndrome type I. *Clin J Pain.* 1998;14(2):143–147.

59. IASP Subcommittee on Taxonomy. Pain terms: a list with definitions and notes on usage. *Pain.* 1979;6:249–252.

60. Fordyce WE, Roberts AH, Sternbach RA. The behavioral management of chronic pain: a response to critics. *Pain.* 1985;22:113–125.

61. McCracken LM, Turk DC. Behavioral and cognitive-behavioral treatment for chronic pain. Outcome, predictors of outcome and treatment process. *Spine.* 2002;27(22):2564–2573.

62. Jensen IB, Bergstrom G, et al. A randomized controlled component analysis of a behavioral medicine rehabilitation program for chronic spinal pain: are the effects dependent on gender? *Pain.* 2001;91:65–78.

63. Kho KH. The impact of acupuncture on pain in patients with reflex sympathetic dystrophy. *Pain Clin.* 1998;8(1):59–61.

64. Jin Y, Wng J, Wang A. Acupuncture in rehabilitation therapies on shoulder hand syndrome: 40 observational cases. *J Clin Acupunct Moxib.* 2007;23(1):14–15.

65. Wu W, Bandilla E, et al. Effects of qigong on late stage complex regional pain syndrome. *Altern Ther Health Med.* 1999;5(1):45–54.

66. Kiralp MZ, Yildiz S. Effectiveness of hyperbaric oxygen therapy in the treatment of complex regional pain syndrome. *Int Med Res.* 2004;32:258–262.

67. Yildiz S, Uzun G, Kiralp MZ. Hyperbaric oxygen therapy in chronic pain management. *Clin Pain Headache Rep.* 2006;10(2):95–100.

CHAPTER 4

Complex Regional Pain Syndrome: Introduction, History, and Physical Examination

MICHAEL J. MEHNERT, MD • VICTOR HSU, MD • GEORGE YOUNG, DO

INTRODUCTION

Complex regional pain syndrome (CRPS) is a challenging neuropathic pain syndrome characterized by severe pain with atypical features. Continuing regional pain that is seemingly disproportionate to the usual course of illness/injury, in time or severity, is a key sign of this disease process. As a clinical entity it has been known by many names. They have evolved from terms such as "causalgia" and "reflex sympathetic dystrophy" (RSD) to the current nomenclature of CRPS type I and type II. Similarly, diagnostic criteria for this complex condition have evolved over time.[1]

Claude Bernard is noted to have documented the first sympathetic pain syndrome in the 1800s, and "causalgia" was first described in American Civil War veterans by Silas Weir-Mitchell. Paul Sudeck described a pain syndrome known as "acute inflammatory bone atrophy" that could spread beyond the initial site of injury and was given the name "Sudeck atrophy."[2,3] In the 1940s the term "reflex sympathetic dystrophy" was used for a sympathetic pain syndrome and entered common clinical usage.[1,4] RSD fell out of favor as a term, as dystrophy was seen in a small percentage of patients and sympathetic and autonomic changes were not consistently delineated as causative factors. Furthermore, the role of a "reflex" in the syndrome was not well identified.[5] In 1994 the International Association for the Study of Pain (IASP) changed the terminology to CRPS type I and type II.[6,7]

CRPS often involves a trauma, but it can occur spontaneously.[8,9] The development of CRPS is not related to the severity of a trauma/injury.[1,8] CRPS type I has been associated with an inciting event (often an injury such as a crush injury or soft tissue injury),[6] whereas type II (similar to the entity previously called "causalgia") has an association with a documented nerve injury, whether penetrating trauma or iatrogenic or surgical in nature.[1]

Classically, syndromes mediated by the sympathetic nervous system had a presenting component of autonomic dysfunction (abnormalities in diaphoresis, perfusion, and trophic changes) and some degree of improvement with neural blockade of the sympathetic supply to the affected area.[9] More recently, pain disproportionate to what should be expected of the injury is the hallmark of this illness, along with atypical symptoms that include disuse, hypersensitivity, sudomotor changes (edema, sweating), and vasomotor changes (skin color/temperature).[1,5] The pain must not be better explained by another diagnosis, and it need not be restricted to a specific nerve territory or dermatome.[1] CRPS symptoms may "spread" over time to other body regions.[10,11] The variety of symptoms (sensory, motor, autonomic, trophic, and others) in patients with CRPS contributes to resistance to typical pharmacologic therapies for other similar/related neuropathic pain syndromes.[12-14] A multimodal approach to clinical treatment is generally employed.

Although our understanding of CRPS continues to improve and evolve,[15] deficiencies in the methodology of published studies have been a limiting factor.[16] Evidence-based reviews of the CRPS literature have cited a need for more high-quality research.[1,17]

EPIDEMIOLOGY AND DEMOGRAPHICS

CRPS is often, but not always, associated with a traumatic injury.[9] It is more commonly associated with fractures,[8,9] followed by sprain injuries and then elective surgery. There is no one particular injury that regularly or reliably leads to the development of CRPS and there is not a direct correlation with the severity of an injury and the onset of CRPS.[9,10] The upper limb is more affected by CRPS than the lower limb. Data on the incidence are variable, ranging from 5.46 new cases per 100,000 persons per year[18,19] to 26.2 new cases per 100,000 persons per year.[9,18] Women are more affected than men.[1,3,4] Peak incidence is 61–70 years old (possibly related to elderly patients having a greater fracture risk).[9,10]

As a disease entity, CRPS has a relatively low prevalence; this and variable clinical presentations may contribute to limited epidemiologic data.[18]

Regarding risk factors, immobilization may be the greatest risk factor[15,20] and may explain the "shoulder-hand syndrome" that has been described after a stroke without a traumatic injury. Postmenopausal women have also been found to be at increased risk for CRPS type I.[9] One literature review also concluded that female sex (postmenopausal females in particular), ankle intradislocations or intraarticular fractures, distal radius fractures, immobilization, and intense pain in the early phases after trauma may be risk factors for CRPS type I.[18,21] CRPS more commonly occurs after a wrist fracture, with a reported incidence of 1%–37%.[18,22–25]

Prior studies[18,26,27] and recent literature reviews[28,29] do not demonstrate an association of psychiatric conditions with CRPS 1.

COURSE/PROGNOSIS

CRPS generally develops within 6 weeks after an inciting event.[7] It has previously been described as having an initial acute stage ("warm" or "hot") of up to 6 months and then a later "cold" stage.[15,18,30] The acute stage, lasting less than 6 months, presents with a painful, red, warm, sweaty, and swollen affected limb with increased hair growth. Over time the chronic stage develops; the swelling resolves, the skin becomes thin and cold, and the nails become brittle and pitted with decreased hair growth (trophic changes). Muscle atrophy with contractures and fibrosis can occur.

A disease course that involves three distinct phases of CRPS has also been described. Again, an *acute stage* with pain and sensory abnormalities with allodynia, hyperalgesia, and vasomotor/sudomotor dysfunction has been postulated. This is followed by a *dystrophic stage* with persistent sensory and vasomotor symptoms and motor and trophic changes over the next 3–6 months and finally an *atrophic stage*, where there are progressive vasomotor, motor, and trophic changes but the pain and sensory abnormalities seem to decrease ("burn out").[8] More recently, these "phases" have not been validated clinically.[1] Instead, more recent subgroup analysis has demonstrated that it is more likely that there are instead three different *subtypes* of CRPS: (1) a vasomotor-predominant, relatively limited syndrome, (2) a similarly limited syndrome with sensory

abnormalities and pain predominating, and (3) a subtype that more closely resembles "classic" RSD.[1,22,31–33] The second subtype may be a synonym for CRPS type II ("causalgia"), and the third subtype may have the greatest degree of trophic change and bone-density change despite having a shorter pain duration.

Overall the burden of illness with CRPS is large and can be quite limiting for patients. CRPS generally requires long-term intensive medical treatment with a significant negative impact on the quality of life.[17,34,35] Prognostic factors are not well defined. Resolution does occur, and it is less probable to do so over time. Resolution rates of up to 74% during the first year and up to 36% within the first 6 years have been reported.[15,19,36] Complications (other than pain and the associated sequelae) often include limited range of motion and/or contractures, and abnormal sensation.[8]

PATHOPHYSIOLOGY

The exact mechanism underlying CRPS as an illness is unknown, but the knowledge gap seems to be narrowing. The disease process seems to be elusive and complicated and likely multifactorial.[18,37] A repeated hypothesis for this illness involves a central sensitization component and a peripheral sensitization component.[15]

The inciting event, when present, provokes an acute stage reaction with a "classic" inflammatory response, but perhaps more importantly a "neurogenic" inflammatory response. Patients with CRPS have increased proinflammatory cytokines locally and systemically (including cerebrospinal fluid) that are responsible for localized edema, warmth, and erythema.[8,18] The role of inflammation is supported by mechano-heat-insensitive C-fibers, which have been found to have a neurosecretory role, where the nociceptors actually release neuropeptides via an axon reflex.[2] Substance P release may correlate with swelling/edema, and calcitonin-gene-related peptide can induce vasodilation.[2] Serum markers of sedimentation rates, autoimmune antibody titers, and cell counts are generally normal.[15]

Chronic activation of the afferent C-fibers from a noxious stimulus has been proposed as a mechanism for subsequent peripheral sensitization and reduction in the threshold for activation.[6,38] It has been postulated that peripheral sensitization may be related to chronic neurogenic inflammation. Markers such as interleukin (IL)-6 and tumor necrosis factor α were elevated in the affected limb,[6,39] and increased serum levels of substance P and IL-8 were also found in patients with CRPS.[40]

The neurotransmitter *N*-methyl D-aspartate (NMDA) has been implicated as a factor in central sensitization. NMDA receptors may make afferent nerves more sensitive to transmitter release and thus may cause action potentials to be produced with lower levels of neurotransmitters, resulting in enhanced nociceptive transmission. In this theory, the NMDA receptors can change the plasticity of the neural tissues.[41]

Central sensitization has also been shown in a study that demonstrated cortical somatosensory organizational changes in patients with CRPS[42,43]; these changes were reversible with resolution of symptoms. Functional MRI changes have demonstrated a difference in side-to-side cortical processing of mechanical stimuli.[2] These maladaptive features are some of the functional and structural changes identified in CRPS.[15] The presence of well-recognized features of the disease, including myoclonus/dystonia/tremor, malperceptions of one's own limb, paresis/weakness, and diffuse, nondermatomal sensory loss, also support a central nervous system (CNS) component.

A study evaluating for "spread" of CRPS type I[11] identified different patterns of spread (contiguous, independent/diffuse, and mirror imaging) and also postulated that localized pathology could be a likely explanation for contiguous spread. A CNS component (including aberrant CNS regulation of neurogenic inflammation) along with increased susceptibility was postulated to contribute to independent or mirror-image spread of the disease process.[11]

CRPS is considered a type of autonomically mediated pain, which often has a sympathetic component to it, although CRPS can be sympathetically independent.[44-47] CRPS with sympathetically mediated pain can be diagnosed by a positive response (pain relief) with sympathetic neural blockade.[46] Autonomic symptoms (particularly the sudomotor changes in the affected body part, with initial warmth and edema and later cooling) are likely due to an inability of the vessels to constrict or dilate.[48] Enhanced sympathetic activity may be a factor in the excitation of nociceptive fibers and development of pain; however, the association of sympathetic and afferent coupling is not well understood.[2]

HISTORY AND PHYSICAL EXAMINATION FINDINGS

As the diagnosis of CRPS is largely based on clinical findings, a thorough history and physical examination is critical, specifically in terms of findings that may correlate with diagnostic criteria.[1,5,18,49-51] Signs and symptoms in CRPS that are important on examination,

particularly for diagnostic purposes, are classified as (1) sensory, (2) vasomotor, (3) sudomotor/edema, and (4) motor/trophic. History and physical examination should focus on an evaluation of these systems and help ensure that a key criterion to diagnose CRPS, the absence of a better explanation for symptoms, is met.[50] In addition, the clinical presentation of CRPS is variable from patient to patient and a complete assessment is necessary to make a correct diagnosis (see Boxes 4.1 and 4.2).

BOX 4.1

History and Physical Findings in Patients With Complex Regional Pain Syndrome (CRPS)

A 1993 study of 829 patients[32] identified a variety of symptoms and findings in patients with CRPS, including:
  Pain (most important)
  Asymmetric temperature
  Skin color changes
  Limited movement
  Muscle spasms
  Pseudoparalysis
  Paresis
  Atrophy (skin, muscle, and bone)
  Hyperhidrosis
  Changes in hair and nail growth

Data from Veldman PH, Reynen HM, Arntz IE, Goris RJ. Signs and symptoms of reflex sympathetic dystrophy: prospective study of 829 patients. *Lancet.* 1993;342:1012–1016.

BOX 4.2

Frequency of Signs and Symptoms in Complex Regional Pain Syndrome

Burning or stinging pain	81%
Hyperesthesia with common mechanical stimuli	65%
Asymmetry of color in the affected limb	87%
Asymmetry of temperature in affected limb	79%
Asymmetry of hidrosis	53%
Trophic changes/abnormal growth:	
Skin	24%
Hair	21%
Nail	18%
Limb edema	80%
Limited limb range of motion	80%
Limb weakness	75%
Tremors/clonic activity/"jumping" of limb	20%

Data from Harden RN, Bruehl SP. Diagnosis of complex regional pain syndrome. *Clin J Pain.* 2006;22(5):415–419 and Harden RN, Bruehl S, Galer BS, et al. Complex regional pain syndrome: are the IASP diagnostic criteria valid and sufficiently comprehensive? *Pain.* 1999;83:211–219.

A patient with CRPS generally has a recent structural injury, and this should be a key point of history taking in suspected patients. History should also include an evaluation of the patient's painful symptoms, including the character and type of pain. Pain is the cardinal symptom of CRPS and is often described as burning or stinging but can be a tearing type of pain, generally deep in the affected limb. Questions about epicritic or neuropathic pain may help to identify symptoms, and patients may report hyperesthesia such as pain from clothing or bed sheets against the injured limb. Environmental changes and temperature sensitivity from air circulation or bathing may be reported. The clinician should evaluate for pain that is present only when evoked (mechanical or thermal stimuli can evoke pain) as well as pain that is spontaneous.

Sensory deficits are also often noted. A detailed history of sensory abnormalities to ascertain for allodynia, hyperalgesia, and decreased sensation is imperative, and mechanical and thermal hyperalgesia are often associated with CRPS.[15]

Reports of swelling and erythema may be present, and other pertinent history includes an evaluation for a limb that is warm or cold. Skin color change, temperature change, and hyperhidrosis are important history points. Symptoms of perceived abnormal hair/nail changes and motor weakness and limited range of motion are also helpful and are salient points of the diagnostic criteria.[50]

Sympathetic/autonomic changes may not be present in all patients and may not be a constant or causative factor, again suggesting that CRPS does not always involve a sympathetic component.[1]

With regards to additional history taking, the evaluation should focus on the patient's functional status and possible decreased mobility/movement disorders, as well as the impact of the symptoms on the patient's activity. A substantial number of patients with CRPS report significant disability,[15,52] and in a survey of 55 patients,[52] 80% reported sleep disturbance and 75% reported substantial interference with work and recreational activities as a result of their disease.

Physical examination should include a detailed neurologic and musculoskeletal examination of all four limbs, including sensation (positive factors such as allodynia and negative factors such as loss of sensation), strength, range of motion, and reflexes. Applying a light stimulus that is nonpainful (brushing with a hand/light touch or a soft object) may help to identify allodynia. Inspection will often allow the clinician to appreciate recent traumatic injury, erythema, atrophy, trophic changes, and hyperhidrosis. Circumferential limb measurements and side-to-side measurement may be helpful. Palpation and skin temperature changes to evaluate for hyper- or hypothermia should be performed when CRPS is suspected, again with side-to-side comparisons. Clinical criteria for *signs* of CRPS require that they be present at the time of diagnosis.[50] Physical signs may be intermittent, and reevaluation of patients is necessary to evaluate for any sudomotor changes that may "come and go." Actual "dystrophy" may be relatively infrequent and present in perhaps only 15% of cases.[5]

Four subgroups of CRPS have been identified based on an analysis of symptoms of hypersensitivity and clinical signs.[1,53,54] These include (1) a grouping with allodynia, hyperesthesia, and hyperalgesia symptoms, (2) a group dominated by temperature asymmetry and color-change signs and symptoms, (3) a grouping of asymmetrical sweating and edema signs/symptoms, and (4) a fourth category dominated by decreased range of motion, motor dysfunction, and trophic change signs/symptoms. The clinical meaning of these different categories of CRPS presentations is somewhat unclear; however, the presence of the fourth group in particular may suggest that some CRPS signs/symptoms that could be useful for diagnosis may have been previously underappreciated.

REFERENCES

1. Harden RN, et al. Complex regional pain syndrome: practical diagnostic and treatment guidelines, 4th ed. *Pain Med.* 2013;14:180–229.
2. Maihöfner C, Seifert F, Markovic K. Complex regional pain syndromes: new pathophysiological concepts and therapies. *Eur J Neurol.* 2010;17:649–660.
3. Sudeck P. Über die akute entzundliche Knochenatrophie. *Arch Klin Chir.* 1900;62:147–156.
4. Evans J. Reflex sympathetic dystrophy. *Surg Clin N Am.* 1946;26:780–790.
5. Harden RN, Bruehl SP. Diagnosis of complex regional pain syndrome. *Clin J Pain.* 2006;22(5):415–419.
6. Simon J, McAuliffe M. Complex regional pain syndrome – lower limb. In: Simon J, et al., eds. *Interventional Spine Procedures: A Case-Based Approach.* Philadelphia – New Delhi: Jaypee Brothers Medical Publishers; 2014:105–114.
7. Field J. Complex regional pain syndrome: a review. *Eur J Hand Surg.* 2013, Jul; 38(6): 616–626.
8. Baerga-Varela L, et al. PM&R Knowledge Now: Complex Regional Pain Syndrome Part 1: Essentials of Assessment and Diagnosis. http://me.aapmr.com/kn.
9. de Mos M, et al. The incidence of complex regional pain syndrome: a population based study. *Pain.* 2006;129: 12–20.

10. Bussa M, et al. The incidence of complex regional pain syndrome type I: a comprehensive review. *Acta Anaesthesiol Scand.* 2015;59(6):685–697.
11. Maleki J, et al. Patterns of spread in complex regional pain syndrome, type I (reflex sympathetic dystrophy). *Pain.* 2000;88:259–266.
12. Gahardoni R, et al. Repetitive transcranial magnetic stimulation in chronic pain: a review of the literature. *Arch Phys Med Rehabil.* 2015;96(4 suppl 2):S156–S172.
13. Wasner G, Schattschneider J, Binder A, Baron R. Complex regional pain syndrome: diagnostic, mechanism, CNS involvement and therapy. *Spinal Cord.* 2003;41:61–75.
14. Baron R, et al. Diagnostic tools and evidence-based treatment of complex regional pain syndrome. In: Campbell JN, ed. *IASP Refresher Courses on Pain Management.* Pain 2005: An Update Review: Refresher Course Syllabus; Seattle: IASP PR; 2005:293–306.
15. Marinus J, et al. Clinical features and pathophysiology of complex regional pain syndrome. *Lancet Neurol.* 2011;10:637–648.
16. Wilson PR. Introduction to CRPS special issue. *Pain Med.* 2010;11:1209–1211.
17. Perez RS, et al. Evidence based guidelines for complex regional pain syndrome type 1. *BMC Neurol.* 2010;10(20):1–14.
18. Bussa M, et al. Adult complex regional pain syndrome type I: a narrative review. *PM R.* 2016;23:S1934–S1482.
19. Sandroni P, et al. Complex regional pain syndrome type I: incidence and prevalence in Olmstead county; a population-based study. *Pain.* 2003;103:199–207.
20. Schwartzmann RJ, McLellan TL. Reflex sympathetic dystrophy: a review. *Arch Neurol.* 1987;44:555–561.
21. Ponce T, Shipton EA, William J, Mulder RT. Potential risk factors for the onset of complex regional pain syndrome type I: a systematic literature review. *Anesthesiol Res Pract.* 2015:956539.
22. Bickerstaff DR, Kanis JA. Algodystrophy: an under-recognized complication of minor trauma. *Br J Rheumatol.* 1994;33:240–248.
23. Cooney WP, Dobyns JH, Linscheid RL. Complications of colles' fractures. *J Bone Joint Surg Am.* 1980;62:613–619.
24. Atkins RM, Duckworth T, Kanis JA. Features of algodystrophy after colles' fracture. *J Bone Joint Surg.* 1990;72-B:105–110.
25. Atkins RM, Duckworth T, Kanis JA. Algodystrophy following colles' fracture. *J Hand Surg Br.* 1989;14:161–164.
26. Beerthuizen A, et al. The association between psychological factors and development of complex regional pain syndrome type I (CRPS 1) – a prospective multicenter study. *Eur J Pain.* 2011;15:971–975.
27. de Mos M, et al. Medical history and the onset of complex regional pain syndrome (CRPS). *Pain.* 2008;139:458–466.
28. Lohnberg A, Altmaier EM. A review of psychosocial factors in complex regional pain syndrome. *J Clin Psychol Med Settings.* 2013;20:247–254.
29. Beerthuizen A, et al. Is there an association between psychological factors and the complex regional pain syndrome type I (CRPS 1) in adults? A systemic review. *Pain.* 2009;145:52–59.
30. Janig W, Baron R. Complex regional pain syndrome: mystery explained? *Lancet.* 2003;2:687–697.
31. Bruehl S, Harden RN, Galer BS, et al. Complex regional pain syndrome: are there distinct subtypes and sequential stages of the syndrome? *Pain.* 2002;95:119–124.
32. Veldman PH, Reynen HM, Arntz IE, Goris RJ. Signs and symptoms of reflex sympathetic dystrophy: prospective study of 829 patients. *Lancet.* 1993;342:1012–1016.
33. Zyluk A. The natural history of post-traumatic reflex sympathetic dystrophy. *J Hand Surg Br.* 1998;23:20–23.
34. Geertzen JH, et al. Reflex sympathetic dystrophy of the upper extremity – a 5.5-year follow-up. Part I. Impairments and perceived disability. *Acta Orthop Scand Suppl.* 1998;279:12–18.
35. Geertzen JH, et al. Reflex sympathetic dystrophy of the upper extremity – a 5.5-year follow-up. Part II. Social life events, general health and changes in occupation. *Acta Orthop Scand Suppl.* 1998;279:19–23.
36. de Mos M, et al. Outcome of the complex regional pain syndrome. *Clin J Pain.* 2009;25:590–597.
37. de Mos M, Sturkenboom MC, Huygen FJ. Current understandings on complex regional pain syndrome. *Pain Pract.* 2009;9:86–89.
38. Pappagallo M, Rosenberg AD. Epidemiology, pathophysiology, and management of complex regional pain syndrome. *Pain Pract.* 2001;1:11–20.
39. Munnikes RJ, et al. Intermediate stage complex regional pain syndrome type I is unrelated to proinflammatory cytokines. *Mediators Inflamm.* 2005;2005(6):366.
40. Schinkel C, et al. Inflammatory mediators are altered in the acute phase of posttraumatic complex regional pain syndrome. *Clin J Pain.* 2006;22(3):235.
41. Kuner R. Central mechanisms of pathological pain. *Nat Med.* 2010;16:1258–1266.
42. Maihöfner C, Handwerker H, Neundörfer B, Birklein F. Cortical reorganization during recovery from complex regional pain syndrome. *Neurology.* 2004;63(4):693.
43. Pleger B, et al. Sensorimotor retuning in complex regional pain syndrome parallels pain reduction. *Ann Neurol.* 2005;5(3):425.
44. Kaelin DL, Adams JS. PM&R Knowledge Now: Autonomically Mediated Pain-Autonomic Pain Syndromes. http://me.aapmr.org/kn/.
45. Mehnert MJ, Simon J, McAuliffe M. Complex regional pain syndrome – upper limb. In: Simon J, et al., eds. *Interventional Spine Procedures: A Case-Based Approach.* Philadelphia – New Delhi: Jaypee Brothers Medical Publishers; 2014:115–124.
46. Stanton-Hicks M, Janig W, Hassenbusch S, Haddox JD, Boas R, Wilson P. Reflex sympathetic dystrophy: changing concepts and taxonomy. *Pain.* 1995;63:127–133.
47. Raja SN, Treede RD, David KD, Campell JN. Systemic alpha-adrenergic blockade with phentolaine: a diagnostic test for sympathetically maintained pain. *Anesthesiology.* 1991;74:691–698.

48. Wasner G, et al. Vascular abnormalities in reflex sympathetic dystrophy (CRPS I): mechanisms and diagnostic value. *Brain.* 2001;124:587–599.
49. Galer BS, Brueh S, Harden RN. IASP diagnostic criteria for complex regional pain syndrome: a preliminary empirical validation study. *Clin J Pain.* 1998;14:211–219.
50. Harden RN, Bruehl S, Perez RS, et al. Validation of proposed diagnostic criteria (the "Budapest criteria") for complex regional pain syndrome. *Pain.* 2010;150:268–274.
51. Harden RN, Bruehl S, Stanton-Hicks M, Wilson PR. Proposed new diagnostic criteria for complex regional pain syndrome. *Pain Med.* 2007;8:326–331.
52. Galer BS, Henderson J, Perander J, Jensen MP. Course of symptoms and quality of life measurement in complex regional pain syndrome: a pilot survey. *J Pain Symptom Manage.* 2000;20:286–292.
53. Harden RN, Bruehl S, Galer BS, et al. Complex regional pain syndrome: are the IASP diagnostic criteria valid and sufficiently comprehensive? *Pain.* 1999;83:211–219.
54. Bruehl S, Harden RN, Galer BS, et al. External validation of IASP diagnostic criteria for complex regional pain syndrome and proposed research diagnostic criteria. International association for the study of pain. *Pain.* 1999;81:147–154.

CHAPTER 5

Complex Regional Pain Syndrome Diagnostic Criteria

ANUPAM SINHA, DO • HARLA K. O'DONNELL, DO • MADHURI DHOLAKIA, MD

Complex regional pain syndrome (CRPS) has evolved over the years not only in its nomenclature, but also in its diagnostic criteria. It was first described by Dr. Silas Weir Mitchell in the American Civil War as "causalgia," describing the chronic burning pain soldiers experienced after neurologic injuries following gunshot wounds. It was later described throughout the 20th century as reflex sympathetic dystrophy, as it was thought to be a pain syndrome linked to a sympathetic nervous system disorder. This terminology was eventually thought to be a misrepresentation of the disorder for multiple reasons. First, the term "reflex" implied the involvement of a complex, multisynaptic process, yet this has not been characterized. In addition, the sympathetic nervous system was considered a primary mediator of pain; however, it is not involved in all stages of disease progression. Lastly, "dystrophy" is not present in all cases. Thus, in 1994, the disorder was renamed "complex regional pain syndrome" or CRPS by the International Association for the Study of Pain (IASP).[1]

As described by Harden et al., there had been a trend of "diagnostic chaos," warranting a clear consensus regarding diagnostic criteria. The IASP held the Schloss Rettershof Conference in 1988, followed by the Orlando Conference in 1994, during which the first definitive diagnostic criteria for CRPS were developed (Box 5.1).[2]

The IASP/Orlando criteria were based on professional consensus and did not include clinical or systematic validation. These guidelines suggest two different types of CRPS: CRPS type I (without nerve injury) and CRPS type II (with nerve injury). The guidelines also suggest two main subgroups of signs and symptoms: one group of criteria with pain, allodynia, or hyperalgesia and the other group of criteria with edema, skin changes, or sudomotor activity. A subsequent survey of 123 patients showed that the signs and symptoms of CRPS could more accurately be categorized into one of four groups (Table 5.1).[4]

The four subsets in Table 5.1 were obtained through statistical factor analysis, which involved the grouping of conceptually, and in this case pathophysiologically, linked factors. This analysis suggested two main flaws in the IASP/Orlando criteria, which contributed to overdiagnosis of CRPS and decreased specificity.[5] First, motor dysfunction and trophic symptoms (Factor 4 in Table 5.1) were commonly experienced by patients, yet had not been included in the original IASP/Orlando criteria. Second, vasomotor and sudomotor signs were better grouped as two independent, statistically separate criteria, whereas the IASP/Orlando criteria grouped these signs as a single criteria.

The IASP/Orlando criteria were further analyzed for their ability to distinguish the syndrome from other neuropathic pain syndromes. An analysis of 48 patients with previously diagnosed neurologic conditions of

---

BOX 5.1
International Association for the Study of Pain (Orlando) Diagnostic Criteria for Complex Regional Pain Syndrome

1. The presence of an inciting noxious event or cause of immobilization
2. Continuing pain, allodynia, or hyperalgesia with which the pain is disproportionate to any inciting event
3. Evidence at some time of edema, changes in skin, blood flow, or abnormal sudomotor activity in the region of pain
4. The diagnosis is excluded by the existence of conditions that would otherwise account for the degree of pain and dysfunction.

Type I: without evidence of major nerve damage.
Type II: with evidence of major nerve damage.

Data from Merskey H, Bogduk N. *Classification of Chronic Pain: Descriptions of Chronic Pain Syndromes and Definitions of Pain Terms*, 2nd ed. Seattle, WA: IASP Press; 1994.

TABLE 5.1
Factors Resulting From Principal Components Factor Analysis of Diagnostic and Associated Signs and Symptoms of Complex Regional Pain Syndrome

Factor 1	Factor 2	Factor 3	Factor 4
Hyperalgesia signs (0.75)	Temperature asymmetry symptoms (0.68)	Edema signs (0.69)	Decreased range of motion signs (0.81)
"Hyperesthesia" symptoms (0.78)	Color change signs (0.67)	Sweating asymmetry signs (0.62)	Decreased range of motion symptoms (0.77)
Allodynic signs (0.44)	Color change symptoms (0.52)	Edema symptoms (0.61)	Motor dysfunction signs (0.77) Motor dysfunction symptoms (0.61) Trophic symptoms (0.52) Trophic signs (0.51)

From Harden RN, Bruehl S, Galer BS, et al. Complex regional pain syndrome: are the IASP diagnostic criteria valid and sufficiently comprehensive? *Pain*. 1999;83:211–219; with permission.

BOX 5.2
Clinical Diagnostic Criteria (the "Budapest Criteria") for CRPS

To make the clinical diagnosis, the following criteria must be met:
1. Continuing pain, which is disproportionate to any inciting event
2. Must report at least one symptom in three of the following categories:
   - Sensory: Reports of hyperesthesia and/or allodynia
   - Vasomotor: Reports of temperature asymmetry and/or skin color changes and/or skin color asymmetry
   - Sudomotor/Edema: Reports of edema and/or sweating changes and/or sweating asymmetry
   - Motor/Trophic: Reports of decreased range of motion and/or motor dysfunction (weakness, tremor, dystonia) and/or trophic changes (hair, nail, skin)
3. Must display at least one sign at the time of evaluation in two or more of the following categories:
   - Sensory: Evidence of hyperalgesia (to pinprick) and/or allodynia (to light touch and/or temperature sensation and/or deep somatic pressure and/or joint movement)
   - Vasomotor: Evidence of temperature asymmetry (>1°C) and/or skin color changes and/or asymmetry
   - Sudomotor/Edema: Evidence of edema and/or sweating changes and/or sweating asymmetry
   - Motor/Trophic: Evidence of decreased range of motion and/or motor dysfunction (weakness, tremor, dystonia) and/or trophic changes (hair, nail, skin)
4. There is no other diagnosis that better explains the signs and symptoms

From Harden N, Oaklander AL, Burton AW, et al. Complex regional pain syndrome: practical diagnostic and treatment guidelines, 4th edition. *Pain Med*. 2013;14:180–229; with permission.

either CRPS (by IASP/Orlando criteria) or diabetic neuropathy was performed by Galer et al. Eighteen patients preemptively met IASP/Orlando guidelines for CRPS, whereas the other 30 patients had diabetic neuropathy. Both patients and physicians took a 10-item questionnaire evaluating symptoms. Data analysis suggested a gross overdiagnosis of CRPS when utilizing the Orlando criteria.[6] A similar, yet larger, study (n = 123) by Harden et al.[4] confirmed that the Orlando criteria had strong sensitivity (0.98); however, specificity was lacking (0.36). These results were disheartening, because in clinical practice, the ability to differentiate

other causes of pain from CRPS is imperative. A lower specificity, and hence a greater risk of overdiagnosis, could result in inappropriate and potential harmful interventions to those patients who have been misdiagnosed as having CRPS.

The IASP reconvened in Budapest in 2003 with intentions to develop guidelines with greater specificity. The Budapest clinical criteria (Box 5.2) required patients to have at least two of four positive sign categories (present at the time of diagnosis) and three of four positive symptom categories. This requirement increased the specificity of CRPS diagnosis to 0.69,

> **BOX 5.3**
> **Subtypes of Complex Regional Pain Syndrome (CRPS)**
>
> - CRPS I (old name: reflex sympathetic dystrophy)
> - CRPS II (old name: causalgia): defined earlier with electrodiagnostic or other definitive evidence of a major nerve lesion
> - CRPS-NOS (not otherwise specified): partially meets CRPS criteria; not better explained by any other condition.[3]

Data from Harden N, Oaklander AL, Burton AW, et al. Complex regional pain syndrome: practical diagnostic and treatment guidelines, 4th edition. *Pain Med.* 2013;14:180–229.

while maintaining a sensitivity of 0.85. In addition to clinical criteria, research criteria were also developed. The purpose of the research criteria was to provide a reliable method to eliminate false positives in those patients involved in future studies. These criteria required patients to meet all four of the positive symptom categories in addition to two of the four positive sign categories. The research criteria yielded a sensitivity of 0.75 and a specificity of 0.96.[7]

The Budapest criteria also categorize patients (Box 5.3) based on the absence or presence of a major nerve lesion, CRPS type I and type II, respectively. An additional category, CRPS-NOS (not otherwise specified),

was added to include the approximately 15% of patients who had previously met the IASP/Orlando criteria but did not meet the Budapest criteria.[8]

REFERENCES

1. Iolascon G, et al. Complex regional pain syndrome (CRPS) type I: historical perspective and critical issues. *Clin Cases Miner Bone Metab.* 2015;12(suppl 1):4–10.
2. Harden N, Oaklander AL, Burton AW, et al. Complex regional pain syndrome: practical diagnostic and treatment guidelines, 4th ed. *Pain Med.* 2013;14:180–229.
3. Merskey H, Bogduk N. *Classification of Chronic Pain: Descriptions of Chronic Pain Syndromes and Definitions of Pain Terms.* 2nd ed. Seattle, WA: IASP Press; 1994.
4. Harden RN, Bruehl S, Galer BS, et al. Complex regional pain syndrome: are the IASP diagnostic criteria valid and sufficiently comprehensive? *Pain.* 1999;83:211–219.
5. Harden RN, Bruehl S, Perez RS, et al. Validation of proposed diagnostic criteria (the "Budapest criteria") for complex regional pain syndrome. *Pain.* 2010;150:268–274.
6. Galer BS, Bruehl S, Harden RN. IASP diagnostic criteria for complex regional pain syndrome: a preliminary empirical validation study. *Clin J Pain.* 1998;14:48–54.
7. Harden R, Bruehl S, Perez R, et al. Validation of proposed diagnostic criteria (the "Budapest criteria") for complex regional pain syndrome. *Pain.* 2010;11:1115–1125.
8. Harden RN, Bruehl S, Stanton-Hicks M, Wilson PR. Proposed new diagnostic criteria for complex regional pain syndrome. *Pain Med.* 2007;8:326–331.

CHAPTER 6

Diagnostic Testing in Complex Regional Pain Syndrome

MADHURI DHOLAKIA, MD • ANUPAM SINHA, DO

The diagnosis of complex regional pain syndrome (CRPS) is made, primarily, based on the previously mentioned clinical criteria. However, diagnostic testing can be utilized to support the diagnosis of CRPS and/or to rule out other diagnoses.

THREE-PHASE BONE SCAN

In cases of acute to subacute CRPS, the three-phase bone scan (TPBS) typically shows an increased radiotracer uptake in the affected limb in all three phases. In cases of chronic CRPS, the uptake is reduced in all three phases.[1] When nerve trauma precedes the development of CRPS (CRPS type 2), TPBS performed within the first 5 months of symptom onset may show an increased uptake in the mineralization (third) phase in joints not affected by the initial trauma.[2]

However, the sensitivity and specificity for TPBS in the diagnosis of CRPS is low; studies have found that when CRPS is diagnosed using the Budapest Criteria, the sensitivity of TPBS is 40%–55.1% and the specificity is 76.6%–93.5%.[3,4] Therefore, a negative TPBS does not exclude the diagnosis of CRPS.

TPBS can be helpful, however, in ruling out malignancy, metabolic bone disease, fracture, heterotopic ossification, or infection in patients with limb pain, edema, and/or erythema.

SKIN TEMPERATURE MEASUREMENT (THERMOMETRY AND THERMOGRAPHY)

Skin temperature is an indicator of skin blood flow. Skin temperature should be measured at several corresponding points on the affected and contralateral limb and on several different occasions using an infrared thermometer. Alternately, skin temperature can be assessed via infrared thermography (IRT). The standard protocol for infrared thermography includes acclimating the patient in a room warmed to 23 °C and relative humidity 50% for 20 min without clothing. IRT images are then obtained using a computer-assisted infrared camera that detects infrared energy emitted from the surface of the body.[5]

A limb temperature difference of >1 °C between the affected and unaffected limb is significant.[6] Temperature in the affected limb can be increased or decreased compared with the unaffected side. Note that skin temperature is dynamic; therefore, the presence of symmetric thermometric or thermographic findings does not exclude the diagnosis of CRPS.[5–7] Gulevich et al.[8] found a 93% sensitivity and 89% specificity of infrared thermography for the diagnosis of CRPS type 1; however, it should be noted that this study was performed before the creation of the Budapest Criteria.

IMAGING

MRI or CT is useful only in assessing for other pathology, not for confirming the diagnosis of CRPS. Plain X-rays may show patchy osteopenia of the affected extremity. If one hand is involved, both hands can be imaged on the same radiograph (side-by-side comparison film) to assess for loss of bone density. The sensitivity of plain X-ray in CRPS is less than 30%.[2]

SYMPATHETIC NERVE BLOCK

Historically, immediate and transient relief from pain and dysesthesia after sympathetic nerve block (stellate ganglion block or lumbar sympathetic block) was considered to be supportive of a diagnosis of CRPS. However, the role of the sympathetic nervous system in CRPS has, more recently, been called into question. The vasomotor and sudomotor dysfunction commonly seen in acute CRPS (edema, increased temperature of the affected limb) seems to be multifactorial, because of both increased levels of circulating neuropeptides (substance P, calcitonin gene related peptide) causing "neurogenic inflammation" and pain, and alterations in the sympathetic nervous system.[9] There is evidence that central inhibition of cutaneous sympathetic vaso-constrictor neurons in CRPS causes increased limb edema and warmth, as well as pain via sensitization of nociceptors to catecholamines (sympathetic-afferent coupling).[9] In addition, pain in CRPS is likely due, at least in part, to central sensitization. Because pain in CRPS may or may not be sympathetically mediated, response to a sympathetic nerve block, although some-times a helpful part of the workup, cannot be used independently to substantiate or exclude the diagnosis of CRPS.

ELECTRODIAGNOSTIC TESTING

Electrodiagnostic testing can be helpful in excluding peripheral or entrapment neuropathy or confirming the presence of a nerve injury (CRPS type 2). However, this type of testing is often uncomfortable and, for a patient with allodynia, may be impossible to tolerate. Some authors, therefore, discourage the use of electro-diagnostic testing in cases of suspected CRPS.[10] Cer-tainly electrodiagnostic testing is most appropriate in these cases when the results will potentially alter the patient's treatment options.

SWEAT TESTING

Altered sudomotor function is a common symptom of CRPS.[11] Sweating can be increased or decreased in the affected limb compared with the unaffected limb.[12] Several tests can be used to measure sweat output. Sub-jective sweat testing can be performed by applying an indicator starch powder to the affected and unaffected limbs. The indicator changes color when exposed to sweat. The resting sweat output (RSO) and quantita-tive sudomotor axon reflex test (QSART) also measure sweat output of the affected and unaffected limb but are not widely available to clinicians. The RSO test is performed with the limbs at rest, whereas the QSART measures sweat output in response to an iontophoresis cholinergic challenge (acetylcholine or methacholine). One study found that, when performed together, the RSO test and QSART are 98% specific for the diagnosis of CRPS.[13]

REFERENCES

1. Park S, Yang C, Kim C, et al. Patterns of three-phase bone scintigraphy according to the time course of complex re-gional pain syndrome type 1 after a stroke or traumatic brain injury. *Clin Nucl Med.* 2009;34(11):773–776.
2. Birklein F, O'Neill D, Schlereth T. Complex regional pain syndrome an optimistic perspective. *Neurology.* 2015;84(1):89–96.
3. Moon JY, Park SY, Lee SC, et al. Analysis of patterns of three-phase bone scintigraphy for patients with complex regional pain syndrome diagnosed using the proposed research criteria (the 'Budapest criteria'). *Br J Anaesth.* 2012;108(4):655–661.
4. Wertli MM, Brunner F, Steurer J, et al. Usefulness of bone scintigraphy for the diagnosis of complex regional pain syn-drome 1: a systematic review and Bayesian meta-analysis. *PLoS One.* 2017;12. e0173688.
5. Cho CW, Nahm FS, Choi E, et al. Multicenter study on the asymmetry of skin temperature in complex regional pain syndrome: an examination of temperature distribution and symptom duration. *Medicine.* 2016;95:52.
6. Krumova EK, Frettloh J, Klauenberg S, et al. Long-term skin temperature measurements: a practical diagnostic tool in complex regional pain syndrome. *Pain.* 2008;140:8–22.
7. Rho RH, Brewer RP, Lamer TJ. Complex regional pain syndrome. *Mayo Clin Proc.* 2002;77:174–180.
8. Gulevich SJ, Conwell TD, Lane J. Stress infrared telether-mography is useful in the diagnosis of complex regional pain syndrome, type 1 (formerly reflex sympathetic dys-trophy). *Clin J Pain.* 1997;13(1):50–59.
9. Marinus J, Moseley GL, Birklein F, et al. Clinical features and pathophysiology of complex regional pain syndrome. *Lancet Neurol.* 2011;10(7):637–648.
10. Harden RN, Oaklander AL, Burton AW. Complex regional pain syndrome: practical diagnostic and treatment guide-lines. *Pain Med.* 2013;14:180–229.
11. Birklein F, Sittl R, Spitzer A, et al. Sudomotor function in sympathetic reflex dystrophy. *Pain.* 1997;69:49–54.
12. Sandroni P, Low PA, Ferrer T, et al. Complex regional pain syndrome 1 (CRPS 1): prospective study and laboratory evaluation. *Clin J Pain.* 1998;14(4):282–289.
13. Chelimsky TC, Low PA, Naessens JM. Value of autonomic testing in reflex sympathetic dystrophy. *Mayo Clin Proc.* 1995;70(11):1029–1040.

FURTHER READING

1. Freedman M, Greis AC, Marino L, et al. Complex regional pain syndrome diagnosis and treatment. *Phys Med Rehabil Clin N Am.* 2014;25:291–303.

CHAPTER 7

A Physiotherapeutic, Biopsychosocial Approach to the Management of Patients With Peripheral Neuropathic Pain and Complex Regional Pain Syndrome

JOHN BARBIS, MA, PT

Pain is the behavioral response of the nervous system to incoming sensory information that the mind interprets as a perceived or actual existential threat to the individual or body part.[1-3] Woolf[3] describes three classifications of pain:

1. "An early-warning physiological protective system, essential to detect and minimize contact with damaging or noxious stimuli";
2. "Sensory sensitivity after unavoidable tissue damage, this pain assists in the healing of the injured body part by creating a situation that discourages physical contact and movement";
3. "Pathological pain, which is not a symptom of some disorder but rather a disease state of the nervous system, can occur after damage to the nervous system (neuropathic pain), but also in conditions in which there is no such damage or inflammation (dysfunctional pain)."

Pain in all of its forms is a whole-organism experience marshaling both affective and effective responses that produce changes in perception, individual behavior, social interaction, and multiple physiologic functions.[3-6] In the management of pain, including neuropathic pain, it is insufficient to focus solely on the location of the pain or incoming nociceptive information.[1,4,6]

Neuropathic pain is an important and costly[5,7] subset of pain. Given the number and variety of traumatic and pathologic entities that can damage or injure the nervous system, neuropathic pain in its entirety can encompass a multitude of diagnoses. Although there is dispute about its precise incidence, there is agreement that most acute neuropathies of the peripheral nervous system caused by injury, compression, or traction forces resolve spontaneously, with most patients experiencing no to minimal residual symptoms or dysfunction.[8,9] Even patients with disease-produced pain, such as shingles, find their symptoms resolve either significantly or fully.[10] The percentages vary, but only a minority of patients with acute neuropathic pain progress to a persistent pain state.[3,11] Acute peripheral nerve injuries have the potential to recruit multiple protective systems, including the immune, autonomic, and endocrine systems, along with behavioral changes to initially protect the organism and hasten healing.[3,11] Most patients with complex regional pain syndrome (CRPS)-like symptoms experienced immediately after a recent injury (the first two classifications described by Woolf)[3] see their symptoms resolve.[3,12,14]

MANAGEMENT OF ACUTE NEUROPATHIC PAIN

In the management of acute nociceptive neuropathic pain where there is an ongoing mechanical insult occurring to a specific nerve or group of nerves, the elimination of the actual existential threat to the neural tissue is only the first and often the most easily accomplished component of management. For the rehabilitation specialist who may have a role in the elimination of the tissue threat and/or who is responsible for the care after that threat is managed, the difficult work of preventing the multifactorial effects (Box 7.1) of that existential threat response becomes the focus of care.

43

> **BOX 7.1**
> **Potential Secondary Problems That Can Develop With Neuropathic Pain**
>
> - Motor changes: weakness, dystonia, muscle atrophy[12-14]
> - Sensory changes: anesthesia, hyperesthesia, paresthesias, allodynia, hyperpathia, etc.[3,12-14]
> - Structural changes in the spinal cord and brain: dorsal root ganglion, dorsal horn, microglial distribution, sensory cortex, motor cortex, limbic structures[2,3,15-18]
> - Increased activity of the autonomic nervous system producing swelling, alterations of blood flow, osteoporosis, dermatologic change[12-14]
> - Elevated stress response with increased endocrine activity[14,19,20,21]
> - Impaired function, including activities of daily living, gait, recreational activities, work capabilities[5,14,22-24]
> - Behavioral changes, including increased depression, anxiety, fear avoidance behaviors, sleep disturbance[14,22-26]
> - Cognitive deficits: ability to focus and concentrate, body part recognition, left/right recognition[9,14,16,23,26]
> - Family, social, and employment difficulties[9,14-16,23,26]
> - Sexual dysfunction[14,21]

Pain suppression and modulation, including physical modalities and electrical stimulation, can play significant roles in management.[4,6,8,23] The sole reliance on this approach, however, may delay needed interventions and develop patient dependence.[14,25,28,29] More comprehensive approaches recognize the need to complement the use of traditional chemical or interventional techniques with those that educate and train patients to avoid those activities and address those beliefs that can inhibit physical recovery of the nerve and function. The prevention of pathologic pain as described by Woolf[3] and proactive intervention to prevent behavioral, social, and physiologic changes that can adversely affect recovery are essential. Any of the effects in Box 7.1 can inhibit or make recovery more difficult.

There is no clinically proven intervention that can stop the continuing neural output from a damaged or sensitized neural membrane or proven techniques to hasten the healing of a nerve. Medication, physical modalities, interventional procedures, and braces/immobilizers may provide transient reductions in pain, but patients often experience insufficient relief from these interventions.[4,8,23,29]

EARLY MANAGEMENT OF CRPS-LIKE SYMPTOMS

Most patients who have experienced a traumatic injury to a peripheral nerve experience a period of elevated autonomic, neuroimmune, and/or endocrine responses. These are normal responses to injury and are necessary for healing of the nerve and resolve in a few weeks or months.[3,11,12,30] Even though early hyperprotective responses generally resolve, patients should be evaluated for the presence of increased risk for CRPS II. Although there is no literature outlining or documenting the effectiveness of a preventative program for CRPS II or persistent neuropathic pain, there are interventions that address the risk factors and take advantage of models from other acute health problems and recent studies from which a potential program can be developed.

Studies indicate that early introduction of movement and neural stimulation can reduce the adverse neuroimmune changes seen with CRPS in mice. Grace[31] demonstrated that early introduction of the use of a running wheel after nerve injury prevented an elevated neuroimmune response seen in rats that rested. Leung[32] demonstrated that early introduction of exercise after injury in mice increased the percentage of resident macrophages that produce antiinflammatory interlukin-10, causing a reduction in pain. Matsuo[32] demonstrated that TENS Transcutaneous Nerve Stimulation applied immediately after nerve damage in mice reduced the neuroimmune response in the spinal cord compared with no intervention. In addition, Matsuo[32] found that if TENS was delayed by a week, the reductive effect was lost.

The evidence against prolonged immobilization, rest, and overprotective instructions after nerve injury is growing.[11,14,34,35] Rehabilitation programs that introduce education, behavioral support, exercise, and movement early in care have shown success in the treatment of spinal pain,[36] joint replacement,[37] heart surgeries,[38] and other problems.[37,39] Hopefully early treatment of acute neuropathic pain using increased activity, education, exercise, and activities that stimulate neural activity can prevent the progression of what is a normal response to injury to the development of a persistent chronic pain problem and CRPS.

MANAGEMENT OF PERSISTENT NEUROPATHIC PAIN

The evaluation and treatment procedures used in the management of persistent neuropathic pain are the same as those for acute neuropathic pain; however, the focus of care moves from prevention and recovery to remediation. The care plan is more multidimensional and integrative.[6,14,29,40] Examination procedures include those that identify the problems that have prevented the resolution of the pain.[6,8,14,40] The resolution of the problems identified in Box 7.1 is often more important to the long-term recovery and function of patients than the recovery from the physical impairments of the nerve injury. The coordinated intervention of a well-trained team of professionals is often needed.[6,8,14,29]

MANAGEMENT OF CRPS

CRPS presents a special case and management problem within the context of persistent neuropathic pain management. An intensive, interdisciplinary, and integrated approach to care is needed for patients with CRPS.[14] Counseling,[14,24,26] stress management,[14,24] pain education,[14,41] and supervised, graded activity programs[14,41-45] can be effective interventions. Graded motor imagery (GMI)[46] is a system developed by Moseley and Butler that organizes several neuroplasticity-based interventions into a logical structure. Clinical studies demonstrate its benefit for patients with CRPS.[14,41-45]

DEVELOPMENT OF A TREATMENT PLAN

Kerstman[7] writes, "Neuropathic pain is a clinical diagnosis and requires a systematic approach to assessment, including a detailed history, physical examination, and appropriate diagnostic testing." Because of the complexity of most neuropathic pain presentations, significant information is required before a rehabilitation program can be developed. Psychometric,[14,24-26,47] central sensitivity,[6,14,48] functional,[4,14] and neurodynamic[48-50] testing provides additional information beyond the classic physical examination.

There are three important questions that need to be answered before the rehabilitation plan can be developed. The answers to these three questions along with information gathered from classic and neurodynamic assessments are critical to the choice and sequencing of the treatment procedures, the level of intensity of their application, and insight to how the treatments can be modified to improve their effectiveness.

Question 1: How Dangerous Is This Pain?

It is self-evident that treatment is more cautiously performed and more closely monitored if the physical condition indicates that there is the potential for continuing damage to the nerve. Where there is a threat to the nerve by mechanical compression or traction, ischemia, disease, or treatment of a systemic pathology, the signs and symptoms that patients report have to be assumed to be nociceptive and indicators of potential existential threats to tissue. As a result, it is important for providers to discern the differences between those signs and symptoms that are indicative of true tissue threat and those that may be due to the triggering of a hypersensitive nervous system and fear-based behaviors.

For many patients with persistent neuropathic pain, the threat to neural tissue is no longer an issue. Patients are left with pain that is no longer produced by a continuing insult to the nerve but is produced by hypersensitive neural membranes, sensitized sensory processing mechanisms, and/or fear-based and learned responses to perceived environmental threats.[2,3,14,47] Care for these patients addresses the behavioral components that trigger the pain and retrains the nervous system to discriminate between dangerous and nondangerous sensory information. For these patients, tissue threat is deemphasized as the source of their pain. The focus of care shifts to restructuring patient behaviors, thoughts, and fears associated with pain.[2,8,11,25] For many patients the strict categorization of their sign and symptom patterns into acute or persistent neuropathic pain is not possible. During the recovery a patient's condition changes, requiring frequent reassessments of the patient's status.

Question 2: How Irritable Is the Condition?

Maitland[51] defined the levels of irritability as tools to grade the intensity of the application of musculoskeletal mobilization/manipulation techniques and exercise. Butler[49] expands Maitland's ideas using irritability as a guide to the treatment of neural pathologies. Irritability is rated on a continuum from high (minor activities produced an increased sign or symptom response that took a prolonged period to return to the original state after activity) to nonirritable (significant activity may produce an increased sign or symptom response, with a rapid return to the original state). There are three components that need to be considered in the gradation of irritability: level of activity, patient response, and duration of that response. Irritability is often considered to be an indicator of the potential ease or difficulty with which activity produces a localized inflammatory response.[49,50] Tracking the duration of the enhanced patient response after activity can be considered as a way of gauging the inflammatory character of the condition.

In 1961, Lishman [52] described a "latency" characteristic to neuropathic pain. This characteristic is familiar to clinicians caring for patients with neuropathic pain. An activity may produce a transitory increase in discomfort during its performance that quickly resolves. Over the next 6–12 h, however, symptoms ramp up and remain elevated for 12–24 h before slowly degrading to baseline levels over the next 24–36 h. Clinicians often dismiss these patient reports because the patient demonstrated no increased discomfort when they left the office.

This pattern of symptom behavior can be correlated to the pattern of increased neuroimmune activity seen after stimulation by chemical, mechanical, behavioral, or neural triggers.[1,3,27] Even after microglia decrease their elevated response, they remain in a heightened "alert" state so that lower intensity triggers can stimulate the response.[27] Defining the level of patient irritability to activity and correctly grading the degree of engagement or challenge in treatment prevent unneeded patient discomfort and lower the potential of increased central sensitization during the treatment process. Irritability is a key component for deciding the type of therapeutic interventions to be used as the condition improves.

Clinicians and patients can use the irritability concept to grade the treatment program to prevent a neural flare response. Patients need to understand that this heightened response is not an indicator of actual tissue damage but its production cannot be ignored. If the treatment plan or activity levels continue to produce this hyperprotective response, the central nervous system (CNS) becomes more sensitized and the protective response is produced at progressively lower stress levels.[1,2] This is a treatment response that must be avoided. The often used phrase "No pain, No gain" is only partially correct. The disciplined, controlled production of pain at activity levels below those that produce the neural flare is required to produce the restructuring of the CNS and tissue healing.

Question 3: What Are the Triggers That Produce a Change in the Patient's Status?

Patients' appraisals of threat and safety are important to the quality of treatment outcomes. Fear avoidance behaviors, depressive behaviors, dependency, kinesiophobia, rumination, and maladaptive thought loops all increase as threat perception caused by pain increases.[14,22,45,47,53] Structural changes can develop in cortical areas that are involved in threat appraisal.[2,16,18] The heightened threat appraisals also cause increased stress responses, increasing sympathetic nervous and endocrine system activities.[1,14,20,21] The same changes can adversely affect the healing of neural tissue and general health status.[1,14,20,21] Finding those entities that trigger the threat response is an important component of the initial evaluation. A thorough subjective examination facilitated by the use of Motivational Interviewing[54] can uncover many of them. The metaphors, adjectives, and verbs that patients use to describe their pain are powerful indicators of how patients view their pain and appraise harm from it.[2] Altering patient stories and language are powerful treatment tools.[2,41,55] Psychometric testing and pain questionnaires can be used as initial screening tools to assess the patient's psychological, threat appraisal, and pain states.[24,26,46] They can provide guidance in exposing those triggers that raise or lower threat appraisals.

During the examination, practitioners risk becoming so focused on finding the threat or pain triggers that they fail to appraise those activities, beliefs, and ideations that trigger reductions in pain and encourage self-efficacy. Uncovering these during the initial examination and ongoing treatment can provide powerful tools to help patients self-regulate their pain, feel safe as new treatments are introduced or the program is advanced, and encourage patient independence.[2] Finding and teaching patients to use these positive triggers can reinforce the therapeutic relationship between the provider and patient. Safety triggers are used not only to assist the patient in controlling the stress response but also to activate the placebo response. Research has demonstrated the power of trust and belief in activating both the placebo and nocebo responses.[56,57]

SELECTION AND IMPLEMENTATION OF THE THERAPEUTIC INTERVENTIONS

Each patient reacts differently to the tissue injury because of past events, beliefs, and social pressures. The secondary problems that develop as a result of the pain can produce recovery time frames that are measured not in weeks but in months and years.[2,7,10] As a result, care plans need to be developed to meet the individual needs of each patient and not around strict protocols.[2,14,43] Classic rehabilitation models in which patients are seen for an hour of intensive physical therapy three times per week for a few weeks do not address the specific needs of patients with neuropathic pain. More appropriate rehabilitation models shift the emphasis of care away from intensive periods of therapist-focused care of limited durations to models that recognize both the importance of patient-centered care and more realistic time frames that are required for

---

BOX 7.2
Questions to Be Answered by an Educational Curriculum Designed for Patients With Neuropathic Pain

1. What happens during an injury to a nerve and how does the nerve heal?
2. What is pain and how can it be effectively reduced and abolished?
3. How do all of the components of the treatment plan work and fit together into a coordinated plan, including medications?
4. How can danger and safety triggers be used to encourage recovery?
5. Why will every treatment intervention require a positive approach, positive reinforcement, persistence, discipline, and patience?
6. Why are grading of activity and pacing important?
7. Why must periods of excessive activity and prolonged symptom elevation be avoided?
8. Why are adequate sleep, good nutrition, and stress control important to the recovery?

BOX 7.3
Techniques to Normalize Sensory Processing

- Visualization of application of various stimuli to the skin
- Observation of application of various stimuli to another person or nonpainful part of the body
- Left/right discrimination training
- Mirror therapy
- Sensory discrimination including two-point discrimination training
- Desensitization

Adapted from Butler D, Moseley GL. *Explain Pain*. Adelaide, Australia: Noigroup Publications; 2013; with permission.

BOX 7.4
Neuromotor and Functional Training Techniques

- Visualization of movement or activity
- Observation of another's performance of the movement or activity
- Left/right discrimination training
- Mirror therapy
- Virtual reality training
- Graded gait or movement training
- Non-load-bearing to load-bearing exercise
- Graded performance of activities of daily living, recreational activities, work, or other activities

Adapted from Butler D, Moseley GL. *Explain Pain*. Adelaide, Australia: Noigroup Publications; 2013; with permission.

---

recovery. Rehabilitation programs that emphasize quality patient education, encourage positive behavioral changes, and improve the brain's ability to discriminate dangerous from nondangerous sensory input have been shown reduce pain and return patients to full and active lives.[2,14,24,42,44]

INTERVENTION CATEGORIES

Patient Education and Promotion of Self-efficacy

Patient education is the bedrock upon which the treatment plan is built. It can provide the information and behavioral change rationales that can improve the effectiveness of the other interventions.[41,55,56] It is also an important intervention that has been shown to be effective in treating pain.[14,41,45,55] The abolishment of pain would be most patients' initial goal, but often that is not a reasonable outcome in neuropathic pain.[4,6,19] Returning patients to active and productive lifestyles then becomes the primary goal of care.

An educational curriculum for the treatment of neuropathic pain should answer the questions posed in Box 7.2. Because each patient with neuropathic pain is different, the curriculum is adjusted to the needs and problems of each specific patient. Research has demonstrated that patients can understand quite complicated concepts when those concepts are packaged in a curriculum that demonstrates a direct relation to their health status and future well-being.[41,55] The support for the use of patient education as an effective intervention for the treatment of pain is extensive.[14,41,45,54] Within the clinical literature, however, those programs that have curricula that are designed to assist the patient to change the concept of their condition are more successful than those that just supply information.[2,41]

Neuroplasticity-Based Interventions

Neuroplasticity is the process that adapts the nervous system's connectivity and structure to changes in the body's internal and external environment. It is responsible not only for learning but also for persistent pain. As the nervous system adapts, those changes producing persistent pain can remain even after the noxious input stops. Research has demonstrated that the activities in Boxes 7.3 and 7.4 can produce neuroplastic changes in the CNS that can reduce pain.

The normalization of sensory processing includes a number of activities (Box 7.3) that provide safe and controlled stimuli to the sensory system to retrain it to correctly discriminate normal, safe sensations from those that are dangerous. The activities included in neuromotor and functional training (Box 7.4) provide controlled stimuli to the motor control system to reduce the effects of pain and fear-based inhibitions of strength and function. Many of the interventions involved in the two categories are the same because they target similar neural structures and work to integrate the sensory and motor systems. GMI[46] integrates the sensory and motor techniques into one system.

Boxes 7.3 and 7.4 list the techniques in order of increasing perceived threat or challenge to the sensory or motor control systems. This gradation of challenge offers the opportunity to adapt the intervention program to the status of the patient. For the patient with CRPS or intense neuropathic pain who avoids cutaneous contact or is afraid to move, visualization, observation, left/right discrimination training, mirror therapy, and virtual reality training can engage central sensory and motor activity without touching or moving the painful area. Patients are often surprised how these activities can provoke pain. When this occurs, clinicians will need to select a technique that produces less challenge and use the experience as a teaching moment. It is important to emphasize that no damage was done to the tissue and that pain can be produced without direct tissue threat.

The application rules in Box 7.5 provide guidance for the use of these interventions with patients of varying levels of irritability and impairment. As the patient's status changes, the application rules provide guidance that allows the care plan to keep pace with those changes. Patient education concepts are an integral component of these interventions and are important in providing patients with the understanding and support to gain the maximum benefit for the interventions.

Neural Mobilization

Neural mobilization techniques involve both clinician- and patient-performed repeated movements of the extremities and spine to move specific nerves.[49] The techniques can be varied to move specific sections of a nerve and apply graded tension to the nerve.[40,48,49,62] The techniques can be used to improve the mobility of the nerve within the nerve bed, decrease the sensitivity of the nerve to motion, potentially improve the vascular/nutritional status of the nerve, and teach the patient how to avoid excessive stress on the nerve during

---

BOX 7.5

Application Rules for Intervention Used in the Treatment of Neuropathic Pain

1. The techniques chosen should be performed at intensity and rate of repetition that is just below or minimally engages the threat response and does not produce a neural flare.
2. All techniques should be preceded by a short period of mental rehearsal.
3. The techniques should be performed mindfully focusing on the quality of the performance.
4. Techniques should be performed at a consistent intensity, five to six times per day for time periods that engage but do not exceed the threat assessment and produce a neural flare.
5. Occasional flares should be expected. When they occur, patients should understand that no damage has been done to the tissue.
6. Performance of the program should be consistent: Patients need to avoid doing more when feeling good and less when symptoms are elevated.
7. A positive upbeat attitude should be maintained when performing the techniques.
8. Patients should experience a sense of accomplishment or even provide themselves a reward at the end of each session.

---

movement and maintenance of specific postures.[48,49,50] Neural mobilization techniques need to be used carefully, particularly with those patients whose conditions are highly irritable. Sustained stretching techniques are to be avoided because they can interrupt intraneural vascular function and irritate the nerve. Clinicians should receive specific training in the use of this technique before attempting its use.

Bracing/Taping

Bracing can be an effective intervention to assist in decreasing neural tension or compression that can irritate or damage neural tissues. It is often part of the initial management of a nerve injury or after peripheral nerve surgery. Bracing, however, needs to be used carefully. Prolonged immobilization and the failure to incorporate frequent periods of graded neural motion during the use of the brace can be harmful.[14,34,35] Bracing should be combined with a graded activity or neural mobilization program.

The use of athletic or other forms of tape to adjust posture, reduce tension/compression on peripheral nerves, or limit extremity movements to protect nerves can be valuable in providing temporary pain relief for a highly irritable nerve. Tape can be used as a biofeedback tool to assist the patient in learning new postures and movement patterns that produce less stress on the neuropathy.[63] Taping should be seen as a temporary tool and used cautiously. Taping can be irritating to the skin when applied for periods of longer than 24 h or repetitively or the patient is allergic to the tape.[63]

Stress Management Programs

Stress management techniques can improve the effectiveness of other interventions.[14,23] Mindfulness meditation, relaxation training, biofeedback, or hypnosis can be integrated into the treatment program to address the emotional stresses associated with performance of the care plan, especially when new challenges are presented to patients.

CONCLUSION—BUILDING RESILIENCY

McEwan[64] defines resilience as "achieving a positive outcome in the face of adversity." A biopsychosocial approach to the management of neuropathic pain focuses on addressing those elements in a patient's presentation that sap their resiliency. Persistent neuropathic pain can be severe, affecting many aspects of a patient's life. Even when neuropathic pain is successfully treated, it can recur.[2,4,5,7] Clinicians often focus on solving immediate patient problems and consider their care accomplished when patients reach established goals or plateau at levels below expectations. Patients with persistent pain need to be coached, counseled, and instructed to deal with the multiple problems created by pain. Clinicians also need to prepare patients for potential recurrences of pain, even though the neuropathy itself has resolved.[2] The brain and neuroimmune system remember.[2,27] As a result, a biopsychosocially based care plan is not complete until the patients have achieved a degree of resiliency.

Building that resiliency requires clinicians to focus on the long-term goals of guiding patients to be able to maintain a productive life while continuing to experience symptoms and developing the self-efficacy to manage the symptoms should they return. Patient self-efficacy, independence, confidence, and life and self-care skills are all necessary components in the development of a patient who is resilient when faced with pain. Each individual component of the care plan is an essential component that supports the resilient patient who will be able to remain involved in life in the face of persistent neuropathic pain or self-manage recurrent episodes.

REFERENCES

1. Butler DS. *The Sensitive Nervous System*. Adelaide, Australia: Noigroup Publications; 2000.
2. Butler D, Moseley GL. *Explain Pain*. Adelaide, Australia: Noigroup Publications; 2013.
3. Woolf CJ. Review series introduction: what is this thing called pain? *J Clin Invest*. 2010;120(11):3742–3744. http://dx.doi.org/10.1172/JCI45178.3742.
4. Gilron I, Watson CPN, Cahill CM, Moulin DE. Neuropathic pain: a practical guide for the clinician. *CMAJ*. 2006; 175(3):265–275. http://dx.doi.org/10.1503/cmaj.060146.
5. O'Connor AB. Neuropathic pain. *Pharmacoeconomics*. 2009;27(2):95–112. http://dx.doi.org/10.2165/00019053-200927020-00002.
6. Chen H, Lamer TJ, Rho RH, et al. Contemporary management of neuropathic pain for the primary care physician. *Mayo Clin Proc*. 2004;79(12):1533–1545. http://dx.doi.org/10.4065/79.12.1533.
7. Kerstman E, Ahn S, Battu S, Tariq S, Grabois M. Neuropathic pain. In: *Handbook of Clinical Neurology*. 2013: 175–187. http://dx.doi.org/10.1016/B978-0-444-52901-5.00015-0.
8. Hanewinckel R, Ikram MA, Van Doorn PA. Peripheral neuropathies. In: *Strategies*. ; 2016:263–282. http://dx.doi.org/10.1016/B978-0-12-802973-2.00015-X.
9. Moseley GL. Graded motor imagery for pathologic pain: a randomized controlled trial. *Neurology*. 2006;67 (12):2129–2134. http://dx.doi.org/10.1212/01.wnl.0000249112.56935.32.
10. Taylor RS. Epidemiology of refractory neuropathic pain. *Pain Pract*. 2006;6(1):22–26. http://dx.doi.org/10.1111/j.1533-2500.2006.00054.
11. Birklein F, Schlereth T. Complex regional pain syndrome-significant progress in understanding. *Pain*. 2015;156 (Suppl.). http://dx.doi.org/10.1097/01.j.pain.0000460344.54470.20.
12. Staunton H. Sudeck atrophy. *Ir Med J*. 1994;99(10):313–315. http://www.ncbi.nlm.nih.gov/pubmed/17274178.
13. Huge V, Lauchart M, Magerl W, et al. Complex interaction of sensory and motor signs and symptoms in chronic CRPS. *PLoS One*. 2011;6(4):e18775. http://dx.doi.org/10.1371/journal.pone.0018775.
14. Society DP, Medicine I. *Updated Guidelines Complex Regional Pain Syndrome Type 1 Initiative: Netherlands Society of Anaesthesiologists*; November 2014.
15. Reinersmann A, Landwehrt J, Krumova EK, Ocklenburg S, Güntürkün O, Maier C. Impaired spatial body representation in complex regional pain syndrome type 1 (CRPS I). *Pain*. 2012;153(11):2174–2181. http://dx.doi.org/10.1016/j.pain.2012.05.025.
16. Parsons LM. Integrating cognitive psychology, neurology and neuroimaging. *Acta Psychol (Amst)*. 2001;107(1–3):155–181. http://www.ncbi.nlm.nih.gov/pubmed/11388134.
17. Moseley GL, Flor H. Targeting cortical representations in the treatment of chronic pain: a review. *Neurorehabil Neural Repair*. 2012;26(6):646–652. http://dx.doi.org/10.1177/1545968311433209.

18. Swart CM, Stins JF, Beek PJ. Cortical changes in complex regional pain syndrome (CRPS). *Eur J Pain.* 2009;13(9):902–907. http://dx.doi.org/10.1016/j.ejpain.2008.11.010.

19. Generaal E, Vogelzangs N, Macfarlane GJ, et al. Biological stress systems, adverse life events and the onset of chronic multisite musculoskeletal pain: a 6-year cohort study. *Ann Rheum Dis.* 2016;75(5):847–854. http://dx.doi.org/10.1136/annrheumdis-2014-206741.

20. Herman JP, Mcklveen JM, Solomon MB, Carvalho-Netto E, Myers B. Neural regulation of the stress response: glucocorticoid feedback mechanisms. *Braz J Med Biol Res.* 2012;45(4):292–298. http://dx.doi.org/10.1590/S0100-879X2012007500041.

21. Chapman CR, Tuckett RP, Song CW. Pain and stress in a systems perspective: reciprocal neural, endocrine, and immune interactions. *J Pain.* 2008;9(2):122–145. http://dx.doi.org/10.1016/j.jpain.2007.09.006.

22. de Jong JR, Vlaeyen JWS, de Gelder JM, Patijn J. Pain-related fear, perceived harmfulness of activities, and functional limitations in complex regional pain syndrome type I. *J Pain.* 2011;12(12):1209–1218. http://dx.doi.org/10.1016/j.jpain.2011.06.010.

23. Jensen MP, Day MA, Miró J. Neuromodulatory treatments for chronic pain: efficacy and mechanisms. *Nat Rev Neurol.* 2014;10(3):167–178. http://dx.doi.org/10.1038/nrneurol.2014.12.

24. Bean DJ, Johnson MH, Heiss-Dunlop W, Lee AC, Kydd RR. Do psychological factors influence recovery from complex regional pain syndrome type 1? A prospective study. *Pain.* 2015;156(11):2310–2318. http://dx.doi.org/10.1097/j.pain.0000000000000282.

25. Clay FJ, Newstead SV, Watson WL, Ozanne-Smith J, Guy J, McClure RJ. Bio-psychosocial determinants of persistent pain 6 months after non-life-threatening acute orthopaedic trauma. *J Pain.* 2010;11(5):420–430. http://dx.doi.org/10.1016/j.jpain.2009.12.002.

26. Wijma AJ, van Wilgen CP, Meeus M, Nijs J. Clinical biopsychosocial physiotherapy assessment of patients with chronic pain: the first step in pain neuroscience education. *Physiother Theory Pract.* 2016;32(5):368–384. http://dx.doi.org/10.1080/09593985.2016.1194651.

27. Grace PM, Hutchinson MR, Maier SF, Watkins LR. Pathological pain and the neuroimmune interface. *Nat Rev Immunol.* 2014;14(4):217–231. http://dx.doi.org/10.1038/nri3621.

28. Grace PM, Strand KA, Galer EL, et al. Morphine paradoxically prolongs neuropathic pain in rats by amplifying spinal NLRP3 inflammasome activation. *Proc Natl Acad Sci USA.* 2016;113(24):E3441–E3450. http://dx.doi.org/10.1073/pnas.1602070113.

29. Jones RCW, Lawson E, Backonja M. Managing neuropathic pain. *Med Clin North Am.* 2016;100(1):151–167. http://dx.doi.org/10.1016/j.mcna.2015.08.009.

30. Bean DJ, Johnson MH, Kydd RR. The outcome of complex regional pain syndrome type 1: a systematic review. *J Pain.* 2014;15(7):677–690. http://dx.doi.org/10.1016/j.jpain.2014.01.500.

31. Grace PM, Fabisiak TJ, Green-Fulgham SM, et al. Prior voluntary wheel running attenuates neuropathic pain. *Pain.* 2016;157(9):2012–2023. http://dx.doi.org/10.1097/j.pain.0000000000000607.

32. Leung A, Gregory NS, Allen L-AH, Sluka KA. Regular physical activity prevents chronic pain by altering resident muscle macrophage phenotype and increasing interleukin-10 in mice. *Pain.* 2016;157(1):70–79. http://dx.doi.org/10.1097/j.pain.0000000000000312.

33. Matsuo H, Uchida K, Nakajima H, et al. Early transcutaneous nerve stimulation reduces hyperalgesia and decreases activation of spinal glial cells in mice with neuropathic pain. *Pain.* 2014;155(9):1888–1901. http://dx.doi.org/10.1016/j.pain.2014.06.022.

34. Guo TZ, Wei T, Li WW, Li XQ, Clark JD, Kingery WS. Immobilization contributes to exaggerated neuropeptide signaling, inflammatory changes, and nociceptive sensitization after fracture in rats. *J Pain.* 2014;15(10):1033–1045. http://dx.doi.org/10.1016/j.jpain.2014.07.004.

35. Pepper A, Li W, Kingery WS, Angst MS, Curtin CM, Clark JD. Changes resembling complex regional pain syndrome following surgery and immobilization. *J Pain.* 2013;14(5):516–524. http://dx.doi.org/10.1016/j.jpain.2013.01.004.

36. Koes B, van Tulder M, Lin C, Macedo L, McAuley J, Maher C. An updated overview of clinical guidelines for the management of non-specific low back pain in primary care. *Eur Spine J.* 2010;19(12):2075–2094. http://dx.doi.org/10.1007/s00586-010-1502-y.

37. Koksal I. Efficacy of rapid recovery protocol for total knee arthroplasty: a historical prospective study. *Acta Orthop Traumatol Turc.* 2015;23(5):45. http://dx.doi.org/10.3944/AOTT.2015.14.0353.

38. Tschakert G, Kroepfl JM, Mueller A, et al. Acute physiological responses to short-and long-stage high-intensity interval exercise in cardiac rehabilitation: a pilot study. *J Sport Sci Med.* 2016;15(1):80–91. http://dx.doi.org/10.1136/openhrt-2015-000369.

39. Kroll HR. Exercise therapy for chronic pain. *Phys Med Rehabil Clin N Am.* 2015;26(2):263–281. http://dx.doi.org/10.1016/j.pmr.2014.12.007.

40. Basson A, Olivier B, Ellis R, Coppieters M, Stewart A, Mudzi W. The effectiveness of neural mobilizations in the treatment of musculoskeletal conditions: a systematic review protocol. *JBI Database Syst Rev Implement Rep.* 2015;13(1):65–75. http://dx.doi.org/10.11124/jbisrir-2015-1401.

41. Moseley GL, Butler DS. Fifteen years of explaining pain: the past, present, and future. *J Pain.* 2015;16(9):807–813. http://dx.doi.org/10.1016/j.jpain.2015.05.005.

42. Bowering KJ, Connell NEO, Tabor A, et al. The effects of graded motor imagery and its components on chronic pain: a systematic review and meta-analysis. *J Pain.* 2013;14(1):3–13. http://dx.doi.org/10.1016/j.jpain.2012.09.007.

43. Daly AE, Bialocerkowski AE. Does evidence support physiotherapy management of adult complex regional pain syndrome type one? A systematic review. *Eur J Pain.* 2009;13(4):339–353. http://dx.doi.org/10.1016/j.ejpain.2008.05.003.

44. Moseley GL. Graded motor imagery is effective for long-standing complex regional pain syndrome: a randomised controlled trial. *Pain.* 2004;108(1–2):192–198. http://dx.doi.org/10.1016/j.pain.2004.01.006.

45. Smart KM, Wand BM, O'Connell NE. Physiotherapy for pain and disability in adults with complex regional pain syndrome (CRPS) types I and II. In: Smart KM, ed. *Cochrane Database of Systematic Reviews.* Chichester, UK: John Wiley & Sons, Ltd; 2016. http://dx.doi.org/10.1002/14651858.CD010853.pub2.

46. Moseley GL, Butler DS, Beames T, Giles T. *The Graded Motor Imagery Handbook.* Adelaide, Australia: Noigroup Publications; 2012.

47. Sullivan MJL, Adams H. Psychosocial treatment techniques to augment the impact of physiotherapy interventions for low back pain. *Physiother Can.* 2010;62(3):180–189. http://dx.doi.org/10.3138/physio.62.3.180.

48. Hall TM, Elvey RL. Nerve trunk pain: physical diagnosis and treatment. *Man Ther.* 1999;4(2):63–73. http://dx.doi.org/10.1054/math.1999.0172.

49. Butler DS. *Mobilisation of the Nervous System.* 2nd ed. Philadelphia: Churchill Livingstone; 1999.

50. Nee R, Butler D. Management of peripheral neuropathic pain: integrating neurobiology, neurodynamics, and clinical evidence. *Phys Ther Sport.* 2006;7(1):36–49. http://dx.doi.org/10.1016/j.ptsp.2005.10.002.

51. Maitland GD. *Peripheral Manipulation.* 3rd ed. London: Butterworths; 1990.

52. Lishman W, Russell W. The brachial neuropathies. *Lancet.* 1961;2(7209):941–947. http://www.ncbi.nlm.nih.gov/pubmed/14465787.

53. Sullivan MJL, Adams H, Rhodenizer T, Stanish WD. A psychosocial risk factor–targeted intervention for the prevention of chronic pain and disability following whiplash injury. *Phys Ther.* 2006;86(1):8–18. http://www.ncbi.nlm.nih.gov/pubmed/16386058.

54. O'Halloran PD, Blackstock F, Shields N, et al. Motivational interviewing to increase physical activity in people with chronic health conditions: a systematic review and meta-analysis. *Clin Rehabil.* 2014;28(12):1159–1171. http://dx.doi.org/10.1177/0269215514536210.

55. Moseley GL. Evidence for a direct relationship between cognitive and physical change during an education intervention in people with chronic low back pain. *Eur J Pain.* 2004;8(1):39–45.

56. Bystad M, Bystad C, Wynn R. How can placebo effects best be applied in clinical practice? A narrative review. *Psychol Res Behav Manag.* 2015;8:41–45. http://dx.doi.org/10.2147/PRBM.S75670.

57. Kaptchuk TJ, Friedlander E, Kelley JM, et al. Placebos without deception: a randomized controlled trial in irritable bowel syndrome. In: Boutron I, ed. *PLoS One.* 2010;5(12):e15591. http://dx.doi.org/10.1371/journal.pone.0015591.

58. Moseley GL, Gallace A, Spence C. Is mirror therapy all it is cracked up to be? Current evidence and future directions. *Pain.* 2008;138(1):7–10. http://dx.doi.org/10.1016/j.pain.2008.06.026.

59. Flor H, Denke C, Schaefer M, Grüsser S. Effect of sensory discrimination training on cortical reorganisation and phantom limb pain. *Lancet.* 2001;357(9270):1763–1764. http://dx.doi.org/10.1016/S0140-6736(00)04890-X.

60. Moseley GL, Wiech K. The effect of tactile discrimination training is enhanced when patients watch the reflected image of their unaffected limb during training. *Pain.* 2009;144(3):314–319. http://dx.doi.org/10.1016/j.pain.2009.04.030.

61. Moseley GL. Using visual illusion to reduce at-level neuropathic pain in paraplegia. *Pain.* 2007;130(3):294–298. http://dx.doi.org/10.1016/j.pain.2007.01.007.

62. Coppieters MW, Butler DS. Do "sliders" slide and "tensioners" tension? An analysis of neurodynamic techniques and considerations regarding their application. *Man Ther.* 2008;13(3):213–221. http://dx.doi.org/10.1016/j.math.2006.12.008.

63. Kase K, Wallis J, Kase T. *Clinical Therapeutic Applications of the Kinesio Taping Method.* Tokyo: Ken Ikai Co. Ltd; 2003.

64. McEwen BS, Gray JD, Nasca C. Recognizing resilience: learning from the effects of stress on the brain. *Neurobiol Stress.* 2015;1(1):1–11. http://dx.doi.org/10.1016/j.ynstr.2014.09.001.

CHAPTER 8

Complex Regional Pain Syndrome: Pharmacotherapy

GEORGE W. YOUNG, DO • MICHAEL J. MEHNERT, MD

INTRODUCTION

Complex regional pain syndrome (CRPS) poses a significant challenge to the treating clinician. Not only is CRPS difficult to recognize and diagnose, but there is also paucity of effective, evidence-based treatments for the condition. CRPS typically presents with pain out of proportion to the mechanism of injury, with varying degrees of motor and sensory changes, sudomotor activity, vasomotor activity, autonomic dysfunction, and atrophy of the affected region. Because of the various pain pathways hypothesized in driving the syndrome, multiple medications in different classes are usually necessary for effective control. Not only does this help to minimize medication side effects by enabling lesser doses of medication, but also multiple pain pathways are blocked, which improves efficacy of treatment. This chapter focuses on oral and topical pharmacotherapy prescribed for the treatment of CRPS.

ANTIINFLAMMATORIES

Injury to an extremity, such as fracture or sprain, or injury to a nerve commonly precedes the development of CRPS. Exaggerated local inflammation of the injured tissue is postulated to play a role in the development of CRPS.[1] Cytokines, including interleukin (IL)-1, tumor necrosis factor-α, and nerve growth factor, are elevated and sensitize the local tissue, whereas calcitonin gene-related peptide and substance P mediate the pain response.[2,3] This theory has popularized the utilization of antiinflammatory medications in the treatment of CRPS.

Corticosteroids reduce inflammation by inhibiting cytokines and pain mediators. Their utility in the treatment of CRPS has been questioned. Often they are not offered when a fracture is involved, as there is fear of delayed bone healing with the initiation of glucocorticoids; however, one small case report showed efficacy in the setting of a fracture without adverse events.[4] There is evidence supporting the utilization of corticosteroids

in the treatment of CRPS. Most studies suggest that the steroid be started in the first 3 months of appearance of symptoms, with a high dose tapered to a lower dose over 2 weeks and then a slow taper off of the steroid for a total treatment length of 4–12 weeks.[4–7] The use of steroids for the treatment of chronic CRPS (>3 months) has less support.[8] Steroid treatment in CRPS following stroke is supported by multiple studies that led to improvement in pain and function.[9–11] Complications are listed in Table 8.1. Caution is advised in the treatment of patients with diabetes, hypertension, glaucoma, or a history of gastrointestinal (GI) bleed/ulceration. Long-term exposure to corticosteroids carries a risk of osteoporosis and cataract formation.

Nonsteroidal antiinflammatory drugs (NSAIDs) are widely used in the treatment of pain. They work by blocking the cyclooxygenase (COX) pathway and the formation of prostaglandins that mediate the inflammatory response. NSAIDs may block prostaglandins at the spinal level, suppressing the nociceptive pathway.[1] Nonselective NSAIDs block both COX-1 and COX-2. Diclofenac 50 mg twice a day for 1 month showed improvement in pain and hand function in one study.[12] Selective NSAIDs block only COX-2 and gained popularity because of a better GI safety profile. However, there is lack of evidence for their use in CRPS.[13] Complications are listed in Table 8.1. NSAIDs are associated with an increased risk of cardiovascular events. It is recommended that kidney function, liver function, and blood pressure be monitored with the continued use of NSAIDs.

Free radical scavengers are utilized to reduce the inflammatory response by eliminating free radicals released during the inflammatory response. Dimethylsulfoxide 50% in a fatty cream and N-acetylcysteine tablets lead to improvement in pain and function in patients with CRPS.[14,15] A study performed by Zyluk et al. revealed a positive outcome with the use of mannitol in patients with CRPS, but their study had

TABLE 8.1
Antiinflammatory Medications

Medication	Dosage	Complications
CORTICOSTEROIDS		
Prednisone	5–60 mg/day po	Facial flushing, hot flashes, GI upset, swelling, insomnia, weight gain, hyperglycemia, HTN, nausea/vomiting, dizziness, and emotional lability
Prednisolone	5–60 mg/day po divided qd-qid	
Methylprednisolone	4–48 mg/day po divided qd-qid	GI bleed, GI perforation/ulceration, adrenal insufficiency, Cushing syndrome, diabetes mellitus, pseudotumor cerebri, psychosis, avascular necrosis, and myopathy
Dexamethasone	0.75–9 mg/day po divided q6-12h	Osteoporosis, cataracts, immunosuppression (long-term use)
NONSELECTIVE NSAIDS		
Ibuprofen	200–800 mg po tid-qid	GI upset, constipation, fluid retention, headache, diarrhea, nausea/vomiting, rash, dizziness, ALT/AST elevation, BUN elevation, photosensitivity
Diclofenac	50 mg po tid	
Etodolac	200–400 mg po q6-8h	GI bleeding, GI perforation/ulcer, MI, stroke, thromboembolism, HTN, CHF, nephrotoxicity, hepatotoxicity, bronchospasm, Stevens-Johnson syndrome
Fenoprofen	300–600 mg po tid-qid	
Indomethacin	25–50 mg po bid-tid	
Ketoprofen	50 mg po q6-8h	
Ketorolac	10 mg po q4-6h	
Meloxicam	7.5–15 mg po qd	
Nabumetone	1000-2000 mg/day po divided qd-bid	
Naproxen	250–500 mg po q12h	
Oxaprozin	1200 mg po qd	
Piroxicam	20 mg po qd	
Sulindac	150–200 mg po bid	
Tolmetin	200–600 mg po tid	
Celecoxib (COX-2 inhibitor)	200 mg po divided qd-bid	
FREE RADICAL SCAVENGERS		
Dimethylsulfoxide	50% cream to affected extremity 5×/day	Skin reaction, rash, headache, dizziness, drowsiness, strong odor
N-acetylcysteine	600 mg effervescent tablets po tid	Nausea/vomiting, diarrhea or constipation, potential bronchospasm in asthmatics
Vitamin C	500 mg po daily for 50 days after wrist fracture	Nausea/vomiting, dyspepsia, diarrhea, headache

ALT, alanine transaminase; *AST*, aspartate transaminase; *BUN*, blood urea nitrogen; *CHF*, congestive heart failure; *GI*, gastrointestinal; *HTN*, hypertension; *MI*, myocardial infarction; *NSAID*, nonsteroidal antiinflammatory drug.

no placebo group and patients were coadministered dexamethasone.[16,17] Prevention of CRPS with daily vitamin C has been studied in patients with wrist fractures, and a lower incidence of CRPS was found in the treatment group.[18,19] The above-mentioned treatments were well tolerated and did not result in significant side effects.

ANTIEPILEPTICS

Gabapentin is widely used for the treatment of neuropathic pain. It also has an indication for controlling partial seizures. It is hypothesized to work by binding to the α2δ subunit of the voltage-gated calcium channel, thus decreasing the release of excitatory neurotransmitters.[20] Treatment of painful diabetic neuropathy and

TABLE 8.2
Antiepileptic Medications

Medication	Dosage	Complications
Gabapentin	300–1200 mg po tid	Somnolence, dizziness, fatigue, dry mouth, peripheral edema, weight gain, gastro-intestinal upset, tremor Depression, suicidal ideation, and withdrawal seizure (abrupt discontinuation)
Pregabalin	150–600 mg po divided bid-tid	Dizziness, somnolence, dry mouth, peripheral edema, blurred vision, weight gain, constipation Suicidality, depression, withdrawal seizure (abrupt discontinuation)
Carbamazepine	200–400 mg po bid	Dizziness, drowsiness, urticaria, nausea/vomiting, constipation, ataxia, rash, blurred vision, tremor, speech difficulty Aplastic anemia, fatal dermatologic reaction, hepatotoxicity, thrombocytopenia, leukopenia, hyponatremia, Syndrome of inappropriate antidiuretic hormone secretion (SIADH)
Oxcarbazepine	300–1200 mg po bid	Fatigue, dizziness, ataxia, and nausea/vomiting, tremor, diplopia, balance difficulty Hyponatremia, SIADH, toxic epidermal necrolysis, thrombocytopenia, leukopenia, pancreatitis
Topiramate	50–400 mg po divided bid	Weight loss, somnolence, nausea, diarrhea, paresthesias, tremor Metabolic acidosis, osteoporosis, hypokalemia, suicidality, hyperthermia

postherpetic neuralgia are two proven uses for gabapentin.[21,22] Two randomized controlled trials of gabapentin have been performed in the population with CRPS. The larger study included 307 patients, of which 85 had the diagnosis of CRPS, and the smaller study included 58 patients with CRPS. The first study revealed a small but statistically significant reduction in pain in the gabapentin-treated group.[23] The second study led to early but only short-term reduction in pain in the treatment group. However, gabapentin did provide long-term improvement of sensory deficits in the affected limb.[24]

Gabapentin is commonly prescribed three times a day with a maximum dose of 3600 mg/day. The initial dose is low and is titrated upward until there is a positive therapeutic effect. Complications are listed in Table 8.2.

Pregabalin is a newer antiepileptic medication with a similar mechanism of action as gabapentin.[20] It has gained popularity because of its twice daily dosing and linear pharmacokinetics that allows faster titration. Pregabalin has supporting evidence for its use in painful diabetic neuropathy and postherpetic neuralgia.[25,26] Research on this agent is lacking in the population with CRPS. One case report revealed resolution of pain within 2 days of initiating pregabalin in a patient who failed to improve after treatment with physical therapy, gabapentin, and multiple stellate ganglion blocks.[27] The side-effect profile of pregabalin (see Table 8.2) is similar to that of gabapentin and tolerated well.

Sodium channel antagonists are another treatment consideration. Carbamazepine is approved by the US Food and Drug Administration (FDA) for the treatment of trigeminal neuralgia. A small study showed support in treating the population with painful diabetic neuropathy.[28] Carbamazepine was compared with morphine in treating CRPS after the spinal cord stimulator of a patient with CRPS was turned off. Carbamazepine given 600 mg/day led to a delayed and reduced level of pain after 8 days, and there was no effect in the morphine group.[29] Larger studies need to be performed before conclusions can be drawn. Complications are listed in Table 8.2.

Oxcarbazepine has a similar mechanism of action as carbamazepine but has not been studied in the population with CRPS. There is one placebo-controlled trial that led to a reduction of pain in 146 patients with painful diabetic neuropathy treated with a maximum daily dose of 1800 mg.[30] Side effects and adverse events are listed in Table 8.2. Syndrome of inappropriate antidiuretic hormone secretion (SIADH) and hyponatremia may develop in patients treated with both carbamazepine and oxcarbazepine.

Topiramate is employed as an anticonvulsant as well as for migraine prophylaxis. Its exact mechanism of action is unknown, but it is thought to block sodium channels, antagonize γ-aminobutyric acid activity, block glutamate receptors, and inhibit carbonic anhydrase.[31] One study revealed efficacy in treatment of painful diabetic neuropathy.[32] When treatment is initiated, the dosage should be started at a low level and titrated slowly to a maximum dose of 400 mg/day. Complications are listed in Table 8.2.

TABLE 8.3
Antidepressant Medications

Medication	Dosage	Complications
TRICYCLIC ANTIDEPRESSANTS		
Nortriptyline	25–150 mg po qhs	Drowsiness, dry mouth, dizziness, constipation, blurred vision, nausea/vomiting, confusion, urinary retention, weight gain, libido changes, tremor
Amitriptyline	25–100 mg po qhs	Hypotension, cardiac arrhythmia, suicidality, extrapyramidal symptoms
Desipramine	25–200 mg po qd	
Doxepin	25–300 mg po qhs	
SEROTONIN-NOREPINEPHRINE REUPTAKE INHIBITORS		
Duloxetine	30–60 mg po qd	Nausea, headache, dry mouth, fatigue, constipation, dizziness, decreased libido, tremor
Venlafaxine	75–225 mg po div bid-tid	Suicidality, depression exacerbation, withdrawal symptoms if abruptly discontinued
	75–225 mg ER po qd	

ANTIDEPRESSANTS (TABLE 8.3)

Tricyclic antidepressants (TCAs), such as nortriptyline, amitriptyline, and desipramine, have been used extensively in the treatment of neuropathic pain.[33] Elevated levels of norepinephrine and serotonin inhibiting the dorsal horn and partial sodium channel blockade[34] are the proposed analgesic mechanisms of action. Their use in the treatment of CRPS is by convention and based on expert opinion. A low starting dosage is recommended with a slow titration. An adequate trial can take up to 2 months before considering treatment failure. Common side effects are listed in Table 8.3.

The serotonin-norepinephrine reuptake inhibitors (SNRIs), including venlafaxine and duloxetine, have been shown to benefit patients with neuropathic pain with the added potential of treating concomitant depression. Venlafaxine was shown to be equally effective to imipramine (TCA) in the treatment of painful polyneuropathy.[35] Patients with painful diabetic neuropathy benefited from treatment with duloxetine in a multicenter trial.[36] SNRIs have not been studied in the population with CRPS but have been used anecdotally. Side effects and complications are listed in Table 8.3.

Selective serotonin reuptake inhibitors (SSRIs) are not beneficial in the treatment of neuropathic pain.[37] They can be considered in treating underlying depression in the population with chronic pain.

BISPHOSPHONATES

Bisphosphonates are potent osteoclast inhibitors that block bone resorption and are used in the management of osteoporosis, Paget disease, and cancer-related bone pain. Patients with CRPS commonly present with osteopenia in the affected limb and increased uptake of radiotracer on three-phase bone scan. Originally, interest in using bisphosphonates in the treatment of patients with CRPS was based on slowing bone resorption. However, newer theories suggest that high levels of bisphosphonates in local tissue prevent the production of hydroxyapatite crystals, reducing lactic acid production and modulating the local inflammatory response.[38,39]

Five randomized controlled trials (Table 8.4) in the population with CRPS have been performed to date. Four of these studies investigated intravenous bisphosphonates, and one investigated an oral bisphosphonate.[40-44] The doses administered in each study were close to the recommended doses for bone metabolism disorders such as Paget disease or cancer-related bone pain, which is significantly higher than the dose used in treating osteoporosis. Dosing regimens were varied and follow-up was up to 3 months. All studies showed a positive outcome, with the treatment groups reporting less pain than the control group. Limitations of the studies include a small, heterogeneous patient population, various CRPS diagnostic criteria, and different outcome measures. The disease was chronic in all but one study.[45]

Common side effects of bisphosphonates include musculoskeletal pain, abdominal pain, and acid reflux. Serious adverse events include osteonecrosis of the jaw, atypical femur fracture, and gastric/duodenal ulcer. It is recommended that patients take a drug holiday after 5 years of treatment. Although the available data are weak, the use of bisphosphonates in treating CRPS is supported particularly in those patients with osteopenia. Because of the higher cost associated with intravenous administration, efficacy has to be supported with future studies.

TABLE 8.4
Randomized-Controlled Trials Investigating Bisphosphonate Treatment in CRPS, Type 1

Investigator	Treatment Regimen	Number of Subjects	Follow-Up Length	Additional Treatments
Adami et al.[40]	Alendronate 7.5 mg IV daily × 3 days versus IV placebo	20	4 weeks	Physical therapy, calcitonin nasal spray, analgesics (unspecified)
Manicourt et al.[41]	Alendronate 40 mg po daily × 8 weeks versus oral placebo	40	24 weeks	Physical therapy
Robinson et al.[42]	Pamidronate 60 mg IV × 1 dose versus IV placebo	27	3 months	Paracetamol, codeine, paracetamol/dextropropoxyphene
Varenna et al.[43]	Neridronate 100 mg IV q3 days × 4 doses versus IV placebo	82	40 days	NSAIDs, paracetamol
Varenna et al.[44]	Clodronate 300 mg IV daily × 10 days versus IV placebo	32	180 days	None

IV, intravenous; *NASID*, nonsteroidal antiinflammatory drug.
Data from Adami S, Fossaluzza V, Gatti D, Fracassi E, Braga V. Bisphosphonate therapy of reflex sympathetic dystrophy syndrome. *Ann Rheum Dis*. 1997;56(3):201–204, Manicourt DH, Brasseur JP, Boutsen Y, Depreseux G, Devogelaer JP. Role of alendronate in therapy for post-traumatic complex regional pain syndrome type I of the lower extremity. *Arthritis Rheum*. 2004;50(11):3690–3697, Robinson JN, Sandom J, Chapman PT. Efficacy of pamidronate in complex regional pain syndrome type I. *Pain Med*. 2004;5(3):276–280, Varenna M, Adami S, Rossini M, et al. Treatment of complex regional pain syndrome type I with neridronate: a randomized, double-blind, placebo-controlled study. *Rheumatol Oxf*. 2013;52(3):534–542, and Varenna M, Zucchi F, Ghiringhelli D, et al. Intravenous clodronate in the treatment of reflex sympathetic dystrophy syndrome. A randomized, double blind, placebo controlled study. *J Rheumatol*. 2000;27(6):1477–1483.

CALCITONIN

Calcitonin inhibits osteoclastic activity and has analgesic properties leading to its use in the population with CRPS. Unfortunately, there is no data to support its use in CRPS. Multiple studies investigated intranasal and intramuscular injections of calcitonin in the treatment of CRPS and found no benefit.[46–49] A recent editorial by Benzon calls for the calcitonin studies to be repeated with validated diagnostic criteria and larger sample sizes.[50] Intranasal administration is cost-effective and well tolerated, with the most common side effects being epistaxis and nasal irritation. Salmon allergy precludes the use of calcitonin.

OPIOIDS

Opioid usage is controversial in the population with chronic, nonmalignant pain. The utility of opioids in chronic neuropathic pain conditions is less than in acute and subacute nociceptive pain conditions.[51] Studies show that controlled-release oxycodone in painful diabetic neuropathy and transdermal fentanyl in neuropathic pain improve pain scores and quality of life.[52,53] However, these studies were short term (<12 weeks). The fentanyl study had a 2-year follow-up, and only 9 of 30 (30%) patients were still using fentanyl; pain relief was moderate to good in five of the nine remaining patients. There are no studies that demonstrate that opioids

control neuropathic pain on a long-term basis. Opioids should be considered second- or third-line agents and prescribed in combination with adjunct agents for neuropathic pain conditions such as CRPS. Traditional opioids produce their analgesic effect by blocking the μ-, δ-, and κ-opioid receptors in the central nervous system (CNS). Before initiating opioid treatment, risk screening patients with measures such as the opioid risk tool or brief risk inventory is recommended.[54,55]

Common side effects associated with opioids include nausea, vomiting, constipation, drowsiness, and cognitive impairment. Caution should be used when combining opioids with benzodiazepines and alcohol. Adverse events include respiratory depression, dependency, addiction, and death. Opioid-induced hyperalgesia (OIH) is a state of hypersensitivity in patients on long-term opioid therapy, which would not bode well in CRPS. Treatment of OIH consists of discontinuing the opioid, rotating to a different opioid class, or adding adjunct medication to suppress the hyperalgesia.[56,57] Opioid tolerance is a physiologic change where an opioid has less analgesic effect over time. Opioid abuse is defined as a compulsive, destructive behavior of using opioids for a nontherapeutic purpose or a dose higher than is medically necessary for an analgesic effect.[58] Opioid use disorder diagnostic criteria are listed in Box 8.1. Long-term opioid therapy

---

BOX 8.1
Opioid Use Disorder Diagnostic Criteria[58]

A problematic pattern of opioid use leading to clinically significant impairment or distress, as manifested by at least two of the following, occurring within a 12-month period:

1. Opioids are often taken in larger amounts or over a longer period than was intended.
2. There is a persistent desire or unsuccessful efforts to cut down or control opioid use.
3. A great deal of time is spent in activities necessary to obtain the opioid, use the opioid, or recovering from its effects.
4. Craving, or a strong desire or urge to use opioids.
5. Recurrent opioid use resulting in a failure to fulfill major role obligations at work, school or home.
6. Continued opioid use despite having persistent or recurrent social or interpersonal problems caused or exacerbated by the effects of opioids.
7. Important social, occupational, or recreational activities are given up or reduced because of opioid use.
8. Recurrent opioid use in situations in which it is physically hazardous.

9. Continued opioid use despite knowledge of having a persistent or recurrent physical or psychological problem. That is likely to have been caused or exacerbated by the substance.
10. Tolerance, as defined by either of the following:
    a. A need for markedly increased amounts of opioids to achieve intoxication or desired effect.
    b. A markedly diminished effect with continued use of the same amount of an opioid.
    Note: This criterion is not considered to be met for those taking opioids solely under appropriate medical supervision.
11. Withdrawal, as manifested by either:
    • Opioid withdrawal syndrome (three or more of the following): Dysphoria, nausea/vomiting, muscle aches, runny nose, dilated pupils, diaphoresis, diarrhea, yawning, fever, insomnia
    • Opioids (or a closely related substance) are taken to relieve or avoid withdrawal symptoms.
    Note: This criterion is not considered to be met for those individuals taking opioids solely under appropriate medical supervision.

Reprinted with permission from the *Diagnostic and Statistical Manual of Mental Disorders*, 5th ed., (Copyright 2013). American Psychiatric Association.

---

may have hormonal effects, including decreased testosterone levels, decrease libido, and irregular menses.[59]

Tramadol and tapentadol differ from other opioids, as they inhibit norepinephrine reuptake as well as bind to the μ-opioid receptor.[60] This has led to the investigation of their use in treating neuropathic pain conditions. Results have been favorable for both tramadol and tapentadol in treating neuropathic pain.[61-63] However, these studies are all short term (<12 weeks), so efficacy for long-term treatment has not been supported. Side-effect profiles are similar to those of traditional opioids. Caution needs to be exercised when these drugs are used in combination with SNRIs and SSRIs to avoid serotonin syndrome, which is a serious reaction that leads to cognitive impairment, hyperthermia, seizures, muscle breakdown, tremors, and potentially death.

Methadone not only provides analgesia by binding to the opioid receptors, but also works as an *N*-methyl-D-aspartate (NMDA) receptor antagonist. Thus methadone has come under investigation in treating neuropathic pain. A Cochrane review found limited evidence supporting the use of methadone in treating chronic, non-cancer-related pain.[64] Small studies and case series have shown positive trends supporting the use of methadone in treating neuropathic pain.[65,66] Methadone has extensive oral bioavailability;

it is metabolized by the cytochrome P-450 system and can prolong the QT interval. Obtaining an electrocardiogram during and shortly after initiating methadone treatment is strongly advised. Drug-drug interactions are important to consider, as blood levels of medication can change with medications that compete with the cytochrome P-450 system. The half-life is variable between 8 h and 2 days, so dosage should be started low and titrated slowly to avoid accidental overdose. Care should also be taken when converting from an alternative opioid to methadone, as the daily morphine dose changes the conversion ratio. Because of the stigma of methadone being used for the treatment of drug addiction, patients with pain may be reluctant to use the medication in fear of being labeled an addict. Methadone may provide an alternative to traditional opioids in the treatment of CRPS, but stronger studies need to be performed and clinicians should take time to become familiar with the risks and special considerations unique to prescribing methadone.

N-METHYL-D-ASPARTATE ANTAGONISTS

Animal models pose evidence that drugs blocking the NMDA receptors may reduce neuropathic pain.[67,68] This finding led to the hypothesis that NMDA receptor antagonists would be beneficial in treating chronic neuropathic pain conditions, including CRPS. There is considerable interest in ketamine delivered intravenously or intrathecally, and this is discussed in the next chapter on CRPS interventions. This section focuses on oral options, including dextromethorphan, memantine, and amantadine.

Dextromethorphan is widely used as a cough suppressant and weakly binds to the NMDA receptor. A few studies have supported its efficacy in reducing pain from diabetic neuropathy but not postherpetic neuralgia.[69,70] The total daily dose used in these studies was 400 mg/day. A study in chemotherapy-induced peripheral neuropathy in 40 patients with breast cancer, at a maximum daily dose of 90 mg/day, showed improved pain at 4 weeks compared with placebo.[71] The studies available are of low quality, small sample size, and short term and not in the population with CRPS.

Memantine is an NMDA receptor antagonist commonly prescribed for Alzheimer dementia. Data do not support the use of memantine in treating diabetic neuropathy or postherpetic neuralgia.[70,72] A case series consisting of six patients with unilateral upper extremity CRPS showed reduced pain at 6 months after treatment with 30 mg/day of memantine and concomitant physiotherapy.[73]

Amantadine is prescribed in the treatment of influenza A and parkinsonism. Twenty-six patients with chronic low back pain were treated with 100 mg/day of amantadine and had a reduction in pain and decreased sensitivity to heat.[74] There have been no other studies in the population with chronic neuropathic pain that reproduce these results.

NMDA receptor antagonists have significant side effects at higher doses, which limit their utility in the population with neuropathic pain, such as CRPS. Side effects include confusion, hallucinations, somnolence, and nausea. These agents carry a risk of abuse because of their potential euphoric and hallucinatory effects. Further data are needed to support their usage in the population with CRPS.

CALCIUM CHANNEL BLOCKERS
Nifedipine is a calcium channel blocker (CCB) commonly prescribed for the treatment of hypertension, but it is also used in Raynaud phenomenon, which is characterized by cold intolerance and vasospasm. This observation led to a case series that showed a reduction of pain in 9 of 13 patients with CRPS treated with oral nifedipine.[75] A retrospective study of 124 patients with CRPS, 35 treated with nifedipine, showed a reduction in pain in 60% of patients with acute pain and 30%

of patients with chronic pain.[76] Common side effects include headache, dizziness, lightheadedness, and nausea. CCBs need further support with placebo-controlled clinical trials to recommend their usage in CRPS.

α-ADRENERGIC RECEPTOR ANTAGONISTS
Blocking the sympathetic nervous system through anesthetic block and surgery has been used in the treatment of CRPS. α-Adrenergic receptor antagonists have been a target of study in the population with neuropathic pain and CRPS. Unfortunately, oral, transdermal, and epidural clonidine show no benefit and are not well tolerated.[77] Phenoxybenzamine, an irreversible α-blocker used in the treatment of pheochromocytoma, has been supported in two case series that evaluated its usage in the population with acute CRPS. The most common side effect is orthostatic hypotension. α-Adrenergic receptor antagonists are considered third-line agents for the treatment in CRPS until stronger data are available.

TOPICAL AGENTS
Patients with CRPS have hypersensitivity and an exaggerated pain response to sensory stimulus. Topical agents have gained popularity in treating painful neuropathic pain conditions, as they can be applied locally to the affected area, which limits side effects compared with enteral and parenteral drug administration. The Lidocaine 5% patch is FDA approved in the treatment of postherpetic neuralgia and supported by multiple studies.[78] In an open-label study, 16 patients, including 6 patients with CRPS, were treated with the Lidocaine 5% patch as an add-on to their current treatment regimen.[79] Moderate to significant pain relief was seen in all patients with CRPS. Randomized-controlled trials have yet to be conducted to strongly support the usage of Lidocaine 5% patches in CRPS. Utilizing topical anesthetics on a patient's lower extremities could result in gait instability and loss of proprioception.

Capsaicin is naturally found in chili peppers. It is a vanilloid that is thought to work by binding and activating the transient receptor potential cation channel subfamily V member 1 (TRPV1), thus activating nociceptive nerve endings. With repeat usage, cutaneous nociceptive neurons desensitize and degenerate.[80] Capsaicin also releases substance P, which depletes its supply and reduces pain impulse transmission. When applied, topical capsaicin induces a burning sensation that is tolerated poorly by patients with neuropathic pain. Capsaicin 8% patch is FDA approved for the treatment of postherpetic neuralgia. A local anesthetic needs to be applied to the treatment area before applying the patch in order to tolerate. It has been shown to be effective in the treatment of painful diabetic peripheral neuropathy.[81] In a prospective study of 10 patients (two patients with CRPS), 5%–10% capsaicin cream was applied between one and eight times to the affected limb.[82] Regional anesthesia was needed to tolerate the treatment. Of 10 patients, 9 responded to treatment, with the two patients with CRPS showing >50% improvement in pain. Double-blind, placebo-controlled trials need to be conducted before conclusions can be drawn regarding high-dose capsaicin in the treatment of CRPS.

Ketamine is an NMDA antagonist used in the treatment of CRPS. Owing to its potential of intolerable side effects when administered intravenously, intrathecally, and epidurally, ketamine has been studied in a topical gel form. One case study investigated the use of 10–20 mg of ketamine gel on the affected area of five patients with neuropathic pain.[83] Three of the five patients had CRPS; one patient reported pain relief because of the treatment and one reported increased flexibility in the limb without pain reduction. Stronger studies are needed to support the usage of transdermal ketamine for CRPS. Ketamine is anecdotally mixed with local anesthetics, NSAIDs, clonidine, gabapentin, baclofen, and other agents in compounded pain creams for the treatment of various painful conditions. A retrospective study of 13 patients with CRPS treated with a cream containing ketamine 10%, pentoxifylline 6%, clonidine 0.2%, and dimethyl sulfoxide 6%–10% showed greater than 50% pain reduction in 69% of patients.[84] There is currently no strong evidence to support the usage of compounded pain creams in CRPS.

ANTI–TUMOR NECROSIS FACTOR MEDICATIONS

Injured tissue causes inflammatory release of cytokines, including tumor necrosis factor (TNF), which are hypothesized to be pivotal in the development of CRPS.[1] Interest in anti-TNF agents started after thalidomide was used to treat multiple myeloma in a patient with CRPS and the CRPS symptoms significantly improved after the treatment began.[85] Thalidomide was taken off the market in the 1960s because of its teratogenicity but has regained FDA approval for the treatment of erythema nodosum leprosum, multiple myeloma, and other cancers/immunologic conditions. A second case report in a patient with both Behçet disease and CRPS showed resolution of the CRPS pain after administration of thalidomide at a dose of 100–400 mg/day was started.[86] Schwartzmann et al. wrote an editorial on their clinical experience using thalidomide in 42 patients, of which 13 (31%) had moderate to excellent pain relief 1 month after starting thalidomide.[87] Lenalidomide is a thalidomide derivative with enhanced antiinflammatory and immunomodulatory properties of thalidomide but reduced toxicity. A Phase II randomized study was performed using lenalidomide in 184 patients with CRPS for 12 weeks; there was no difference between the treatment group and the placebo group, with a 16.1% response rate in both groups.[88]

Special precautions need to be taken before prescribing thalidomide because of its teratogenicity. Special certification is needed for prescribing physicians, and a patient-physician agreement form must be signed before starting treatment. Female patients must have a negative pregnancy test, use contraception 4 weeks before through 4 weeks after finishing treatment, and immediately stop the medication if they become pregnant. Male patients must agree to use latex/synthetic condoms with sexual contact and not donate sperm until 4 weeks after discontinuing treatment. Patients are not allowed to donate blood during the administration through 4 weeks after stopping thalidomide. Complications include birth defects, deep vein thrombosis, pulmonary embolism, and peripheral neuropathy. Side effects include somnolence, rash, constipation, and numbness. Stronger research is needed to support the usage of this medication, which has strict prescribing guidelines and serious side effects, in the population with CRPS.

Anti-TNF monoclonal antibodies have been studied in the treatment of CRPS, including infliximab and adalimumab. A case report of two patients with CRPS treated with infliximab for 4 weeks showed a reduction of TNF-α and IL-6 levels in blister fluid and reduced pain, edema, and temperature with improved motor function in the affected limb.[89] These results were not replicated in a double-blind placebo-controlled trial using infliximab in 13 patients with CRPS.[90] There was no statistical difference in skin blister cytokine levels or pain reduction, and the study was discontinued prematurely because of patient recruitment difficulties. A case series of 10 patients with CRPS treated with adalimumab failed to demonstrate improvement in pain intensity.[91] Because these agents are immunosuppressive and myelosuppressive, data do not support routine use in CRPS.

CANNABINOIDS

Cannabis has been used medicinally for millenniums. Cannabinoid has been of interest recently because of the legalization of marijuana, both medicinal and recreational, in select states. Approved diagnoses for medicinal marijuana vary from state to state. Patients can be arrested if they travel to another state with their medication or while under the influence of the medication. Airports fall under federal jurisdiction, so it is illegal to carry or to be found under the influence of medicinal marijuana. Experimental animal studies reveal that cannabinoids possess analgesic properties.[92] The mechanism is through activation of cannabinoid receptors, CB1 and CB2, in the CNS and peripheral nervous system. Activation of the CB1 receptor is responsible for the mood-altering effects of cannabis; however, it also has multiple nociceptive effects throughout the body when active. The CB2 receptor activation produces no cognitive alteration and plays a pivotal role in decreasing the CNS response to inflammation, mitigating the nociceptive response.[93]

Cannabinoids are available in multiple forms, including edibles, tablets, topicals, inhaled vapor, and inhaled smoke. The literature supports their use in neuropathic pain conditions.[94,95] Common side effects include dizziness, nausea, fatigue, intoxication-type feeling, vomiting, and diarrhea. Most studies to date are of low quality, with varied cannabinoid preparations and delivery routes. Further high-quality studies are needed to make strong recommendations for the use of cannabinoids in the treatment of neuropathic pain and to assess for long-term patient safety and addiction potential.

CONCLUSION

CRPS is a challenging neuropathic pain condition that is often refractory to traditional pain treatments. Multimodal treatment is strongly recommended in the population with CRPS. Multiple medication options exist, but few have strong supporting evidence. Corticosteroids are supported in the acute phase of the disease. Gabapentin has low-quality evidence and pregabalin has not been studied for CRPS, but are commonly prescribed because of their safety profile and tolerability. Bisphosphonates have supporting evidence during the acute phase of CRPS. Chronic opioid therapy should be used cautiously because of the risk of addiction and OIH. Second- and third-line agents can be considered after failure to initial treatment options. The prescribing physician should become familiar with the complexity and potential adverse events of these medications or refer to a specialist/CRPS treatment center.

REFERENCES

1. Geisslinger G, Muth-Selbach U, Coste O, et al. Inhibition of noxious stimulus-induced spinal prostaglandin E2 release by flurbiprofen enantiomers: a microdialysis study. *J Neurochem.* 2000;74(5):2094–2100.
2. Birklein F, Schmelz M. Neuropeptides, neurogenic inflammation and complex regional pain syndrome (CRPS). *Neurosci Lett.* 2008;437(3):199–202.
3. Huygen FJ, De Bruijn AG, De Bruin MT, Groeneweg JG, Klein J, Zijlstra FJ. Evidence for local inflammation in complex regional pain syndrome type 1. *Mediators Inflamm.* 2002;11(1):47–51.
4. Winston P. Early treatment of acute complex regional pain syndrome after fracture or injury with prednisone: why is there a failure to treat? A case series. *Pain Res Manag.* 2016;2016:7019196.
5. Atalay NS, Ercidogan O, Akkaya N, Sahin F. Prednisolone in complex regional pain syndrome. *Pain Physician.* 2014;17(2):179–185.
6. Christensen K, Jensen EM, Noer I. The reflex dystrophy syndrome response to treatment with systemic corticosteroids. *Acta Chir Scand.* 1982;148(8):653–655.
7. Fischer SG, Zuurmond WW, Birklein F, Loer SA, Perez RS. Anti-inflammatory treatment of complex regional pain syndrome. *Pain.* 2010;151(2):251–256.
8. Barbalinardo S, Loer SA, Goebel A, Perez RS. The treatment of longstanding complex regional pain syndrome with oral steroids. *Pain Med.* 2016;17(2):337–343.
9. Braus DF, Krauss JK, Strobel J. The shoulder-hand syndrome after stroke: a prospective clinical trial. *Ann Neurol.* 1994;36(5):728–733.
10. Kalita J, Misra U, Kumar A, Bhoi SK. Long-term prednisolone in post-stroke complex regional pain syndrome. *Pain Physician.* 2016;19(8):565–574.
11. Kalita J, Vajpayee A, Misra UK. Comparison of prednisolone with piroxicam in complex regional pain syndrome following stroke: a randomized controlled trial. *QJM.* 2006;99(2):89–95.
12. Lee SK, Yang DS, Lee JW, Choy WS. Four treatment strategies for complex regional pain syndrome type 1. *Orthopedics.* 2012;35(6):e834–e842.
13. Breuer AJ, Mainka T, Hansel N, Maier C, Krumova EK. Short-term treatment with parecoxib for complex regional pain syndrome: a randomized, placebo-controlled double-blind trial. *Pain Physician.* 2014;17(2):127–137.
14. Perez RS, Zuurmond WW, Bezemer PD, et al. The treatment of complex regional pain syndrome type I with free radical scavengers: a randomized controlled study. *Pain.* 2003;102(3):297–307.
15. Zuurmond WW, Langendijk PN, Bezemer PD, Brink HE, de Lange JJ, van loenen AC. Treatment of acute reflex sympathetic dystrophy with DMSO 50% in a fatty cream. *Acta Anaesthesiol Scand.* 1996;40(3):364–367.
16. Perez RS, Pragt E, Geurts J, Zuurmond WW, Patijn J, van Kleef M. Treatment of patients with complex regional pain syndrome type I with mannitol: a prospective, randomized, placebo-controlled, double-blinded study. *J Pain.* 2008;9(8):678–686.
17. Zyluk A, Puchalski P. Treatment of early complex regional pain syndrome type 1 by a combination of mannitol and dexamethasone. *J Hand Surg Eur Vol.* 2008;33(2):130–136.

18. Zollinger PE, Tuinebreijer WE, Breederveld RS, Kreis RW. Can vitamin C prevent complex regional pain syndrome in patients with wrist fractures? A randomized, controlled, multicenter dose-response study. *J Bone Joint Surg Am.* 2007; 89(7):1424–1431.

19. Zollinger PE, Tuinebreijer WE, Kreis RW, Breederveld RS. Effect of vitamin C on frequency of reflex sympathetic dystrophy in wrist fractures: a randomised trial. *Lancet.* 1999;354(9195):2025–2028.

20. Fink K, Dooley DJ, Meder WP, et al. Inhibition of neuronal Ca(2+) influx by gabapentin and pregabalin in the human neocortex. *Neuropharmacology.* 2002;42(2):229–236.

21. Backonja M, Glanzman RL. Gabapentin dosing for neuropathic pain: evidence from randomized, placebo-controlled clinical trials. *Clin Ther.* 2003;25(1):81–104.

22. Rowbotham M, Harden N, Stacey B, Bernstein P, Magnus-Miller L. Gabapentin for the treatment of postherpetic neuralgia: a randomized controlled trial. *JAMA.* 1998;280(21): 1837–1842.

23. Serpell MG. Gabapentin in neuropathic pain syndromes: a randomised, double-blind, placebo-controlled trial. *Pain.* 2002;99(3):557–566.

24. van de Vusse AC, Stomp-van den Berg SG, Kessels AH, Weber WE. Randomised controlled trial of gabapentin in complex regional pain syndrome type 1 [ISRCTN84121379]. *BMC Neurol.* 2004;4:13.

25. Dworkin RH, Corbin AE, Young Jr JP, et al. Pregabalin for the treatment of postherpetic neuralgia: a randomized, placebo-controlled trial. *Neurology.* 2003;60(8):1274–1283.

26. Rosenstock J, Tuchman M, LaMoreaux L, Sharma U. Pregabalin for the treatment of painful diabetic peripheral neuropathy: a double-blind, placebo-controlled trial. *Pain.* 2004;110(3):628–638.

27. Saltik S, Sozen HG, Basgul S, Karatoprak EY, Icagasioglu A. Pregabalin treatment of a patient with complex regional pain syndrome. *Pediatr Neurol.* 2016;54:88–90.

28. Rull JA, Quibrera R, Gonzalez-Millan H, Lozano Castaneda O. Symptomatic treatment of peripheral diabetic neuropathy with carbamazepine (tegretol): double blind crossover trial. *Diabetologia.* 1969;5(4):215–218.

29. Harke H, Gretenkort P, Ladleif HU, Rahman S, Harke O. The response of neuropathic pain and pain in complex regional pain syndrome I to carbamazepine and sustained-release morphine in patients pretreated with spinal cord stimulation: a double-blinded randomized study. *Anesth Analg.* 2001;92(2):488–495.

30. Dogra S, Beydoun S, Mazzola J, Hopwood M, Wan Y. Oxcarbazepine in painful diabetic neuropathy: a randomized, placebo-controlled study. *Eur J Pain.* 2005;9(5): 543–554.

31. Shank RP, Gardocki JF, Streeter AJ, Maryanoff BE. An overview of the preclinical aspects of topiramate: pharmacology, pharmacokinetics, and mechanism of action. *Epilepsia.* 2000;41(suppl 1):S3–S9.

32. Raskin P, Donofrio PD, Rosenthal NR, et al. Topiramate vs placebo in painful diabetic neuropathy: analgesic and metabolic effects. *Neurology.* 2004;63(5):865–873.

33. Sindrup SH, Jensen TS. Pharmacologic treatment of pain in polyneuropathy. *Neurology.* 2000;55(7):915–920.

34. Sudoh Y, Cahoon EE, Gerner P, Wang GK. Tricyclic antidepressants as long-acting local anesthetics. *Pain.* 2003;103 (1–2):49–55.

35. Sindrup SH, Bach FW, Madsen C, Gram LF, Jensen TS. Venlafaxine versus imipramine in painful polyneuropathy: a randomized, controlled trial. *Neurology.* 2003;60(8): 1284–1289.

36. Raskin J, Pritchett YL, Wang F, et al. A double-blind, randomized multicenter trial comparing duloxetine with placebo in the management of diabetic peripheral neuropathic pain. *Pain Med.* 2005;6(5):346–356.

37. Max MB, Lynch SA, Muir J, Shoaf SE, Smoller B, Dubner R. Effects of desipramine, amitriptyline, and fluoxetine on pain in diabetic neuropathy. *N Engl J Med.* 1992;326(19): 1250–1256.

38. Varenna M. Bisphosphonates beyond their anti-osteoclastic properties. *Rheumatol Oxf.* 2014;53(6):965–967.

39. Varenna M, Adami S, Sinigaglia L. Bisphosphonates in complex regional pain syndrome type I: how do they work? *Clin Exp Rheumatol.* 2014;32(4):451–454.

40. Adami S, Fossaluzza V, Gatti D, Fracassi E, Braga V. Bisphosphonate therapy of reflex sympathetic dystrophy syndrome. *Ann Rheum Dis.* 1997;56(3):201–204.

41. Manicourt DH, Brasseur JP, Boutsen Y, Depreseux G, Devogelaer JP. Role of alendronate in therapy for post-traumatic complex regional pain syndrome type I of the lower extremity. *Arthritis Rheum.* 2004;50(11):3690–3697.

42. Robinson JN, Sandom J, Chapman PT. Efficacy of pamidronate in complex regional pain syndrome type I. *Pain Med.* 2004;5(3):276–280.

43. Varenna M, Adami S, Rossini M, et al. Treatment of complex regional pain syndrome type I with neridronate: a randomized, double-blind, placebo-controlled study. *Rheumatol Oxf.* 2013;52(3):534–542.

44. Varenna M, Zucchi F, Ghiringhelli D, et al. Intravenous clodronate in the treatment of reflex sympathetic dystrophy syndrome. A randomized, double blind, placebo controlled study. *J Rheumatol.* 2000;27(6):1477–1483.

45. Giusti A, Bianchi G. Treatment of complex regional pain syndrome type I with bisphosphonates. *RMD Open.* 2015;1 (suppl 1):e000056.

46. O'Connell NE, Wand BM, McAuley J, Marston L, Moseley GL. Interventions for treating pain and disability in adults with complex regional pain syndrome. *Cochrane Database Syst Rev.* 2013;(4):CD009416.

47. Gobelet C, Waldburger M, Meier JL. The effect of adding calcitonin to physical treatment on reflex sympathetic dystrophy. *Pain.* 1992;48(2):171–175.

48. Perez RS, Kwakkel G, Zuurmond WW, de Lange JJ. Treatment of reflex sympathetic dystrophy (CRPS type 1): a research synthesis of 21 randomized clinical trials. *J Pain Symptom Manage.* 2001;21(6):511–526.

49. Tran DQH, Duong S, Bertini P, Finlayson RJ. Treatment of complex regional pain syndrome: a review of the evidence. *Can J Anesth.* 2010;57(2):149–166.

50. Benzon HT, Liu SS, Buvanendran A. Evolving definitions and pharmacologic management of complex regional pain syndrome. *Anesth Analg.* 2016;122(3):601–604.
51. Dellemijn P. Are opioids effective in relieving neuropathic pain? *Pain.* 1999;80(3):453–462.
52. Dellemijn PL, van Duijn H, Vanneste JA. Prolonged treatment with transdermal fentanyl in neuropathic pain. *J Pain Symptom Manage.* 1998;16(4):220–229.
53. Watson CP, Babul N. Efficacy of oxycodone in neuropathic pain: a randomized trial in postherpetic neuralgia. *Neurology.* 1998;50(6):1837–1841.
54. Jones T, Lookatch S, Grant P, McIntyre J, Moore T. Further validation of an opioid risk assessment tool: the brief risk interview. *J Opioid Manag.* 2014;10(5):353–364.
55. Webster LR, Webster RM. Predicting aberrant behaviors in opioid-treated patients: preliminary validation of the opioid risk tool. *Pain Med.* 2005;6(6):432–442.
56. Yi P, Pryzbylkowski P. Opioid induced hyperalgesia. *Pain Med.* 2015;16(suppl 1):S32–S36.
57. Chu LF, Clark DJ, Angst MS. Opioid tolerance and hyperalgesia in chronic pain patients after one month of oral morphine therapy: a preliminary prospective study. *J Pain.* 2006;7(1):43–48.
58. Substance-Related and Addictive Disorders. Diagnostic and Statistical Manual of Mental Disorders, 5th Edition. 2013.
59. Daniell HW. Hypogonadism in men consuming sustained-action oral opioids. *J Pain.* 2002;3(5):377–384.
60. Goncalves L, Friend LV, Dickenson AH. The influence of mu-opioid and noradrenaline reuptake inhibition in the modulation of pain responsive neurones in the central amygdala by tapentadol in rats with neuropathy. *Eur J Pharmacol.* 2015;749:151–160.
61. Hollingshead J, Duhmke RM, Cornblath DR. Tramadol for neuropathic pain. *Cochrane Database Syst Rev.* 2006;(3):Cd003726.
62. Norrbrink C, Lundeberg T. Tramadol in neuropathic pain after spinal cord injury: a randomized, double-blind, placebo-controlled trial. *Clin J Pain.* 2009;25(3):177–184.
63. Vadivelu N, Kai A, Maslin B, Kodumudi G, Legler A, Berger JM. Tapentadol extended release in the management of peripheral diabetic neuropathic pain. *Ther Clin Risk Manag.* 2015;11:95–105.
64. Haroutiunian S, McNicol ED, Lipman AG. Methadone for chronic non-cancer pain in adults. *Cochrane Database Syst Rev.* 2012;11:Cd008025.
65. Gagnon B, Almahrezi A, Schreier G. Methadone in the treatment of neuropathic pain. *Pain Res Manag.* 2003;8(3):149–154.
66. Teixeira MJ, Okada M, Moscoso AS, et al. Methadone in post-herpetic neuralgia: a pilot proof-of-concept study. *Clinics (Sao Paulo, Brazil).* 2013;68(7):1057–1060.
67. Kristensen JD, Karlsten R, Gordh T, Berge OG. The NMDA antagonist 3-(2-carboxypiperazin-4-yl)propyl-1-phosphonic acid (CPP) has antinociceptive effect after intrathecal injection in the rat. *Pain.* 1994;56(1):59–67.
68. Tal M, Bennett GJ. Dextrorphan relieves neuropathic heat-evoked hyperalgesia in the rat. *Neurosci Lett.* 1993;151(1):107–110.
69. Nelson KA, Park KM, Robinovitz E, Tsigos C, Max MB. High-dose oral dextromethorphan versus placebo in painful diabetic neuropathy and postherpetic neuralgia. *Neurology.* 1997;48(5):1212–1218.
70. Sang CN, Booher S, Gilron I, Parada S, Max MB. Dextromethorphan and memantine in painful diabetic neuropathy and postherpetic neuralgia: efficacy and dose-response trials. *Anesthesiology.* 2002;96(5):1053–1061.
71. Martin E, Morel V, Joly D, et al. Rationale and design of a randomized double-blind clinical trial in breast cancer: dextromethorphan in chemotherapy-induced peripheral neuropathy. *Contemp Clin Trials.* 2015;41:146–151.
72. Eisenberg E, Kleiser A, Dortort A, Haim T, Yarnitsky D. The NMDA (N-methyl-D-aspartate) receptor antagonist memantine in the treatment of postherpetic neuralgia: a double-blind, placebo-controlled study. *Eur J Pain.* 1998;2(4):321–327.
73. Sinis N, Birbaumer N, Gustin S, et al. Memantine treatment of complex regional pain syndrome: a preliminary report of six cases. *Clin J Pain.* 2007;23(3):237–243.
74. Kleinbohl D, Gortelmeyer R, Bender HJ, Holzl R. Amantadine sulfate reduces experimental sensitization and pain in chronic back pain patients. *Anesth Analg.* 2006;102(3):840–847.
75. Prough DS, McLeskey CH, Poehling GG, et al. Efficacy of oral nifedipine in the treatment of reflex sympathetic dystrophy. *Anesthesiology.* 1985;62(6):796–799.
76. Muizelaar JP, Kleyer M, Hertogs IA, DeLange DC. Complex regional pain syndrome (reflex sympathetic dystrophy and causalgia): management with the calcium channel blocker nifedipine and/or the alpha-sympathetic blocker phenoxybenzamine in 59 patients. *Clin Neurol Neurosurg.* 1997;99(1):26–30.
77. Kingery WS. A critical review of controlled clinical trials for peripheral neuropathic pain and complex regional pain syndromes. *Pain.* 1997;73(2):123–139.
78. Davies PS, Galer BS. Review of lidocaine patch 5% studies in the treatment of postherpetic neuralgia. *Drugs.* 2004;64(9):937–947.
79. Devers A, Galer BS. Topical lidocaine patch relieves a variety of neuropathic pain conditions: an open-label study. *Clin J Pain.* 2000;16(3):205–208.
80. Anand P, Bley K. Topical capsaicin for pain management: therapeutic potential and mechanisms of action of the new high-concentration capsaicin 8% patch. *Br J Anaesth.* 2011;107(4):490–502.
81. Simpson DM, Robinson-Papp J, Van J, et al. Capsaicin 8% patch in painful diabetic peripheral neuropathy: a randomized, double-blind, placebo-controlled study. *J Pain.* 2017;18(1):42–53.
82. Robbins WR, Staats PS, Levine J, et al. Treatment of intractable pain with topical large-dose capsaicin: preliminary report. *Anesth Analg.* 1998;86(3):579–583.

83. Gammaitoni A, Gallagher RM, Welz-Bosna M. Topical ketamine gel: possible role in treating neuropathic pain. *Pain Med.* 2000;1(1):97–100.

84. Russo MA, Santarelli DM. A novel compound analgesic cream (ketamine, pentoxifylline, clonidine, DMSO) for complex regional pain syndrome patients. *Pain Pract.* 2016;16(1):E14–E20.

85. Rajkumar SV, Fonseca R, Witzig TE. Complete resolution of reflex sympathetic dystrophy with thalidomide treatment. *Arch Intern Med.* 2001;161(20):2502–2503.

86. Ching DW, McClintock A, Beswick F. Successful treatment with low-dose thalidomide in a patient with both Behcet's disease and complex regional pain syndrome type I: case report. *J Clin Rheumatol.* 2003;9(2):96–98.

87. Schwartzman RJ, Chevlen E, Bengtson K. Thalidomide has activity in treating complex regional pain syndrome. *Arch Intern Med.* 2003;163(12):1487–1488. author reply 1488.

88. Manning DC, Alexander G, Arezzo JC, et al. Lenalidomide for complex regional pain syndrome type 1: lack of efficacy in a phase II randomized study. *J Pain.* 2014;15(12):1366–1376.

89. Huygen FJ, Niehof S, Zijlstra FJ, van Hagen PM, van Daele PL. Successful treatment of CRPS 1 with anti-TNF. *J Pain Symptom Manage.* 2004;27(2):101–103.

90. Dirckx M, Groeneweg G, Wesseldijk F, Stronks DL, Huygen FJ. Report of a preliminary discontinued double-blind, randomized, placebo-controlled trial of the anti-TNF-alpha chimeric monoclonal antibody infliximab in complex regional pain syndrome. *Pain Pract.* 2013;13(8):633–640.

91. Eisenberg E, Sandler I, Treister R, Suzan E, Haddad M. Anti tumor necrosis factor – alpha adalimumab for complex regional pain syndrome type 1 (CRPS-I): a case series. *Pain Pract.* 2013;13(8):649–656.

92. Rahn EJ, Hohmann AG. Cannabinoids as pharmacotherapies for neuropathic pain: from the bench to the bedside. *Neurotherapeutics.* 2009;6(4):713–737.

93. Fine PG, Rosenfeld MJ. Cannabinoids for neuropathic pain. *Curr Pain Headache Rep.* 2014;18(10):451.

94. Boychuk DG, Goddard G, Mauro G, Orellana MF. The effectiveness of cannabinoids in the management of chronic nonmalignant neuropathic pain: a systematic review. *J Oral Facial Pain Headache.* 2015;29(1):7–14.

95. Nurmikko TJ, Serpell MG, Hoggart B, Toomey PJ, Morlion BJ, Haines D. Sativex successfully treats neuropathic pain characterised by allodynia: a randomised, double-blind, placebo-controlled clinical trial. *Pain.* 2007;133(1–3):210–220.

CHAPTER 9

Complex Regional Pain Syndrome: Interventional Treatment

DAVID STOLZENBERG, DO • HENRY CHOU, DO • DAVID JANERICH, DO

Interventional pain management procedures for complex regional pain syndrome (CRPS) are often considered when conservative treatment options such as physical therapy (PT), occupational therapy (OT), and/or medications fail to provide adequate pain relief. The literature supports the concurrent use of certain procedures along with medications, modalities, and psychologic treatment to help maximize pain relief and functional restoration.[1,2]

SYMPATHETIC NERVE BLOCKS

The sympathetic nervous system has been implicated in the pathophysiology of CRPS in certain presentations of the syndrome. Thus it may be a useful target for injection therapy.[3,4] Sympathetic nerve blocks (SNBs) have been used for both diagnostic and therapeutic purposes for many years.[5] Historically, some clinicians diagnosed CRPS only if SNB relieved pain.[6] However, it was found that for some patients, there is a lack of response to SNB, which led to the concept of CRPS variants that are not sympathetically mediated (sympathetically independent pain, SIP) and rethinking of the mechanism behind the disorder.[2,6] Overall, there is a lack of universally accepted guidelines in selecting patients for SNB and a lack of high-quality studies to provide significant evidence to support or refute the use of SNB for CRPS.[7] Based on the available literature, along with clinical experiences of many experts, it is believed that patients with CRPS with signs of mechanical allodynia and temperature and color changes of the affected limb are more likely to have a positive response from SNB. In general, the procedure is often recommended for those patients who have pain that limits participation in PT or OT despite adequate oral medications.[4,6]

The primary targets for SNB involve the stellate ganglion (SGB) for upper extremity CRPS and the lumbar sympathetic chain (LSB) for lower extremity CRPS. The stellate ganglion is composed of the inferior cervical ganglion and the first thoracic ganglion. It is typically located anteriorly to the first rib. SGB was traditionally performed "blindly" via palpation of anatomic landmarks, but now it is done via guidance with fluoroscopy, ultrasonography, or computerized tomography. The typical target of the needle is the junction of the vertebral body and uncinate process of C6 (Chassaignac tubercle). An example of the procedure being performed under fluoroscopic guidance is shown in Figs. 9.1–9.4. Both the C6 and C7 vertebrae have been used as targets for injection, but injection at the C6 level has become a more common practice to lessen potential complications such as pneumothorax and vertebral artery puncture.[8] For LSB, the lumbar sympathetic chain ganglia are located along the anterolateral aspect of the first through fourth lumbar vertebral bodies. The target of injection is usually at the inferior portion of the L2 or superior

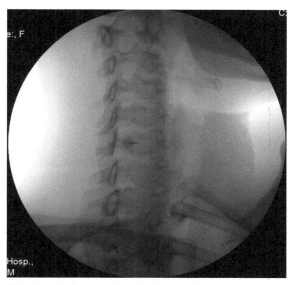

FIG. 9.1 Stellate ganglion block under fluoroscopic guidance—Part 1. (Copyright David Stolzenberg, DO.)

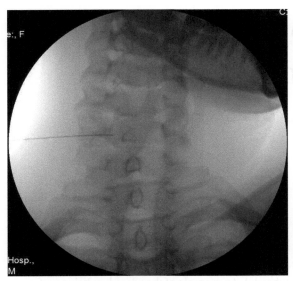

FIG. 9.2 Stellate ganglion block under fluoroscopic guidance—Part 2. (Copyright David Stolzenberg, DO.)

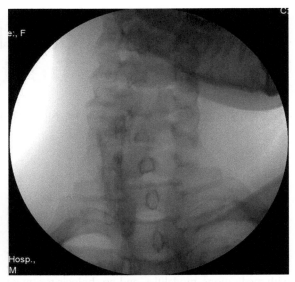

FIG. 9.4 Stellate ganglion block under fluoroscopic guidance—Part 4. (Copyright David Stolzenberg, DO.)

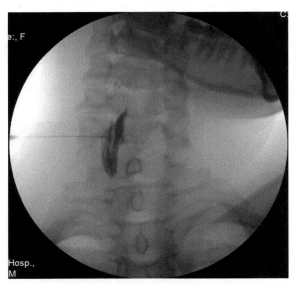

FIG. 9.3 Stellate ganglion block under fluoroscopic guidance—Part 3. (Copyright David Stolzenberg, DO.)

portion of the L3 vertebral body (Figs. 9.5 and 9.6).[8] An example of the procedure being performed under fluoroscopic guidance is shown in figures 9.5 and 9.6. After the needle reaches the target site, a small volume of contrast dye is injected to confirm localized spread and rule out vascular uptake. Then 5–10 mL of local anesthetic is injected, usually lidocaine or bupivacaine, with or without corticosteroid.

Success of the SGB is defined by Malmqvist et al. as: (1) Horner' syndrome, which consists of ptosis (drooping of upper eyelid), anhidrosis (decreased sweating on the affected side of the face), and miosis (constricted pupil); (2) Gutman sign, which is increased skin and upper limb temperature >34 °C (or by 1–3 degrees compared with before the procedure) within 5 min of the block; (3) increased blood flow by more than 50% by laser Doppler flowmetry; (4) abolition of radial and ulnar skin resistance response; (5) increase in the skin resistance level by 13% or more.[4,9,10] However, even in the study by Malmqvist, complete sympathetic blockade of the stellate ganglion meeting all five criteria was met only in 6 of the 54 blocks and only 15 of 54 cases met four of the criteria.[9] This indicates that there is a high rate of incomplete or partial sympathetic blockade in SGB. Another study by Schurmann et al. demonstrated there is difficulty in correlating increased limb temperature, Horner syndrome, and complete sympathetic blockade. In addition, even in patients with complete sympathetic block, the amount of pain relief following the SGB was just slightly more than 50%, further supporting the concept of nonsympathetically mediated CRPS, or SIP.[4] Temperature testing is perhaps the most widely used measurement of sympathetic blockade.[10] Subjective successful responses to a block include

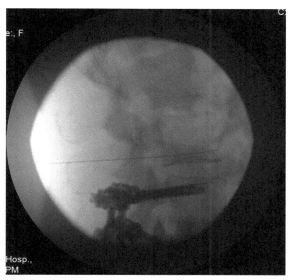

FIG. 9.5 Lumbar sympathetic block under fluoroscopic guidance—Part 1. (Copyright David Stolzenberg, DO.)

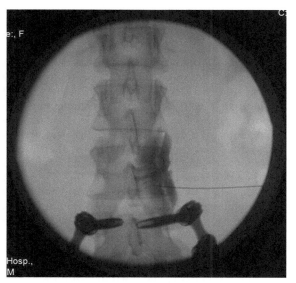

FIG. 9.6 Lumbar sympathetic block under fluoroscopic guidance—Part 2. (Copyright David Stolzenberg, DO.)

patient's report of decreased pain and/or allodynia of the affected limb.

The pain relief from an SNB often lasts longer than the duration of effect of the local anesthetics, and in some cases, it may provide long-lasting relief, although the response duration and efficacy is variable.[4,11,12] Based on the currently available treatment guidelines, patients should immediately begin aggressive PT and OT. The treatments focus on desensitization, normalizing sensation, restoration of range of motion (ROM), and promoting functional use of the affected limb. A successful response would be expected in patients with sympathetically maintained pain (SMP) as compared with those with SIP.[13] Many researchers have studied the effectiveness of the SGB and LSB in CRPS. However, the majority of these are low-quality studies and lack significant numbers of subjects. Price et al. conducted a double-blind crossover study evaluating the use of anesthetic versus saline in SGB and LSB. Analgesia was achieved within 30 min of using both anesthetic and saline, but the anesthetic group with a mixture of lidocaine and bupivacaine resulted in average of 3 days 18 h of analgesia versus 19 h for the saline group.[11] Cepeda and colleagues conducted a systematic review evaluating SNB with local anesthetics. Among the 30 studies that were evaluated, only a few were prospective, randomized, and placebo controlled. In total, over a 1000 patients were included. Overall, 29% of patients had a full response, 41% had partial response, and 32% had no response to SNB. Another review evaluated the results of two additional small randomized, double-blinded, crossover studies. The combined effect of the two trials (23 subjects) produced a relative risk to achieve at least 50% of pain relief for 30 min to 2 h after the sympathetic blockade of 1.17 (95% confidence interval 0.80–1.72).[14] However, the effect of sympathetic blockade on long-term pain relief was inconclusive.[14] A randomized trial of SGB with 0.5% bupivacaine versus guanethidine intravenous (IV) regional block (which in itself lacks strong evidence of efficacy as discussed later) found significant improvement in both groups and no significant difference between SGB and guanethidine IV regional block.[15]

SNBs may be repeated if there is short-term benefit in those patients who had a clear reduction of pain, improved ROM, and increase tolerance to PT and/or OT.[1,2,6] However, there is lack of evidence to support routine extended series of SNB.

The addition of botulinum toxin to LSB has been studied as a potential option to prolong the analgesic duration of the LSB.[16,17] Carroll et al. conducted a small prospective, randomized, double-blind, controlled crossover study of nine patients with refractory CRPS type I. The botulinum toxin enhanced the analgesic effect of LSB. Each patient received two injections, the first with 10 mL of 0.5% bupivacaine and the second with 10 mL of 0.5% bupivacaine plus 75 units of botulinum toxin A. The median time to analgesic failure in patients who received bupivacaine plus botulinum toxin was 71 days compared with less than 10 days when patients received bupivacaine alone.[16] Choi et al. reported similar findings in a case study consisting of two male patients with CRPS after ankle injuries. Pain relief lasted for 2 months after injection of 5 mL of 0.25% bupivacaine plus 5000 IU of botulinum toxin type B compared with only 5 h after injection with bupivacaine alone. Furthermore, there was no further need for opioid pain medications after LSB using botulinum toxin.[17] Despite these promising findings, additional studies with larger sample sizes are required.

Potential complications of SGB and LSB include needle injury to the nearby visceral organs and neurovascular structures. The SGB can cause pneumothorax, hemothorax, and injury to the brachial plexus, trachea, or esophagus. The local anesthetics can cause laryngeal nerve block, resulting in hoarseness of voice, or phrenic nerve block, which can lead to diaphragmatic paralysis with respiratory depression, and hence bilateral SGB is contraindicated.[10] SNB can cause vasodilation of the extremities, which may lead to orthostatic hypotension; thus blood pressure needs to be monitored. Genitofemoral neuritis is a possible complication specific to LSB.[13] As with any injection, infection can occur.

CHEMICAL AND SURGICAL SYMPATHECTOMY

For longer term relief, chemical or surgical sympathectomy has been performed for SMP from CRPS in those patients who receive transient relief from SGB or LSB. Chemical sympathectomy involves using alcohol or phenol injection to denature the proteins of the sympathetic chain ganglion. Outcomes for chemical sympathectomy are variable with uncertain efficacy.[1] Surgical treatment can be performed by open removal or electrocoagulation of the sympathetic chain ganglion or by minimally invasive techniques using stereotactic thermal or laser ablation. The effect of analgesia may last for up to 1 year with radiofrequency ablation. Nerve regeneration is common following both surgical and chemical ablation, and recurrence of symptoms and development of postsympathectomy neuralgia is common. Manjunath et al. randomized 20 patients with lower limb CRPS to either radiofrequency or phenol lumbar sympathectomy and found a statistically significant reduction from baseline in all pain scores for both treatment groups at 4 months' follow-up. Complications of sympathectomy include postsympathectomy neuralgia in up to 50% of patients, as well as hyperhidrosis and persistent Horner syndrome (for SGB).[18] Owing to the poor evidence for long-term

effectiveness coupled with the risk of complications, sympathectomy should be used with great caution and reserved only for patients who have failed other treatments options but responded to SNB.

INTRAVENOUS REGIONAL ANESTHESIA

Intravenous regional anesthesia (IVRA) involves peripheral injection of medication, including sympatholytics, anesthetics, or nonsteroidal antiinflammatory drugs into the affected extremity. IVRA has been used for many years to empirically treat CRPS with a wide variety of substances, including guanethidine, lidocaine, bretylium, clonidine, droperidol, ketanserin, or reserpine.[4] IVRA with guanethidine to treat CRPS was first described by Hannington-Kiff, and the procedure consists of intravenous injection of guanethidine, followed by elevation of the injected arm and then inflation of a tourniquet above the patient's systolic pressure. The tourniquet is then maintained for 15–30 min while the medication bathes the area, then the tourniquet is slowing released. The theory is that this causes displacement of noradrenaline from presynaptic vesicles and prevents the reuptake causing increased blood flow.[13,19] Numerous IVRA trials using guanethidine have been conducted and have been proved to be largely ineffective. Perez et al. conducted a meta-analysis of nine IVRA studies, and six of those included guanethidine.[20] The analysis showed a lack of proven effect of IVRA overall and guanethidine in particular. Other studies have also reported generally negative outcomes. Ramamurthy et al. conducted a double-blind, multicenter randomized control trial comparing IVRA with guanethidine with control of lidocaine in 60 patients with CRPS and found no difference in long-term outcomes.[21] Another study compared low-dose guanethidine with saline and did not find significant differences between the groups. The study had to be terminated because of complications from high-dose guanethidine.[22]

Many other IVRA trials have been done using atropine, guanethidine, lidocaine, bretylium, clonidine, droperidol, ketanserin, and reserpine. Of these agents, only bretylium and ketanserin IVRA have shown some modest efficacy.[22] One retrospective study that evaluated IVRA using lidocaine and ketorolac showed ketorolac had pain-relieving effects.[23] However, a randomized, double-blind crossover study found that lidocaine with ketorolac reduced pain significantly for only 1 day. All other outcome measures found no difference between treatment with lidocaine alone and lidocaine with ketorolac.[24] In summary, based on the available literature, the efficacy of IVRA in treating CRPS is poor.

INTRAVENOUS INFUSION

Various agents have been used for intravenous infusion attempting to treat CRPS. Ketamine has been the most widely utilized and studied. Ketamine, an N-methyl-D-aspartate (NMDA) receptor antagonist, has been used in the treatment of acute and chronic pain, targeting the central sensitization of pain.[25,26] Central sensitization is a phenomenon whereby persistent activation of the nociceptor results in an increased excitatory transmission along the afferent fibers. Over time the continuous and repetitive activation results in modulation of the dorsal root ganglion (DRG) and dorsal horn wide dynamic range (WDR) neurons, which accentuate the responsiveness of the nociceptive pathways. NMDA receptor activation plays a significant role in the accentuated response to repeated noxious stimulation.[25,27]

In a randomized controlled trial by Sigtermans, patients receiving 100 h continuous IV infusion of subanesthetic ketamine had a significantly lower pain score for the first 11 weeks of the study compared with those receiving placebo. However, by week 12 of the study, there was no significant improvement in pain relief. Also, there was no significant improvement in function.[28] Schwartzmann conducted a double-blind placebo-controlled study of 19 patients with CRPS and found that IV infusion of normal saline with ketamine for 4 h daily for 10 days resulted in a significant reduction in weekly pain measures for the duration of the study (12 weeks) and nonsignificant improvements in quantitative sensory testing.[29] Kiefer et al. conducted a nonrandomized, open label, Phase II trial of continuous IV infusion of ketamine at an anesthetic dose for 5 days in 20 patients with refractory CRPS. All patients were sedated during the treatment period. The study showed a significant pain reduction in the Numeric Rating Scale from baseline in all patients at 1 week and at 6 months (8.0 vs. 2, $P < .001$) post infusion. They also found complete remission from CRPS in all patients at 1 month, in 17 of 20 patients at 3 months, and in 16 of 20 patients at 6 months. The study demonstrated efficacy using an anesthetic dose of ketamine, but investigators highlighted safety as a main concern.[30]

Adverse effects of ketamine have been found to include possible liver toxicity, psychotropic side effects, nightmares, insomnia, and hallucinogenic and other psychomimetric effects. Although ketamine is generally safe, there is only low- to moderate-quality evidence showing the efficacy of IV ketamine infusion in treating CRPS.[7,25,26]

SPINAL CORD STIMULATION
Mechanism of Action

Spinal cord stimulation (SCS) is a reversible and nondestructive method of controlling chronic, severe, and intractable pain. SCS involves delivering an electrical field directly over the dorsal columns of the spinal cord to modulate pain generation and processing. It is approved by the US Food and Drug Administration for failed back surgery syndrome (FBSS) and CRPS when there has been a failure or inadequate response to more conservative medical management.

The development of the Gate Control Theory of pain by Wall and Melzack in 1965 led to the first case report of SCS in a human for chronic intractable pain.[31] In 1967 Shealy performed a thoracic laminectomy and sutured an electrode to the dura of a patient with intractable chest and abdominal wall pain from inoperable metastatic lung cancer. The patient had significant pain relief and was quickly off opioid medications. Unfortunately, the patient died shortly thereafter from medical issues unrelated to the procedure.[32] The technology and understanding of its mechanism of action has evolved over time.

The current understanding of the mechanism of pain relief of SCS has been found to be complex and incompletely understood. The Gate Control Theory still serves as a core mechanism of action, but the details are controversial and there are other factors and distinct mechanisms of action. Wall and Melzack theorized that cells of the substantia gelatinosa in the dorsal horn of the spinal cord act as a gate control system, modulating transmission of nerve impulses from the peripheral to central nervous system via inhibitory interneurons. Stimulation of large myelinated afferent αβ fibers effectively "closes the gate" to pain-transmitting small unmyelinated C fibers and small myelinated αδ fibers.[31]

Modulation of neural activity with SCS has been found to occur at several levels of the nervous system, including ascending and descending pathways via peripheral nerves, suppression of dorsal horn WDR neuronal hyperexcitability, supraspinal inhibition, and the sympathetic nervous system.[33,34] In addition, alterations of local neurochemistry have been identified. Cerebrospinal fluid analysis in the area of SCS in animal models has demonstrated an increased release of the inhibitory neurotransmitter γ-aminobutyric acid (GABA). Furthermore, pain relief from SCS can be blocked with a GABA antagonist. Increased glycine, serotonin, and adenosine have also been found, as well as decreased excitatory neurotransmitters of glutamate and aspartate.[33,35] Contributions from endogenous opioid release have not been found to exist, and the pain relief of SCS is not reversed or blocked by naloxone.[36]

Procedure Technique

Placement in the epidural space over the dorsal columns is typically performed in a two-stage process. Initially, a temporary trial is undertaken, whereby a cylindrical lead with multiple electrodes at its tip is placed percutaneously via an introducer needle under fluoroscopic guidance. The target spinal level of placement is guided by the sensory mapping work of Barolat, where the goal is to overlap pleasant paresthesia sensations in the area of the patients' pain.[37] Sedation is diminished so that patients can clearly confirm that paresthesia coverage is present over their appropriate individual painful sites. Intraoperative adjustments of electrode location can be made via repositioning the lead(s). Once the location is optimal, the needle is removed and the electrode is secured to the skin and left in place for the 3- to 7-day trial period (see Figs. 9.7–9.9). An example of the procedure being performed under fluoroscopic guidance is shown in figures 9.7–9.9. The external portion is connected to a controller that allows programming with variations in frequency, pulse width, and amplitude to optimize pain control.

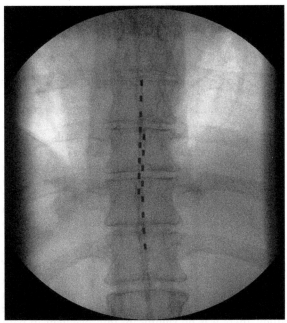

FIG. 9.8 Spinal cord stimulator trial—Part 2. (Copyright David Stolzenberg, DO.)

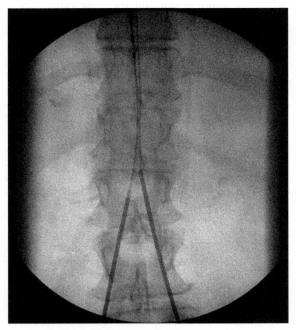

FIG. 9.7 Spinal cord stimulator trial—Part 1. (Copyright David Stolzenberg, DO.)

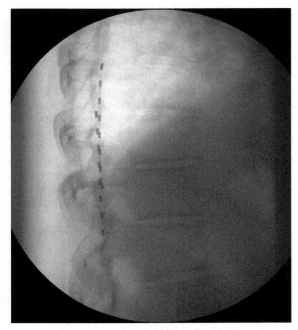

FIG. 9.9 Spinal cord stimulator trial—Part 3. (Copyright David Stolzenberg, DO.)

Anatomic impediments to safe percutaneous cylindrical trial lead placement, typically spinal stenosis or prior posterior spine surgery at the levels where the lead would enter or traverse, necessitate a more invasive surgical trial. This is performed in a similar fashion to a permanent surgical implant via a small laminotomy. A successful trial should have a minimum of 50% pain relief, which has been associated with a higher probability of long-term success. Less than 50% success is highly associated with long-term treatment failure.[38] There should be functional improvements and a decrease in pain medications. After a successful trial, a permanent implant can be performed and the generator is internalized with a surgical pocket in a similar fashion to a pacemaker. The permanent system can utilize similar cylindrical leads used in the trial or a flat paddle lead via laminotomy. The main advantages to surgical paddle leads are the capability of broader stimulation patterns and lower stimulation requirements, which may prolong battery life. Classically they were felt to be more stable with less lead migration and positional effects on stimulation, but that is now controversial because of newer anchoring systems and techniques with percutaneous leads.[39]

Efficacy of SCS in CRPS

Many studies have shown a strong efficacy for SCS in CRPS with regards to reducing pain and improving limb function and quality of life (QOL); however, only a few are of robust methodologic quality. Kemlers' study in the *New England Journal of Medicine* was a prospective randomized controlled trial that evaluated 54 patients with chronic severe pain and functional impairment from CRPS who had failed extensive conservative care. The initial study had a 1-year follow-up, and a subsequent study continued to follow up patients for 5 years.[40,41] Patients were randomized into SCS plus PT (n = 36) or PT alone (n = 18). The PT regimen was standardized and performed for 6 months in both groups. In 24 of 36 patients who underwent SCS trial, greater than 50% relief was obtained, and these patients went on to implantation. Pain and health-related QOL measures improved significantly more in the SCS plus PT group than in the PT alone group at 1 year, although there was no change in function. Of those who underwent implantation, 20 of 24 had 50% pain relief, and a visual analog scale (VAS) decrease of 2.7 at 1 year, whereas pain was slightly increased with PT alone.[40]

Five-year follow-up data revealed similar results, although there was some diminished effectiveness of SCS over time. The difference between groups on intent-to-treat analysis was no longer statistically significant. Nonetheless, those with SCS had a 2.5 VAS improvement versus 1.0 with PT alone, 11 of 20 patients who underwent implantation maintained greater than 50% pain relief, and 95% of patients with SCS would have repeated the treatment for the same results at 5 years.[41]

Another study with a long-term follow-up on 25 patients, averaging 88 months, demonstrated a slight regression of outcome with SCS over time, but the statistical significance remained for improvements in pain on VAS, disability via Oswestry Disability Index (ODI), mood via Beck Depression Inventory (BDI), and other QOL parameters.[42]

Geurts published a large prospective cohort study in 2013 with follow-up data of up to 12 years, with a mean of 5.2 years, on 84 consecutive patients with CRPS after a positive SCS trial. Treatment success was defined as a 30% reduction in pain relief. About 63% of patients who underwent implantation still met this criterion at long-term follow-up. About 59% of patients rated pain as "much" or "very much" improved.[38] In another prospective study, 29 patients with CRPS type I and SMP, proven by response to SNB and negative placebo block, were followed up for 3 years after SCS implantation. Stimulation was periodically turned off during the trial, and full return of pain occurred in all patients during those times. Outcomes included a greater than 80% decrease in deep pain and allodynia, significantly increased function on the pain disability index, grip strength in upper limb CRPS, ability to walk without crutches in lower limb CRPS, and decrease in pain medications, with 17 of 29 no longer requiring any pain medication.[43] Reig followed up 40 patients with SCS for CRPS for an average of 38 months; 47.5% obtained pain relief between 50% and 75%, and 7.5% of patients received greater than 75% relief.[44] Numerous other prospective and retrospective studies report similar outcomes, with between 45% and 80% of patients achieving greater than 50% pain relief with SCS, with results limited by study designs and quality.[45–52]

Optimizing Outcomes of SCS in CRPS

Several factors have been evaluated with regards to predicting and achieving optimal outcomes. Two studies have evaluated the outcomes in CRPS type I with SMP and suggest that SMP responds to SCS better than SIP. Hord performed a multicenter retrospective study of 23 patients who had an adequate SNB and later underwent SCS trial. All sympathetic blocks were confirmed to be technically adequate by temperature elevation in the limb of at least 1°C. The block was considered positive if greater than 50% pain relief was achieved, and these patients were determined to have SMP. All 13 patients who experienced a positive response to SNB had a positive SCS trial, whereas only 3 of 10 patients with a negative SNB had a positive SCS trial. The seven patients with negative SNB had poor pain relief during the SCS trial despite adequate paresthesia coverage. At 9 months' follow-up after permanent SCS implantation, 88% of those with SMP had a greater than 50% pain relief compared with 33% with SIP.[53] Another study described earlier, with all patients having SMP, demonstrated a much greater than typical response with SCS in terms of pain relief and functional improvement.[43]

A shorter duration of time between pain onset and implantation with SCS is strongly associated with positive outcomes. Kumar found that the best SCS outcomes occur within 1 year of onset of CRPS and in the early stages of the disease rather than as a last resort after a protracted course.[42] It has also been demonstrated in a study involving 410 patients with CRPS and other diagnosis, such as FBSS, that if time to SCS treatment was less than 2 years from pain onset, the long-term success rate was 85%, but it declined substantially thereafter and was only 9% if implantation was delayed beyond 15 years.[54]

With regards to outcomes for SCS on upper versus lower limb CRPS, no significant difference has been demonstrated.[47,54] Psychologic factors such as depression and fear avoidance are negative predictive factors. Workers compensation insurance coverage is also a negative predictive factor for pain relief and return-to-work rates as compared with other types of insurers.[54] One study found that an increased severity of allodynia was associated with a lower chance of achieving long-term pain reduction with SCS, whereas no correlation was found with age, baseline pain severity, or gender.[55]

Cost-effectiveness of SCS in CRPS
Several studies have demonstrated that SCS is overall more cost-effective than conventional management over the long term, despite the initial increased costs. Kemler demonstrated that SCS for CRPS becomes less expensive than conventional treatment after 3 years and cost-effective at 2 years.[56] The predicted lifetime cost savings is $60,000 when SCS is used with conventional medical management.[57,58]

Future Innovations in SCS
There are several promising newer variations of SCS, with some theoretical advantages in CRPS, but little to no data specifically in CRPS. DRG stimulation involves the placement of epidural leads directly in the neuroforamen near the DRG relevant to the patient's location

of pain and allows the targeting of discrete body areas that can be difficult to reach or isolate with traditional SCS (i.e., foot).[59,60] Only one study involved patients with CRPS. In a prospective trial of 51 patients with a variety of diagnosis, 39 had positive trials, including 9 with CRPS. At 6 months, foot pain was decreased by greater than 50% in 84.5% of patients compared with 52% for leg or back pain. There was no outcome breakdown by diagnosis.[60]

Novel electrical parameters have also been developed and compared with traditional tonic stimulation, with favorable results in several studies. Both high-frequency and burst stimulation (which provides intermittent brief packets of closely spaced stimulation), provide pain relief without the need for paresthesias in the areas of pain.[61-64] Although the lack of paresthesia in general or outside the painful area seems intuitively advantageous, this type of stimulation has yet to be rigorously tested for efficacy specifically in CRPS. The lack of paresthesia will also allow for future blinded and placebo-controlled studies on SCS, which is not possible with tonic, paresthesia-based, stimulation.

AMPUTATION
Amputation is a controversial treatment option for refractory severe CRPS.[1] A study involving 31 amputations showed that CRPS symptoms recurred in 28 of the residual limbs after amputation. Furthermore, only two patients were able to tolerate prosthesis because of the recurrence of CRPS symptoms post amputation.[65] Interestingly, another retrospective study involving 22 patients with CRPS type I found that most patients experienced reduced pain and increased mobility after amputation. CRPS symptoms recurred in the residual limb in 14% of patients. In 10% of patients, symptoms developed in a different limb.[66] Another study compared pain and depression in 19 patients who underwent amputation for intractable CRPS and 19 patients who did not have the procedure. The results showed that the amputation group consistently reported less pain and depression than those who chose against amputation as a treatment.[67] Overall, the current literature on amputation for CRPS is limited and reports mixed findings. More research is required for amputation to be considered a routine treatment option for CRPS.

INTRATHECAL MEDICATION
Evidence for intrathecal (IT) pain medication efficacy in CRPS is very limited. Several studies have evaluated

the utilization of IT baclofen, a GABA-B agonist, particularly in those with CRPS-associated dystonia given its accepted use in severe refractory spasticity and dystonia. One study with 42 subjects and 12 months' follow-up sought to evaluate the effects of IT baclofen on dystonia, though also noted significant benefits in pain, disability, and quality of life. Of the 36 patients who had IT pumps implanted, there was a high rate of complications and six pumps were explanted during the study period.[68] A follow-up study was designed to determine if the decrease in pain from IT baclofen was independent from the improvement in dystonia. Significantly decreased pain was seen during the first 6 months, and then the pain leveled off, whereas further escalating doses of baclofen further improved dystonia, indicating a separate effect.[69]

REFERENCES

1. Freedman M, Greis AC, Marino L, et al. Complex regional pain syndrome: diagnosis and treatment. *Phys Med Rehabil Clin N Am.* 2014;25(2):291–303.
2. Stanton-Hicks M, Baron R, Boas R, et al. Complex regional pain syndromes: guidelines for therapy. *Clin J Pain.* 1998;14:155–166.
3. Evans J. Sympathectomy for reflex sympathetic dystrophy: report of 29 cases. *JAMA.* 1946;132:620–623.
4. Harden RN, Oaklander AL, Burton AW, et al. Complex regional pain syndrome: practical diagnostic and treatment guidelines, 4th edition. *Pain Med.* 2013;14:180–229.
5. Bonica JJ. *The Management of Pain.* Philadelphia, PA: Lea and Feibiger; 1953.
6. Nelson DV, Stacey BR. Interventional therapies in the management of complex regional pain syndrome. *Clin J Pain.* 2006;22(5):438–442.
7. O'Connell NE, Wand BM, McAuley J, et al. Interventions for treating pain and disability in adults with complex regional pain syndrome- an overview of systematic reviews. *Cochrane Database Syst Rev.* 2013;(4).
8. Furman MB, Lee TS, Berkwits L. *Atlas of Image-Guided Spinal Procedures.* 1st ed. Philadelphia, PA: Elsevier Saunders; 2013.
9. Malmqvist EL, Bengtsson M, Sorensen J. Efficacy of stellate ganglion block: a clinical study with bupivacaine. *Reg Anesth.* 1992;17:340–347.
10. Elias M. Cervical sympathetic and stellate ganglion blocks. *Pain Physician.* 2000;3:294–304.
11. Price D, Long S, Wilsey B, et al. Analysis of peak magnitude and duration of analgesia produced by local anesthetics injected into sympathetic ganglia of complex regional pain syndrome patients. *Clin J Pain.* 1998;14:216–226.
12. Burton A, Conroy B, Sims S, et al. Complex regional pain syndrome type II as a complication of subclavian line insertion (letter). *Anesthesiology.* 1998;89:804.

13. van Eijs F, Stanton-Hicks M, Van Zundert J, et al. Evidence-based interventional pain medicine according to clinical diagnoses. Complex regional pain syndrome. *Pain Pract.* 2011;11:70–87.
14. Cepeda M, Lau J, Carr D. Defining the therapeutic role of local anesthetic sympathetic blockade in complex regional pain syndrome: a narrative and systematic review. *Clin J Pain.* 2002;18:216–233.
15. Bonelli S, Conoscente F, Movilia P, et al. Regional intravenous guanethidine versus stellate ganglion blocks in reflex sympathetic dystrophy: a randomized trial. *Pain.* 1983;16:297–307.
16. Carroll I, Clark JD, Mackey S. Sympathetic block with botulinum toxin to treat complex regional pain syndrome. *Ann Neurol.* 2009;65(3):348–351.
17. Choi E, Cho CW, Kim HY, et al. Lumbar sympathetic block with botulinum toxin type B for complex regional pain syndrome: a case study. *Pain Physician J.* 2015;18:E911–E916.
18. Manjunath PS, Jayalakshimi TS, Dureja GP, et al. Management of lower limb complex regional pain syndrome type 1: an evaluation of percutaneous radiofrequency thermal lumbar sympathectomy versus phenol lumbar sympathetic neurolysis – a pilot study. *Anesth Analg.* 2008;106(2):647–649.
19. Hannington-Kiff JG. Intravenous regional sympathetic block with guanethidine. *Lancet.* 1974;1:1019–1020.
20. Perez R, Kwakkel G, Zuurmond W, et al. Treatment of reflex sympathetic dystrophy (CRPS type I): a research synthesis of 21 randomized clinical trials. *J Pain Symptom Manage.* 2001;21:511–526.
21. Ramamurthy S, Hoffman J, Group GS. Intravenous regional guanethidine in the treatment of reflex sympathetic dystrophy/causalgia: a randomized double blind study. *Anesth Analg.* 1995;81:718–723.
22. Jadad AR, Carroll D, Glynn CJ, et al. Intravenous regional sympathetic dystrophy: a systemic review and a randomized, double-blind crossover study. *J Pain Symptom Manage.* 1995;10:13–20.
23. Hanna MH, Peat SJ. Ketanserin in reflex sympathetic dystrophy. A double-blind placebo controlled cross-over trial. *Pain.* 1989;38:145–150.
24. Eckmann MS, Ramamurthy S, Griffin JG. Intravenous regional ketorolac and lidocaine in the treatment of complex regional pain syndrome of the lower extremity: a randomized, double-blinded, crossover study. *Clin J Pain.* 2011;27(3):203–206.
25. Connolly SB, Prager JP, Harden RN. A systemic review of ketamine for complex regional pain syndrome. *Pain Med.* 2015;16:943–969.
26. Azari P, Lindsay DR, Briones D, et al. Efficacy and safety of ketamine in patients with complex regional pain syndrome: a systematic review. *CNS Drugs.* 2012;26(3):215–228.
27. Kosharskyy B, Almonte W, Shaparin N, et al. Intravenous infusions in chronic pain management. *Pain Phys.* 2013;16(3):231–249.

28. Sigtermans MJ, Hilten JJ, Bauer MC, et al. Ketamine produces effective and long-term pain relief in patients with complex regional pain syndrome type 1. *Pain.* 2009;145(3):304–311.

29. Schwartzman RJ, Alexander GM, Grothusen JR, et al. Outpatient intravenous ketamine for the treatment of complex regional pain syndrome: a double-blind placebo controlled study. *Pain.* 2009;147(1–3):107–115.

30. Kiefer RT, Rohr P, Ploppa A, et al. Efficacy of ketamine in anesthetic dosage for the treatment of refractory complex regional pain syndrome: an open-label phase II study. *Pain Med.* 2008;9(8):1173–1201.

31. Melzack R, Wall P. Pain mechanisms: a new theory. *Science.* 1965;150:971–979.

32. Shealy C, Mortimer J, Resnick J. Electrical inhibition of pain by stimulation of the dorsal columns. Preliminary reports. *J Int Anesth Res Soc.* 1967;46:489–491.

33. Oakley J, Prager J. Spinal cord stimulation: mechanism of action. *Spine.* 2002;22:2574–2583.

34. Linderoth B, Foreman R. Physiology of spinal cord stimulation. Review and update. *Neuromodulation.* 1999;3:150–164.

35. Duggan AW, Fong FW. Bicuculline and spinal inhibition produced by dorsal column stimulation in the cat. *Pain.* 1985;22:249–259.

36. Stiller C-O, Cui J-G, O'Connor WT, et al. Release of GABA in the dorsal horn and suppression of tactile allodynia by spinal cord stimulation in mononeuropathic rats. *Neurosurgery.* 1996;39:367–375.

37. Barolat G, Massaro F, He J, et al. Mapping of sensory responses to epidural stimulation of the intraspinal neural structures in man. *J Neurosurg.* 1993;78:233–239.

38. Geurts J, Smits H, Kemler M, et al. Spinal cord stimulation for complex regional pain syndrome type I: a prospective cohort study with long-term follow-up. *Neuromodulation.* 2013;16:523–529.

39. North R, Kidd D, Olin J, et al. Spinal cord stimulation electrode design: a prospective randomized comparison of percutaneous and insulated paddle electrodes. In: *Abstracts of the 4th International Congress of the International Neuromodulation Society.* 1998:211.

40. Kemler M, Barendse G, van Kleef M, et al. Spinal cord stimulation in patients with chronic reflex sympathetic dystrophy. *N Engl J Med.* 2000;343:618–624.

41. Kemler M, de Vet C, Barendse G, et al. Effect of spinal cord stimulation for chronic complex regional pain syndrome type I. Five-year final follow-up of patients in a randomized controlled trial. *J Neurosurg.* 2008;108:292–298.

42. Kumar K, Rizvi S, Bishop S. Spinal cord stimulation is effective in management of complex regional pain syndrome I: fact or fiction. *Neurosurgery.* 2011;69:566.

43. Harke H, Gretenkort P, Ladleif H, et al. Spinal cord stimulation in sympathetically maintained complex regional pain syndrome type I with severe disability. A prospective clinical study. *Eur J Pain.* 2005;9:363–373.

44. Reig E, Abejan D. Spinal cord stimulation. A 20-year retrospective analysis in 260 patients. *Neuromodulation.* 2009;12:232–239.

45. Oakley J, Weiner R. Spinal cord stimulation for complex regional pain syndrome. A prospective study of 19 patients at two centers. *Neuromodulation.* 2002;1:47–50.

46. Moriyama K, Murakawa K, Uno T, et al. A prospective, open-label, multicenter study to assess the efficacy of spinal cord stimulation and identify patients who would benefit. *Neuromodulation.* 2012;15:7–11.

47. Forouzanfar T, Kemler M,Weber W, et al. Spinal cord stimulation in complex regional pain syndrome: cervical and lumbar devices are comparably effective. *Br J Anaesth.* 2004;92:348–353.

48. Bennett D, Alo K, Oakley J, et al. Spinal cord stimulation for complex regional pain syndrome I. A retrospective multicenter experience from 1995–1998 of 101 patients. *Neuromodulation.* 1999;3:202–210.

49. Calvillo O, Racz G, Didie J, et al. Neuroaugmentation in the treatment of complex regional pain syndrome of the upper extremity. *Acta Orthop Belg.* 1998;1:57–63.

50. Kumar K, Hunter G, Demeria D. Spinal cord stimulation in treatment of chronic benign pain: challenges in treatment planning and present status, a 22-year experience. *Neurosurgery.* 2006;58:481–496.

51. Sears N, Machado A, Nagel S, et al. Long-term outcomes of spinal cord stimulation with paddle leads in the treatment of complex regional pain syndrome and failed back surgery syndrome. *Neuromodulation.* 2011;14:312–318.

52. Olsson G, Meyerson B, Linderoth B. Spinal cord stimulation in adolescents with complex regional pain syndrome type I (CRPS-I). *Eur J Pain.* 2008;12:53.

53. Hord E, Cohen S, Cosgrove G, et al. The predictive value of sympathetic block for the success of spinal cord stimulation. *Neurosurgery.* 2003;53(3):626–632.

54. Kumar K, Wilson J. Factors affecting spinal cord stimulation outcome in chronic benign pain with suggestions to improve success rate. *Acta Neurochir Suppl.* 2007;97:91–99.

55. Van Eijs F, Smits H, Geurts J, et al. Brush-evoked allodynia predicts outcome of spinal cord stimulation in complex regional pain syndrome type 1. *Eur J Pain.* 2010;14:164–169.

56. Kemler M, Raphael J, Bentley A, et al. The cost-effectiveness of spinal cord stimulation for complex regional pain syndrome. *Value Health.* 2010;13:735–742.

57. Taylor R, Buyten J, Buchser E. Spinal cord stimulation for complex regional pain syndrome. A systematic review of the clinical and cost-effectiveness literature and assessment of prognostic factors. *Eur J Pain.* 2006;10:91–101.

58. Kumar K, Rizvi S. Cost-effectiveness of spinal cord stimulation therapy in management of chronic pain. *Pain Med.* 2013;14:1631–1649.

59. Deer T, Grigsby E, Weiner R, et al. A prospective study of dorsal root ganglion stimulation for the relief of chronic pain. *Neuromodulation.* 2012;16:67–71.

60. Liem L, Russo M, Huygen F, et al. A multicenter, prospective trial to assess the safety and performance of the spinal modulation dorsal root ganglion neurostimulator system in the treatment of chronic pain. *Neuromodulation.* 2013;16:471–482.

61. De Ridder D, Vanneste S, Plazier M, et al. Burst spinal cord stimulation: toward paresthesia-free pain suppression. *Neurosurgery.* 2010;66:986–990.
62. De Ridder D, Plazier M, Kamerling N, et al. Burst spinal cord stimulation for limb and back pain. *World Neurosurg.* 2013;80:642–649.
63. Al-Kaisy A, Van Buyten J, Smet I, et al. Sustained effectiveness of 10 kHz high-frequency spinal cord stimulation for patients with chronic low back pain: 24-month results of a prospective multicenter study. *Pain Med.* 2013;15:347–354.
64. Kapural L, Yu C, Doust M, et al. Novel 10-kHz high-frequency therapy (HF10 therapy) is superior to traditional low-frequency spinal cord stimulation for the treatment of chronic back and leg pain: the SENZA-RCT randomized controlled trial. *Anesthesiology.* 2015;123(4):851–860.
65. Dielissen PW, Claassen AT, Veldman PH, et al. Amputation for reflex sympathetic dystrophy. *Bone Joint J.* 1995;77-B:270–273.
66. Krans-Schreuder HK, Bodde MI, et al. Amputation for long-standing, therapy-resistant type-I complex regional pain syndrome. *J Bone Joint Surg.* 2012;94(24):2263–2268.
67. Midbari A, Suzan E, Adler T, et al. Amputation in patients with complex regional pain syndrome: a comparative study between amputees and non-amputees with intractable disease. *Bone Joint J.* 2016;98-B(4):548–554.
68. VanderPlas AA, VanRijn MA, Marinus J, et al. Efficacy of intrathecal baclofen on different pain qualities in complex regional pain syndrome. *Anesth Analg.* 2013;116:211–215.
69. VanRijn MA, Munts AG, Marinus J, et al. Intrathecal baclofen for dystonia of complex regional pain syndrome. *Pain.* 2009;143:41–47.

CHAPTER 10

Diabetic Neuropathic Pain Syndromes

FATIMA Z. SYED, MD, MSC • ERIC SHIFFRIN, MD •
SANYA THOBANI, MD • NAZISH AHMAD, MD

INTRODUCTION

Diabetic neuropathy is a common complication of diabetes. The goal of this chapter is to present the symptoms, understand the demographics, provide differential diagnosis and diagnostic criteria, explore treatment options, and understand disease prognosis. Diabetic amyotrophy is also discussed as a less frequent but potentially debilitating complication of diabetes. It refers to the weakness and pain, particularly along the lumbosacral plexus, which can be associated with diabetes. It can be idiopathic or related to diabetes. Diabetic amyotrophy is also known as Bruns-Garland syndrome, diabetic myelopathy, proximal diabetic neuropathy, diabetic lumbosacral plexopathy, or diabetic lumbosacral radiculoplexus neuropathy. It differs from peripheral neuropathy, which is commonly seen in diabetic patients, because it is specific to the proximal muscles. It can be associated with weakness and excruciating pain. Other causes can be idiopathic.[1]

PRESENTATION

Diabetic polyneuropathy can present at any point in patients with diabetes but is more common in patients who have had poorly controlled diabetes. It results from a loss of myelination in large and small nerve fibers. A decrease in myelination in small fibers can cause impairment in pain, light touch, and temperature. A decrease in myelination in large fibers can cause impairment in vibratory sense and proprioception. Diabetic polyneuropathy follows a stocking-glove-like pattern, but neuropathy can ascend.

DEMOGRAPHICS

Diabetic neuropathy is a common complication of diabetes and is seen most commonly in the West. A landmark study done over 25 years showed that neuropathy most commonly occurs the longer the duration of diabetes, and by 25 years of having diabetes, 50% of people exhibit symptoms of neuropathy.[1] The ethnic background can also influence symptoms. In the United Kingdom, it was seen that patients of South Asian descent often have symptoms of painful neuropathy.[2] It has also been found that the worse the control of diabetes, the more likely the patients are to develop neuropathy.[3] Neuropathy is much more common in patients with type 2 diabetes than in patients with type 1 diabetes.[4]

Diabetic amyotrophy is more commonly seen in patients with long-standing type 2 diabetes. A prospective study on patients with diabetes showed that the mean age of diagnosis was 65 years and the mean duration of diabetes was 4 years when diabetic amyotrophy was diagnosed. These patients did not necessarily have poorly controlled diabetes. In fact, their mean A1C was 7.5. Most patients were older and had diabetes for longer. A gender or ethnic distribution was not seen. Weakness and pain were the main complaints. These patients were found to have weight loss. They ultimately required ambulatory aids, including wheelchair or cane.[5]

DIAGNOSTIC CRITERIA

Many patients are diagnosed with diabetic neuropathy based only on their symptoms, and these may have a poor correlation to clinical neurologic abnormalities on physical examination.[6,7] Historically, the diagnosis of diabetic neuropathy has been based on a set of symptoms and signs, such as loss of vibratory and/or light touch sensation, loss of lower extremity reflexes, and complaints of numbness and burning pain.[8]

The first official meeting regarding diabetic neuropathy took place in 1988, where a group of diabetologists and neurologists proposed a comprehensive set of criteria, called the San Antonio Consensus statement, to diagnose diabetic neuropathy.[9] These criteria were updated in 2009 in Toronto and are summarized in Table 10.1.[10]

TABLE 10.1
Diagnostic Criteria for Diabetic Neuropathy (San Antonio Consensus Statement)

	Minimal Criteria

Possible clinical DSPN	• Presence of symptoms or signs of DSPN:
	 • Symptoms
	   • Decreased sensation
	   • Positive neuropathic sensory symptoms (e.g., "asleep numbness," "prickling" or "stabbing", "burning" or "aching" pain) predominantly in the toes, feet, or legs
	 • Signs
	   • Symmetric decrease of distal sensation
	   • Unequivocally decreased or absent ankle reflexes

Probable clinical DSPN	• A combination of symptoms and signs of distal sensorimotor polyneuropathy with any two or more of the following: • Neuropathic symptoms • Decreased distal sensation • Unequivocally decreased or absent ankle reflexes
Confirmed clinical DSPN	• An abnormal nerve conduction study, and a symptom or symptoms or a sign or signs of sensorimotor • Polyneuropathy
Subclinical DSPN	• No signs or symptoms of polyneuropathy • Abnormal nerve conduction

Data from Tesfaye S, Boulton AJM, Dyck PJ, et al. Diabetic neuropathies: update on definitions, diagnostic criteria, estimation of severity, and treatments. *Diabetes Care* 2010; 33(10):2285-2293.

Although the Toronto criteria are useful for research purposes, they are difficult to apply to clinical practice and are more suited for research. Therefore, several screening tests to diagnose diabetic neuropathy have been developed. The Michigan Neuropathy Screening Instrument (MNSI) is an assessment that has two parts; the first part is a patient questionnaire that requires at least 7 of 13 points to make a diagnosis of neuropathy. The second portion of the questionnaire is scored by a healthcare professional and is based on physical examination findings, with a score of three or more indicating neuropathy.[11,12] The MNSI has been validated as a sensitive screening test for diabetic peripheral neuropathy (DPN) (see Table 10.2).

The diagnosis of diabetic amyotrophy is mainly clinical. If a diabetic patient has proximal weakness and/or pain, diabetic amyotrophy should be considered.[13] Most patients with diabetic amyotrophy are known to have diabetes at diagnosis.[14] Diagnosis of amyotrophy specifically involves a thorough physical examination and evaluation of muscle strength and sensation. Diagnosis also includes electrodiagnostic studies.[15-18]

RISK FACTORS AND PATHOPHYSIOLOGY

The risk factors of neuropathy are not fully understood; they range from hyperglycemia to duration of diabetes, as well as hypertension, blood pressure, lipid levels, and obesity.[19] The vast majority of theories regarding the mechanisms underlying hyperglycemia-induced diabetic neuropathy include vascular damage and focus on five major mechanisms: increased flux of glucose and other sugars through the polyol pathway, increased intracellular formation of advanced glycation end products (AGEs), increased expression of the receptor for AGEs and its activating ligands, activation of protein kinase C (PKC) isoforms, and overactivity of the hexosamine pathway.[20]

Experimental evidence shows that hyperglycemia, glucose toxicity, and impaired insulin signaling act in concert with other risk factors and activate several biochemical pathways that affect cellular metabolism.[19] The changes in blood sugars promote structural changes such as segmental demyelination, axonal loss, and microangiopathy and induce dorsal root ganglia neuronal apoptosis, resulting in subsequent damage to and loss of myelinated and unmyelinated sensory fibers.

TABLE 10.2
Michigan Neuropathy Screening Instrument (MNSI): Questionnaire

1. Are your legs and/or feet numb?	Yes/No
2. Do you ever have any burning pain in your legs and/or feet?	Yes/No
3. Are your feet too sensitive to touch?	Yes/No
4. Do you get muscle cramps in your legs and/or feet?	Yes/No
5. Do you ever have any prickling feelings in your legs or feet?	Yes/No
6. Does it hurt when the bed covers touch your skin?	Yes/No
7. When you get into the tub or shower, are you able to tell the hot water from the cold water?	Yes/No
8. Have you ever had an open sore on your foot?	Yes/No
9. Has your doctor ever told you that you have diabetic neuropathy?	Yes/No
10. Do you feel weak all over most of the time?	Yes/No
11. Are your symptoms worse at night?	Yes/No
12. Do your legs hurt when you walk?	Yes/No
13. Are you able to sense your feet when you walk?	Yes/No
14. Is the skin on your feet so dry that it cracks open?	Yes/No
15. Have you ever had an amputation?	Yes/No

MICHIGAN NEURO`PATHY SCREENING INSTRUMENT (MNSI): EXAMINATION

	Right	Left
Appearance of feet: (Deformity, dry skin, callus, infection, fissure)	Normal = 0 Abnormal = 1	Normal = 0 Abnormal = 1
Ulceration	Absent = 0 Present = 1	Absent = 0 Present = 1
Ankle reflexes	Present = 0 Present/reinforced = 0.5	Present = 0 Present/reinforced = 0.5 Absent = 1
Vibration perception at great toe	Present = 0 Decreased = 0.5 Absent = 1	Present = 0 Decreased = 0.5 Absent = 1
Monofilament	Present = 0 Reduced = 0.5 Absent = 1	Present = 0 Reduced = 0.5 Absent = 1

MNSI, © University of Michigan, 2000; with permission.

Metabolic disorders are the primary cause of diabetic neuropathy. Hyperglycemia, induced through decreased insulin secretion or insulin resistance, is responsible for the enhancement of the polyol pathway activity. This pathway is pathogenic primarily by increasing the turnover of cofactors such as nicotinamide adenine dinucleotide phosphate and nicotinamide adenine dinucleotide, which leads to a decrease in the reduction and regeneration of glutathione, as well as an increase of AGE production and activation of diacylglycerol and PKC isoforms. Depletion of glutathione could be the primary cause of oxidative stress and be related to the accumulation of toxic species.[21,22] Oxidative stress could also be initiated by the autoxidation of glucose and their metabolites, increased intracellular formation of AGEs, increased expression of the receptor for AGEs and their activating ligands, altered mitochondrial function, activation of PKC isoforms, and overactivity of the hexosamine pathway.[21,22]

Microvascular impairment also plays a role in diabetic neuropathic pain (DNP). Nerve ischemia occurs when peripheral perfusion is reduced. An increase in the wall thickness and hyalinization of the basal lamina of vessels that feed the peripheral nerves can cause nerve ischemia.[23,24] Nerve ischemia can further decrease intraepidermal nerve fiber density. This leads to axonal retraction and regeneration and myelin sheath alteration.[22]

In humans, observational studies have shown that hyperglycemia is critical for the development of DNP in both type 1 and type 2 diabetes. Surprisingly, the importance of hyperglycemia as an independent risk factor for diabetic DSP was not confirmed in a randomized controlled trial (RCT) until 1993, when the Diabetes Control and Complications Trial strongly demonstrated that intensive glycemic control is essential to preventing DNP in patients with type 1 diabetes.[19]

The cause of diabetic amyotrophy is likely multifactorial. The proposed mechanisms include metabolic damage from hyperglycemia, ischemic, inflammatory, and immune mediated. Multiple studies have evaluated the type of injury at a pathologic level and have found multifocal fiber loss, perineural thickening, neovascularization, and impaired regeneration of nerve fibers. Experts have questioned hyperglycemia as a cause of diabetic amyotrophy. Studies have found that the majority of patients with diabetic amyotrophy did not have significantly worse glycemic control than those without the disorder. Those with diabetic amyotrophy also usually do not have many of the chronic complications typically associated with poor glycemic control, such as retinopathy or nephropathy. Also, the nerve damage of diabetic amyotrophy is unlike the microvessel disease (deterioration of pericytes and reduplication of basement membranes) associated with chronic hyperglycemia. An alternative explanation implicates an immune-mediated microvasculitis, causing inflammatory injury and microinfarcts of nerves. The degree of inflammation of biopsied nerves in subjects with diabetic amyotrophy has been found to be significantly greater than in healthy controls and in patients with diabetic polyneuropathy. Consequently, the leading explanation as to the cause of diabetic amyotrophy is ischemic injury secondary to a nonsystemic vasculitis of nerve roots, lumbosacral plexus, and peripheral nerves.[19]

DIFFERENTIAL DIAGNOSIS

It is important to consider a differential diagnoses for diabetic neuropathy because similar symptoms may be caused by drug use, such as alcohol, nitrofurantoin, and isoniazid. Heavy metals can also cause distal symmetric neuropathy. Other illnesses, such as pernicious anemia (vitamin B_{12} deficiency), chronic inflammatory demyelinating polyneuropathy, hypothyroidism, paraneoplastic syndromes from malignancy, Sjögren syndrome, vasculitides, Guillian-Barré syndrome, and uremia, need to be excluded through a thorough history, physical examination, and laboratory testing. Various studies have suggested that 10%–50% of individuals with diabetes may have an additional potential cause of a peripheral neuropathy and some may have more than one cause.

DIAGNOSTIC TESTS

The MNSI and other screening assessments have demonstrated the need to combine history with physical examinations findings, to more accurately diagnosis diabetic neuropathy. Studies have shown that "numbness of the feet" is a poor indicator of polyneuropathy in patients with type 2 diabetes. An office neurologic examination is fast and simple but can have substantial variation between providers. It is important to standardize the examination as much as possible. It is recommended that a 128-Hz tuning fork be used when assessing vibration sense, as this has shown to have the best sensitivity for detecting neuropathy. Many prospective studies have confirmed that loss of pressure sensation using the 10-g monofilament is highly predictive of an ensuing foot ulcer. Screening for sensory loss with the 10-g monofilament has been validated in many studies, including the Seattle Diabetic Foot Study. Most experts recommend testing 10 sites on the feet with the monofilament. Using a 10-g monofilament can help predict foot ulceration, as can the Achilles reflex, but both may be insensitive to the early detection of neuropathy. Some experts have proposed that a 1-g monofilament could increase sensitivity of detecting early neuropathy from 60% to 90%. Although the monofilament assessment is an important and the most common way to evaluate diabetic neuropathy, a diagnosis should not rest solely on this test because studies have shown a wide range of sensitivity and specificity in detecting neuropathy.

Diabetic neuropathy involves a slowing of nerve conduction velocity as a result of demyelination and a decrease in nerve action potential amplitudes from a loss of axons. Although nerve conduction studies are the most objective noninvasive measure of neuropathy, in clinical practice they are not typically part of the diagnostic workup for diabetic neuropathy. One reason they are not useful in this context is that small nerve fibers, which are affected early in the disease course of diabetic neuropathy, do not contribute to the sensory action potential detected by routine nerve conduction studies. However, some advocate for their use if the etiology of the neuropathy is uncertain and if the distribution differs from the usual distal symmetric polyneuropathy of diabetes. Electrodiagnostic studies can help establish whether the neuropathy is the result of axonal neuropathy or demyelinating neuropathy, or both (mixed). Normal nerve conduction studies significantly decrease the possibility of peripheral neuropathy, whereas abnormal nerve conduction findings confirm the diagnosis.

Nerve biopsies can be useful when the etiology of a neuropathy is unclear or when treatments such as chemotherapy or drugs for autoimmune disorders are being considered. They are often used to diagnose cases of neuropathy related to vasculitis, sarcoidosis, amyloidosis, and CIDP. These neural biopsies are able to differentiate between causes. Sural and superficial fibular nerves are the ones usually biopsied. Epidermal skin biopsy can be performed in patients in whom small, unmyelinated nerve fibers are suspected to be the cause. Small nerve fiber damage may represent the earliest stages of some peripheral neuropathies and cannot be identified by electrodiagnostic studies. The majority of patients with diabetes experience a distal, symmetric polyneuropathy, and nerve biopsies are not necessary.

TREATMENT
Rehabilitation and Physical Medicine + Function

Multiple studies have proved that optimal glycemic control through diet, exercise, and medication can aid in preventing diabetic complications. Exercise may positively influence the pathologic factors associated with nephropathy by promoting microvascular dilation, reducing oxidative stress, and reducing neurotrophic factors, but it is unknown whether exercise worsens or improves the signs and symptoms of neuropathy.[23] Exercise is a systemic treatment that improves metabolism through multiple mechanisms concurrently and, over the past decade, has been shown to both reduce the risk for diabetic neuropathy and partially reverse its effects on symptoms and axonal integrity.[23]

Large RCTs have established that a combination of aerobic and resistance exercise improves physical fitness, glycemic control, and insulin sensitivity in older adults and in people with diabetes. Exercise has long

been recognized as a part of therapy in the management of diabetes, yet 31% of type 2 diabetic patients fail to participate in basic physical activity, and people with DPN may have difficulty participating in weight-bearing exercise because of pain or absent sensation.[23]

One study implemented an 8-week aerobic exercise intervention in people with type 2 diabetes mellitus and age-matched controls. The study did not find adaptive arterial remodeling but reported an improved vascular endothelial function within 2 weeks of the intervention and this improvement was maintained in both groups at 4, 6, and 8 weeks of the intervention.[24]

Billinger et al. reported that a 16-week aerobic exercise program can improve measures of vascular health in people with DPN. The study showed that aerobic is associated with improvement in peak arterial diameter and faster response time to peak dilation. However, the absolute mean difference in percent FMD was 2.1%, which is below a clinically relevant improvement of 3.6%. Although an absolute difference is seen it is likely not clinically significant. They report that people with DPN can improve measures of vascular health but the improvements may be blunted by the duration and severity of DPN.[25]

A number of small studies have demonstrated that patients with diabetic neuropathy respond positively to physical exercises designed to improve muscle force generation, balance, walking speed, reaction time, and similar measures.[26]

A 4-year trial randomized 78 diabetic participants without baseline neuropathy to usual care or 4 h of observed treadmill walking weekly, designed to achieve 50%–85% of calculated maximum heart rate. No dietary intervention was imposed. Exercisers tolerated the prolonged intervention well but did not show significant change in the body mass index, waist circumference, or lipid profiles. Treadmill walkers had a significantly increased exercise capacity as measured by VO_2max, improved vibration detection, and nerve conduction study indices and were significantly less likely to develop either motor or sensory features of diabetic neuropathy (as measured by clinical evaluation) than controls.[26,27]

Kluding et al. evaluated the effect of an intense 10-week, supervised exercise program with aerobic and resistance training in a cohort of 17 patients (mean age 58 years) with diabetes (mean duration 12.5 years) and neuropathy. Exercise resulted in a significant improvement in HgbA1c but not in weight. Exercise resulted in a significant improvement in neuropathic symptoms as measured by the Michigan Neuropathy Symptom Inventory, pain as measured by the visual analog scale, and epidermal nerve fiber branching at the thigh.[26]

MEDICATION OPTIONS
Glycemic Control

The cornerstone to prevention of diabetic neuropathy is to achieve optimal diabetic control. High-quality evidences support that enhanced glucose control prevents the development of diabetic neuropathy and reduces nerve conduction and vibration threshold abnormalities in both type 1 and type 2 diabetes.[28]

In patients with type 1 diabetes, the DCCT study[2] was by far the largest study and demonstrated a 1.53% per year risk reduction (95% confidence interval [CI] 0.51–2.54) and a relative risk reduction after 5 years of 53% in the primary prevention cohort. The DCCT trial showed that blood glucose levels as close to normal as possible were associated with improved microvascular outcomes. In the secondary prevention cohort, there was a 1.97% per year risk reduction (95% CI 0.90–3.04) and a 52% relative risk reduction. Taking these two cohorts together, there was a 1.74% per year (95% CI 1.00–2.48) risk reduction in the incidence of clinical neuropathy in the intensive optimal glycemic control treatment groups.[29]

In patients with type 2 diabetes, the UKPDS Study Group,[30] where patients were followed up for 15 years, found that there was a modest risk reduction in the incidence of diabetic neuropathy in favor of intensive glycemic control treatment similar to that found by the ACCORD trial.[31] The UKPDS trial was a landmark study which established that intensive therapy for blood glucose control were associated with less microvascular complications. However, this result was only statistically significant at 15 years. This was the largest study with the longest follow-up to date in this patient population other than the Accord trial.

Foot Care

As per American Diabetes Association recommendations, all individuals with peripheral neuropathy should wear proper footwear and examine their feet daily to detect lesions early. Anyone with a foot injury or an open sore should be restricted to non–weight bearing activities.

Painful Diabetic Neuropathy Symptomatic Treatment

Treatment of DPN requires a stable and optimal glycemic control, and as several observational studies have indicated, avoidance of extreme blood glucose fluctuations is also important.[6,32,33]

Once the diagnosis of painful diabetic polyneuropathy is established, the patient should be informed that the condition is sometimes self-limited and may spontaneously resolve in 4–6 months. The main aim is to control pain.[34]

Several agents have shown promising results in RCTs. Meta-analysis of these RCTs shows that several analgesics may be effective for the short-term treatment of painful diabetic neuropathy. Selective serotonin reuptake inhibitors, topical capsaicin, tricyclic antidepressants (TCAs), and anticonvulsants were associated with statistically significant reductions in pain.[35]

The US Food and Drug Administration (FDA) has approved pregabalin, duloxetine, and tapentadol for the treatment of DPN. TCAs, gabapentin, venlafaxine, carbamazepine, topical capsaicin, and tramadol may be considered as additional treatment options.[36]

Evidence-based guidance about the selection of analgesic agents for painful diabetic neuropathy is not definitive. Stepwise approaches and algorithms may be used.

As per the American Academy of Neurology recommendations[37]:

1. If clinically appropriate, pregabalin should be offered for the treatment of PDN (level A).
2. Gabapentin and sodium valproate should be considered for the treatment of PDN (level B).
3. There is insufficient evidence to support or refute the use of topiramate for the treatment of PDN (level U).
4. Oxcarbazepine, lamotrigine, and lacosamide should probably not be considered for the treatment of PDN (level B).

Fig. 10.1 depicts an algorithm for the management of symptomatic DPN.[28]

In clinical trials, treatment is considered successful if patients obtain a 50% reduction in the pain level, accompanied by improvement in sleep, fatigue, depression, and quality of life (Box 10.1).

Anticonvulsants[38,39]

Pregabalin was the first anticonvulsant to be approved by the FDA for the treatment of postherpetic neuralgia, diabetic polyneuropathy, and neuropathic pain after spinal cord injury. It acts by binding to presynaptic voltage-gated calcium channels containing the $\alpha2\delta$ subunit at the level of the brain and spinal cord and cause inhibition of the release of excitatory neurotransmitters.

Gabapentin is the other antiepileptic drug with demonstrated efficacy in the treatment of diabetes. It has a similar mechanism of action to pregabalin with a number needed to treat of 5.8. Gabapentin is licensed for

Symptomatic neuropathy

↓

Exclude nondiabetic etiologies

↓

Stabilize glycemic control

(insulin not always required in type 2 diabetes)

↓

Tricyclic drugs

(e.g., Amitriptyline 25–150 mg before bed)

↓

Anticonvulsants

(e.g., Gabapentin, typical dose 1.8 g/day)

↓

Opioid or opioid-like drug

(e.g., Tramadol, Oxycodone)

↓

Consider pain clinic referral

FIG. 10.1 Algorithm for management of symptomatic diabetic peripheral neuropathy. (Data from Callaghan BC, Little AA, Feldman EL, et al. Enhanced glucose control for preventing and treating diabetic neuropathy. *Cochrane Database Syst Rev*. 2012 Jun 13;(6):CD007543.)

BOX 10.1
Drugs Used to Treat Neuropathic Pain[12,13]

ANTIEPILEPTICS
Pregabalin
Gabapentin
Carbamazepine
Oxcarbamazepine
Valproic acid
Lamotrigine
Lacosamide

ANTIDEPRESSANTS
Duloxetine
Venlafaxine
Amitriptyline
Nortriptyline
Imipramine
Milnaxipran

OPIODS
Oxycodone
Morphine sulfate
Tapentadol
Tramadol

OTHERS
α-Lipoic acid
Capsaicin cream
Lidocaine cream or patch

neuropathic pain in the United Kingdom but not in the United States. Some clinical trials have shown gabapentin and pregabalin to have a better analgesic effect than TCAs or opioids, greater tolerability, and lower risk for toxicity.

Other anticonvulsants, namely, valproic acid and carbamazepine, have shown some degree of effectiveness in reducing DPN pain but need to be used with caution in females of reproductive age group because of teratogenic effects.

Antidepressants[38,39]

Serotonin-norepinephrine reuptake inhibitors (SNRIs): Venlafaxine and duloxetine are also efficacious and are considered first-line drugs for the treatment of DPN. Duloxetine has shown significant improvement in pain over placebo in several RCTs. It also has a known analgesic effect, which can last for several months, and is used as an alternative to pregabalin for pain control.

Reported side effects include nausea, somnolence, and dizziness.

Venlafaxine has a varying mechanism of action at different prescribed doses. It predominantly inhibits serotonin reuptake at low doses and noradrenaline at higher doses. It also helps in the reduction of pain in painful DPN and has minor side effects.

TCAs: TCAs are another class of antidepressants and have been around longer than the SNRIs. Amitriptyline, nortriptyline, and other TCAs have the advantage of once daily dosing.

These drugs have shown similar efficacy in attenuating pain as pregabalin and gabapentin in several meta-analyses. However, these drugs are less popular because of their side effects. The most common side effects include dry mouth, postural hypotension, arrhythmias, cognitive impairment, constipation, and urinary retention, which are more frequently observed with amitriptyline than with nortriptyline treatment.

Opioids

Opioids are considered second- to third-line drugs for the treatment of diabetic neuropathy. Dextromethorphan, oxycodone, and tramadol have demonstrated efficacy in reducing pain and improving quality of life. However, the use of these drugs is limited by their abuse potential. Patients given opioids need to be monitored closely with urine drug screens and electronic medical prescriptions to avoid overuse.[40]

Topical Agents

Capsaicin is a natural product of hot peppers. It demonstrates its analgesic properties by inhibiting substance P, which is an important neurotransmitter in the C fibers responsible for the transmission of pain signals from the peripheral to the central nervous system. In RCTs it has been shown to be moderately effective in reducing pain.[41] Some patients are unable to tolerate it because of increased pain on initial application and local skin irritation. Their use can be considered in patients intolerant to conventional therapy and in whom use of other drugs is limited because of drug interactions.

Lidocaine patches are used focally on painful areas but are less effective for more diffuse pain. These work by inhibiting the sodium channels and decrease the excitability of the peripheral nociceptors. Adverse effects include local skin irritation and contact dermatitis. Lidocaine should be used with care on feet because it worsens sensation and may predispose patients to falls.

α-Lipoic Acid

Oxidative stress is considered an important pathophysiology in painful DPN. α-Lipoic acid is an antioxidant that works by reducing the oxidative stress. It has few side effects as compared with the other agents, including nausea and vomiting. It has shown clinically significant reduction in pain as compared with placebo in several placebo-control trials at three different doses. However, the best tolerated dose was 600 mg/day as higher doses were associated with nausea, vomiting, and vertigo, with no increased benefit.

Other Therapies

Isosorbide dinitrate spray: Nitric oxide causes vasodilation and improves microvascular blood flow. Several placebo-control trials support that this may be efficacious in reducing pain from DPN.

Acetyl-L-carnitine has shown some pain relief but needs further trials to prove its efficacy.

Spinal cord stimulation is used in refractory painful diabetic neuropathy. Electrodes are used to stimulate the dorsal columns of the spinal cord. In a small multicenter RCT involving 60 patients conducted over 6 months, spinal cord stimulation in refractory painful diabetic neuropathy resulted in a significant improvement in pain and quality of life.[42]

Electric nerve stimulation has been reported to have some benefit in a few clinical trials but is not widely available in clinical practice.[43]

Surgical decompression of peripheral nerves (Dellon procedure) is a controversial method that is no longer recommended because of the lack of well-designed trials proving its efficacy.[44]

Prognosis for Pain and Function

The efficacy of pharmacologic and nonpharmacologic treatments is not easily identified and at times is unpredictable. A combination of lifestyle changes, pharmacologic changes, and physical functions shows some improvement but not complete improvement of function. Patients may experience approximately 50% relief. DNP treatment is based mainly on the patient's symptoms, pain level, and tolerance of side effects.[45]

Despite several decades of determined research, medical therapy used to improve peripheral nerve function and promote reinnervation in the setting of diabetic neuropathy remains unavailable.[46] Successful DNP treatment with medication and exercise is limited secondary to the severity of neuropathic pain, the tolerability of exercise and or medication, and a variety of comorbidities that can limit medication and exercise.

The natural course of diabetic amyotrophy is monophasic, with spontaneous recovery without treatment in most cases. It has been proposed that the effectiveness of treatments in various studies could simply be due to the natural course of the disease and not a treatment effect. The mean time to recovery is typically about 3 months and can range from 1 to 18 months. Recovery can often be incomplete, and foot drop, residual weakness, and neuropathic symptoms are common. It is unclear whether early treatment with immunomodulating agents speeds recovery or prevents residual symptoms. Occasionally, patients have recurrent attacks of diabetic amyotrophy, but the recurrence rate is not clear.[47,48]

No treatments have been proved to be effective for diabetic amyotrophy. Given the leading theory that diabetic amyotrophy is caused by an ischemic process due to a microvasculitis, treatments have focused on inhibiting this process. Some studies indicate that diabetic amyotrophy may improve with immune-modulating therapies, including corticosteroids, intravenous immunoglobulin (IVIG), plasma exchange, cyclophosphamide, or combined treatment. The majority of the promising data are derived from case reports and cohort studies. Initial studies assessed the response to prednisone and prednisone with cyclophosphamide in patients with diabetic amyotrophy. There was reported improvement of pain and weakness in patients in both groups. In other studies, patients with diabetic amyotrophy were treated with prednisone or IVIG either alone or in combination with azathioprine or cyclophosphamide. There was improvement in symptoms and activities of daily living in the majority of patients. However, the only randomized controlled study using immunotherapy to treat diabetic amyotrophy had mixed results, and results were reported only in abstract form. The randomized study by Dyck et al. investigated the use of pulse intravenous methylprednisolone in treating diabetic amyotrophy. Although there was some improvement in pain and neuropathic symptoms in the treatment group, there was no significant difference in the neuropathy impairment score, the primary outcome, indicating a lack of effectiveness.

Symptomatic treatment is important given the lack of clear effectiveness of immunotherapy in diabetic amyotrophy. Patients are often unable to work or even perform daily activities of living while symptoms are at their peak. Physical therapy should be recommended, although it has not been proven to speed up recovery or prevent residual weakness and symptoms. Depression is common, given the severe impact that the illness can have. Antidepressant medications and counseling should be prescribed when indicated. Weight loss is very common, and patients may believe they have an undiagnosed cancer or a progressive and permanent illness. Medications used to treat painful neuropathies can be trialed, such as gabapentin, pregabalin, amitriptyline, duloxetine, and venlafaxine. Pain is a major component of the morbidity of diabetic amyotrophy. Physicians should not discount the role of medications to treat pain, including narcotics. Referral to a pain management specialist can help, but the majority of patients are not pain free until disease remission.[49,50]

There is no known way to prevent diabetic amyotrophy. Unlike peripheral neuropathy, patients with better glycemic control have not had reduced risk. The current recommendation is to attempt to meet hemoglobin A1C, blood pressure, and lipid goals for all patients with diabetes. Screening for diabetic neuropathy should occur at outpatient visits, and early referral to neurologists can help diagnosis and differentiate complex and/or severe neurologic complaints and symptoms.[51]

REFERENCES

Section Demographics

1. Pirart J. Diabetes mellitus and its degenerative complications: a prospective study of 4,400 patients observed between 1947 and 1973 (author's transl). *Diabete Metab.* 1977;3:97.
2. Pirart J. Diabetes mellitus and its degenerative complications: a prospective study of 4,400 patients observed between 1947 and 1973 (2nd part) (author's transl). *Diabete Metab.* 1977;3:173.
3. Abbott CA, Malik RA, van Ross ER, et al. Prevalence and characteristics of painful diabetic neuropathy in a large community-based diabetic population in the U.K.. *Diabetes Care.* 2011;34:2220.
4. Young MJ, Boulton AJ, MacLeod AF, et al. A multicentre study of the prevalence of diabetic peripheral neuropathy in the United Kingdom hospital clinic population. *Diabetologia.* 1993;36:150.
5. Sands ML, Shetterly SM, Franklin GM, Hamman RF. Incidence of distal symmetric (sensory) neuropathy in NIDDM. The San Luis Valley Diabetes Study. *Diabetes Care.* 1997; 20:322.

Sections Diagnostic Criteria and Differential Diagnosis

6. Boulton AJ. Management of diabetic peripheral neuropathy. *Clin Diabetes.* 2005;23(1):9–15.
7. Davies M, Brophy S, Williams R, Taylor A. The prevalence, severity, and impact of painful diabetic peripheral neuropathy in type 2 diabetes. *Diabetes Care.* 2006;29(7): 1518–1522.
8. Fateh HR, Madani SP, Heshmat R, Larijani B. Correlation of Michigan neuropathy screening instrument, United Kingdom screening test and electrodiagnosis for early detection of diabetic peripheral neuropathy. *J Diabetes Metab Disord.* 2015;15:8.
9. Franse LV, Valk GD, Dekker JH, Heine RJ, van Eijk JT. 'Numbness of the feet' is a poor indicator for polyneuropathy in type 2 diabetic patients. *Diabet Med.* 2000;17(2):105–110.
10. Freeman R. Not all neuropathy in diabetes is of diabetic etiology: differential diagnosis of diabetic neuropathy. *Curr Diabetes Rep.* 2009;9:423–431.
11. Hughes RA. Peripheral neuropathy. *BMJ.* 2002;324(7335): 466–469.
12. Lozeron P, Nahum L, Lacroix C, Ropert A, Guglielmi J-M, Said G. Symptomatic diabetic and nondiabetic neuropathies in a series of 100 diabetic patients. *J Neurol.* 2000;249:569–575.

13. Mendell JR, Sahenk Z. Clinical practice. Painful sensory neuropathy. *N Engl J Med.* 2003;348(13):1243–1255.

14. Mulder DW, Lambert EH, Bastron JA, Sprague RG. The neuropathies associated with diabetes mellitus. A clinical and electromyographic study of 103 unselected diabetic patients. *Neurology.* 1961;11(4):275–284.

15. Singh R, Kishore L, Kaur N. Diabetic peripheral neuropathy: current perspective and future directions. *Pharmacol Res.* 2014;80:21–35.

16. Tesfaye S, Vileikyte L, Rayman G, et al. Painful diabetic peripheral neuropathy: consensus recommendations on diagnosis, assessment and management. *Diabetes Metab Res Rev.* 2011;27(7):629–638.

17. Vinik AI, Park TS, Stansberry KB, Pittenger GL. Diabetic neuropathies. *Diabetologia.* 2000;43(8):957–973.

18. Willison HJ, Winer JB. Clinical evaluation and investigation of neuropathy. *J Neurol Neurosurg Psychiatry.* 2003;74(suppl 2):ii3–ii8.

Sections Course, Rehab, Prognosis

19. Albers JW. *Diabetic Neuropathy: Mechanisms, Emerging Treatments, and Subtypes.* PMC; 2016.

20. Giacco F, Brownlee M. Oxidative stress and diabetic complications. *Circ Res.* 2010;107(9):1058–1070. http://dx.doi.org/10.1161/CIRCRESAHA.110.223545.

21. Schreiber AK. Diabetic neuropathic pain: physiopathology and treatment. *World J Diabetes.* 2015;6:432–444.

22. Oates PJ. Polyol pathway and diabetic peripheral neuropathy. *Int Rev Neurobiol.* 2002;50:325–392. PMID: 12198816.

23. Malik RA, Tesfaye S, Thompson SD, et al. Endoneurial localisation of microvascular damage in human diabetic neuropathy. *Diabetologia.* 1993;36:454–459. http://dx.doi.org/10.1007/BF00402283. PMID: 8314451.

24. Pavy-Le Traon A, Fontaine S, Tap G, Guidolin B, Senard JM, Hanaire H. Cardiovascular autonomic neuropathy and other complications in type 1 diabetes. *Clin Auton Res.* 2010;20:153–160. http://dx.doi.org/10.1007/s10286-010-0062-X. PMID: 20354891.

25. Balducci S, Iacobellis G, Parisi L, et al. Exercise training can modify the natural history of diabetic peripheral neuropathy. *J Diabetes Complicat.* 2006;20:216–223.

26. Schreuder TH, Green DJ, Nyakayiru J, et al. Time-course of vascular adaptations during 8 weeks of exercise training in subjects with type 2 diabetes and middle-aged controls. *Eur J Appl Physiol.* 2015;115(1):187–196.

27. Billinger SA, Sisante JV, Alqahtani AS, Pasnoor M, Kluding PM. Aerobic exercise improves measures of vascular health in diabetic peripheral neuropathy. *Int J Neurosci.* 2016;127. http://dx.doi.org/10.3109/00207454.2016.1144056.

Section Treatment

28. Callaghan BC, Little AA, Feldman EL, Hughes RA. Enhanced glucose control for preventing and treating diabetic neuropathy. *Cochrane Database Syst Rev.* 2012;(6).

29. The effect of intensive treatment of diabetes on the development and progression of long-term complications in insulin-dependent diabetes mellitus. *N Engl J Med.* 1993;329:977–986.

30. Holman RR, Paul SK, Bethel MA, Matthews DR, Neil HA. 10-year follow-up of intensive glucose control in type 2 diabetes. *N Engl J Med.* 2008;359:1577–1589.

31. Effects of intensive glucose lowering in type 2 diabetes. *N Engl J Med.* 2008;358:2545–2559.

32. Boulton AJM, Vinik AI, et al. Diabetic neuropathies: a statement by the American Diabetes Association. *Diabetes Care.* 2005;28(4).

33. Boulton AJM. *Clin Diabetes.* 2005;23(1):9–15.

34. Boulton AJM, Malik RA, Arezzo JC, Sosenko JM. *Diabetes Care.* 2004;27(6):1458–1486.

35. Griebeler ML, Morey-Vargas OL, Brito JP, et al. Pharmacologic interventions for painful diabetic neuropathy. An umbrella systematic review and comparative effectiveness network meta-analysis. *Ann Intern Med.* 2014;161:639–649.

36. Chamberlain JJ, Rhinehart AS, Shaefer CF, Neuman A. Diagnosis and management of diabetes: synopsis of the 2016 American Diabetes Association Standards of medical care in diabetes. *Ann Intern Med.* 2016;164:542–552. http://dx.doi.org/10.7326/M15-3016.

37. Bril V, England J, Franklin GM, et al. Evidence-based guideline: treatment of painful diabetic neuropathy; American Academy of Neurology.

38. *BMJ*2014;348:g1799.

39. Schreiber AK, Nones CFM, Reis RC, Chichorro JG, Cunha JM. *World J Diabetes.* 2015;6(3):432–444. https://www.ncbi.nlm.nih.gov/pubmed/21482920?dopt=Abstract Neurology 2011.

40. Gaskell H, Derry S, Stannard C, Moore RA. Oxycodone for neuropathic pain in adults. *Cochrane Database Syst Rev.* 2016;(7). http://dx.doi.org/10.1002/14651858.CD010692.pub3. Art. No.: CD010692.

41. Scheffler NM, Sheitel PL, Lipton MN. Treatment of painful diabetic neuropathy with capsaicin 0.075%. *J Am Podiatr Med Assoc.* 1991;81(6):288–293.

42. de Vos CC, Meier K, Zaalberg PB, et al. Pain. *J Int Assoc Study Pain.* 2014;155(11):2426–2431. http://dx.doi.org/10.1016/j.pain.2014.08.031.

43. Hamza MA, White PF, Craig WF, et al. Percutaneous electrical nerve stimulation: a novel analgesic therapy for diabetic neuropathic pain. *Diabetes Care.* 2000;23(3):365.

44. Chaudhry V, Stevens JC, Kincaid J, So YT. Practice advisory: utility of surgical decompression for treatment of diabetic neuropathy: report of the Therapeutics and Technology Assessment Subcommittee of the American Academy of Neurology. *Neurology.* 2006;66(12):1805.

45. Chan YC, Lo YL, Chan ES. Immunotherapy for diabetic amyotrophy. *Cochrane Database Syst Rev.* 2012;6:CD006521.

46. Dyck PJ, Windebank AJ. Diabetic and nondiabetic lumbosacral radiculoplexus neuropathies: new insights into pathophysiology and treatment. *Muscle Nerve.* 2002;25(4):477Y491.

47. Dyck PJB, O'Brien P, Bosch P, et al. The multi-center double-blind controlled trial of IV methylprednisolone in diabetic lumbosacral radiculoplexus neuropathy. *Neurology*. 2006;66(suppl 2):A191.
48. Kawagashirea Y, Watanabe H, Oki Y, et al. Intravenous immunoglobulin therapy markedly ameliorates muscle weakness and severe pain in proximal diabetic neuropathy. *J Neurol Neurosurg Psychiatry*. 2007;78: 899–901.
49. Said G, Goulon-Goeau C, Lacroix C, Moulonguet A. Nerve biopsy findings in different patterns of proximal diabetic neuropathy. *Ann Neurol*. 1994;35: 559–569.

Diabetic Neuropathies

50. Boulton A, Vinik A, Arezzo J, et al. http://care.diabetesjournals.org/content/28/4/956.short.
51. Tamburin S, Zanette G. Intravenous immunoglobulin for the treatment of diabetic lumbosacral radiculoplexus neuropathy. *Pain Med*. 2009;10(8):1476–1480.

FURTHER READING

1. Kluding PM, Pasnoor M, Singh R, et al. The effect of exercise on neuropathic symptoms, nerve function, and cutaneous innervation in people with diabetic peripheral neuropathy. *J Diabetes Complicat*. 2012;26(5):424–429.

CHAPTER 11

HIV-Related Pain Syndromes

SALONI SHARMA, MD • MICHAEL J. MEHNERT, MD

HIV-related neuropathies are the most common neurologic complication of HIV. These neuropathies have increased in frequency as the mortality rate of people with HIV decreases as a result of improved pharmacologic treatments.[1] Neuropathies related to HIV include distal sensory polyneuropathy (DSP), antiretroviral toxic neuropathy, acute inflammatory demyelinating polyneuropathy, and multiple others (Box 11.1). People with HIV may also develop neuropathy related to hepatitis C, diabetes, chemotherapy, vitamin deficiencies, alcohol abuse, and other causes in the non-HIV population. Furthermore, diabetes mellitus and other causes of neuropathy may increase the risk for HIV DSP.[2] The most frequent HIV-related neuropathy is DSP.[3] HIV-related peripheral sensory neuropathy is the focus of this chapter.

PRESENTATION: HISTORICAL AND PHYSICAL FEATURES

The primary complaints are similar to those of other distal neuropathies, including symmetric, distal sensory loss with tingling and/or numbness. Patients may describe sensory loss in the lower limbs or in a glove and stocking distribution. Other complaints are sensitivity to light touch in the feet and distal weakness. Typically, patients describe a progressive onset of symmetric, abnormal sensation in the feet with feelings of walking on rocks, sand, or a sunburned area.[4] The degree of pain may fluctuate and be worse at night as is commonly found in neuropathic pain. It is important to take a full history and note the course, onset, intensity, duration, exacerbating or remitting factors, and associated symptoms. A thorough family history and social history should be reviewed to rule out other causes of these symptoms.

Physical features on examination are distal sensory loss beginning with decreased vibratory sense, hyporeflexia and/or absent reflexes, and possible distal weakness.

DEMOGRAPHICS

In 2001, DSP was reported in 35% of people with HIV.[5] More recently, the prevalence of DSP has been reported

as greater than 50% and both the development and severity of neuropathy are not necessarily correlated to the amount of immunosupression.[6] At the time of autopsy, it has been reported that nearly 100% of patients with AIDS have evidence of neuropathy on biopsy.[7]

DIAGNOSTIC CRITERIA
Course

The course can be progressive and include symptoms ascending proximally and incorporating the upper limbs. If there is a known cause, including medication or an additional neuropathic condition that can be modified or treated, it is important to do so quickly to minimize progression. The differential diagnosis includes other causes of neuropathy as seen in the general population (Box 11.2).

Diagnostic Testing

An assessment tool such as the Brief Peripheral Neuropathy Screen may be used as a quick method to make an initial diagnosis of neuropathy.[8] It is not specific to HIV-related neuropathy. Diagnostic testing should be used to rule out other causes of neuropathy and confirm the diagnosis (Box 11.3).

Treatment

Treatment of neuropathic pain in patients who are HIV positive is challenging for a variety of reasons. It

---

BOX 11.1
Neuropathies Related to HIV

HIV-related peripheral sensory neuropathy
  Distal sensory polyneuropathy
  Antiretroviral toxic neuropathy
Acute inflammatory demyelinating polyneuropathy
Chronic inflammatory demyelinating polyneuropathy
Mononeuritis multiplex
Diffuse infiltrative lymphocytosis syndrome
Progressive polyradiculopathy

BOX 11.2
The Differential Diagnosis for HIV-Related Peripheral Sensory Neuropathy

Diabetic neuropathy
Nutritional neuropathy
Toxic neuropathy
Uremic neuropathy
Vitamin B_{12}-associated neuropathy
Alcoholic neuropathy
Metabolic neuropathy
Paraneoplastic neuropathies
Monoclonal gammopathy
Acute inflammatory demyelinating polyradiculoneuropathy
Chronic inflammatory demyelinating polyradiculoneuropathy
Mononeuritis multiplex
Diffuse infiltrative lymphocytosis syndrome
Progressive polyradiculopathy

BOX 11.3
Diagnostic Tests

Laboratory studies
   HIV RNA viral load
   Complete blood cell count
   Complete metabolic panel
   Hemoglobin A1C
   Thyroid function tests
   Hepatitis workup
   Vitamin B_{12}, folate levels
   Serum, urine protein electrophoresis
Skin biopsy, optional
Electromyography/nerve conduction features include symmetric:
   Lower > upper limbs
   Sensory > motor abnormalities
   Severely decreased sensory and motor amplitudes
   Normal to slightly decreased sensory and motor conduction velocities
   Normal to slightly prolonged sensory and motor distal latencies

requires an approach to each individual patient that includes:

- Treating the HIV illness itself
- Adjusting drug therapy if possible when antiretroviral therapy (ART) drugs are causing/contributing to neuropathy and when concerns about pain medicine interactions with ART drugs exists
- Mitigating/managing other factors that predispose to neuropathy or chronic pain (for example, HIV-infected patients with a history of substance abuse)
- Employing multimodal palliative treatment of neuropathic symptoms (nonpharmacologic and pharmacologic treatments)

HIV infection, itself a chronic condition, is a causative factor for neuropathy, and to complicate things further, treatments required to manage the viral infection (antiviral medications) may be causative agents as well.[9,10] Immunosuppression caused by HIV infection predisposes the patient to other medical comorbidities that can contribute to neuropathy and other painful disorders. Furthermore, in HIV-positive patients with a history of substance abuse there is a higher incidence of chronic pain, and substance abuse itself can increase the risk of neuropathy in certain HIV-positive cohorts.[11]

Mitigating the disease process and controlling the viral load while maintaining optimal CD^{4+} counts may be helpful in minimizing neuropathy and associated symptoms. However, in the age of highly active ART, more recent studies have not shown an association with viral load/CD^{4+} counts and distal symmetric polyneuropathy.[11,12] Careful monitoring for neuropathy caused by drug therapy (specifically reverse-transcriptase inhibitors) is also necessary as part of disease management.[10,11] If possible the offending agent should be removed or adjusted.

Addressing other factors unique to each patient, specifically a history of substance abuse, is also a paramount concern if treatment of neuropathy symptoms via pharmacologic treatments is provided.

HIV-infected patients have a high incidence of distal symmetric polyneuropathy.[11] However, careful diagnostic evaluation should be undertaken to look for myriad other causes of neurologic compromise specific to the HIV-positive patient, including but not limited to herpes zoster or cytomegalovirus infection, tuberculosis, inflammatory demyelinating polyneuropathy (acute or chronic), and central nervous system complications of HIV.[13] Currently available treatment modalities do not reverse painful neuropathy; the focus is on pain relief and palliation with available treatments.[14]

Rehabilitation and Physical Medicine Options
Physical therapy
Physical therapy interventions may be more beneficial for general HIV symptoms such as fatigue and decreased mobility as opposed to neuropathic pain.

Interventions directed at the individual's functional capacity should be undertaken. Neuropathic pain, in general, has been shown to have a significant illness burden on the patient; high pain levels associated with poor function, compromised health status and sleep, and increased anxiety and depression have been documented.[15] An outcomes-measure study of HIV-infected patients found that 27% had a mood disorder and 8.4% reported substance abuse. In this study, pain was considered an independent risk factor for the impairment in mobility, self-care, and usual activities[16] and physiotherapy to address these impairments may be helpful.

Decreased mobility and lack of movement can be due to kinesophobia (fear of movement), and active therapy aimed at not only moving past these fears, but also improving balance, endurance, and posture may be beneficial.[17] Aquatherapy can be considered for the population with neuropathic pain with limited tolerance for land-based therapies.[17,18]

Occupational therapy
In the patient with HIV-associated neuropathic pain, occupational therapy can address functional limitations through several pathways. Goals should include energy conservation techniques for patients with endurance and mobility limitations, as well as body mechanics and environmental modifications. Patients whose pain includes a component of allodynia or hypersensitivity may benefit from a structured graded desensitization program.[17,19] With regards to a patient's work capacity, there may be a role for a work hardening/conditioning program that employs work-specific activities.[17]

Psychiatric/behavioral/hypnosis
HIV-infected individuals with chronic pain often initiate some self-management strategies, including physical activity, social support, and cognitive and spiritual strategies.[20] Brief hypnosis interventions may be beneficial in patients and allow for self-care/participation on behalf of the patient.[21] Cognitive-behavioral therapy (CBT) has been employed for patients with neuropathic pain[18,22] and can be a helpful self-management strategy that allows patients to cope with limiting thoughts of pain and disability. A 2003 randomized controlled trial demonstrated CBT as a useful intervention in the HIV-infected population.[17,23]

Acupuncture has been explored as a treatment modality for HIV-distal sensory neuropathic pain. Studies investigating the use of acupuncture with and without the medication amitriptyline did not demonstrate either intervention as being better than placebo.[24,25]

Orthotics
Orthotics may be helpful in patients with HIV-associated distal symmetric neuropathy who have muscle weakness. They may be beneficial with regards to improved mobility and perhaps function, but there is little evidence suggesting that they reduce neuropathic pain, particularly in HIV-associated neuropathy.

Transcutaneous electrical nerve stimulation
There is little evidence supporting the use of a transcutaneous electrical nerve stimulation unit with regards to HIV-associated neuropathy. It has been tried for acute herpes zoster neuropathy, also without consistent supporting findings, but it does appear to be safe.[26] Passive modalities may facilitate patient participation in therapy[17] but may not provide long-lasting benefit.

Medication Options
As a general rule, pharmacotherapy has been considered the mainstay of treatment for pain attributable to a neuropathy[27] (Box 11.4). It is noteworthy that HIV-infected patients continue to report moderate to severe chronic pain (not solely because of polyneuropathy) and elevated depression symptoms despite

---

BOX 11.4
Medication Options

Nonanalgesics
Anticonvulsants
    $\alpha_2\delta$ Subunit ligands
        Gabapentin
        Pregabalin
    Lamotrigine
    Carbamazepine
Antidepressants
    Tricyclic antidepressants
        Amitriptyline
        Nortriptyline
        Desipramine
    Selective norepinephrine reuptake inhibitors
        Duloxetine
Topicals
    Lidocaine 5%
    Capsaicin 8%
Analgesics
    Nonopiate analgesics
        Tramadol (weak opioid μ-receptor agonist)
        Cannabis
Opiate analgesics

pharmacologic treatment.[28] Specifically, with regards to pain from distal symmetric neuropathies in HIV-positive patients, the more recent literature suggests that commonly used medications are not as effective as they may be for other types of neuropathic pain.[29,30] These findings suggest that an emphasis on nonpharmacologic therapies may be beneficial for HIV-related neuropathic pain.

There exist other challenges with medication management of neuropathic pain that are not unique to the HIV-positive patient. Specifically, there is a lack of randomized controlled trials pertaining to medications and other commonly used nonpharmacologic treatments.[17] Although there are some medications approved by the Food and Drug Administration (FDA) for neuropathic pain, none have been approved for nondiabetic peripheral polyneuropathy or for HIV-associated neuropathy. Off label usage of medications is common, but uniform guidelines are not well established.[17] Given these limitations, a multimodal approach should be considered for patients with HIV-associated neuropathic pain and opioids should be prescribed in accordance with current guidelines to avoid diversion and abuse.

As noted earlier, adjusting ART to minimize iatrogenic neuropathy in HIV-infected patients should be done whenever possible. Prescribers should also be aware that some opioid- and nonopioid analgesics can also alter the blood levels of antiretroviral medications and dosage adjustments may be required.[31]

General Medication Categories
Nonanalgesics
Anticonvulsants

Anticonvulsants, specifically gabapentin, pregabalin, lamotrigine, and carbamazepine, have been successfully used for neuropathic pain. For painful neuropathies they can be considered one of the first-line agents.[32]

Gabapentin, originally an anticonvulsant medication, acts by binding to the $\alpha_2\delta$ subunit of calcium channels to inhibit nociceptive transmitters. Side effects of this medication include somnolence, dizziness, and edema. Pregabalin acts via a similar mechanism but may have better bioavailability, fewer adverse-related events, and the advantage of twice-daily dosing. Pregabalin typically is a more expensive medication.[26] With regards to efficacy, a multicenter randomized trial in HIV-associated neuropathy did not demonstrate a difference between gabapentin and placebo.[33,34] Similarly, a 2010 study comparing pregabalin with placebo did not demonstrate an improved efficacy for pregabalin.[33,35]

Few studies have compared combined drug regimens for neuropathic pain, although a 2005 study of patients with postherpetic neuralgia and diabetic neuropathy showed better analgesia with gabapentin and morphine combined versus single-drug therapy. In this study, lower doses of each medication were utilized with combined therapy but adverse effects were documented.[36,37] However, a similar study has not been done in patient populations with HIV-associated neuropathy.

The anticonvulsant lamotrigine enhances the activity of the inhibitory neurotransmitter γ-aminobutyric acid (GABA) and may reduce painful nociceptive transmissions. It has been studied specifically in patients with HIV-associated neuropathy with some benefit noted, particularly in patients who were also being treated with ART.[33,38] A skin rash was the most common adverse effect.

Carbamazepine is an anticonvulsant medication that is a GABA receptor agonist and that also acts to block voltage-gated sodium channels, leading to decreased neural excitability. It has been shown to have efficacy for neuropathic pain. However, possible leukopenia as a side effect is of particular concern in the HIV-infected patient, where anemia and leukopenia are already more common.[39]

Antidepressants

Antidepressants, specifically the tricyclic antidepressants (TCAs) amitriptyline, nortriptyline, and desipramine have been employed in the past for neuropathic pain and can also be considered one of the first-line treatments. There is the potential advantage of treating depression, which may be present in patients with chronic pain.[32] A study specifically of HIV-infected patients with neuropathy published in 2015 by Dinat et al. did not demonstrate superiority of amitriptyline versus placebo in a randomized, crossover trial of patients in South Africa.[40]

The mechanism of action of TCAs includes blockade of norepinephrine and serotonin reuptake. There is also inhibition of the spinal nociceptive neurons and sodium-channel blockade.[26] TCAs may not be well tolerated in older patients, although overall desipramine and nortriptyline are better tolerated with similar efficacy to amitriptyline. Desipramine is the least sedating, with similar efficacy to amitriptyline.[26] Anticholinergic adverse effects of dry mouth, urinary retention, and orthostatic hypotension are fairly common and can also include constipation, weight gain, and cardiac arrhythmia.[32]

Duloxetine is a selective serotonin and norepinephrine reuptake inhibitor (SSNRI), a different classification of antidepressant. SSNRIs also may be beneficial for neuropathic pain. However, a small group of HIV-infected patients were randomized to either duloxetine and/or methadone or placebo, with little change in neuropathic pain compared with placebo. Some increased adverse effects were documented.[36,41] Duloxetine may have associated nausea but does not require aminotransferase monitoring.[32]

Topicals

Lidocaine (5%) acts by providing local anesthesia of peripheral sensory nerves.[26] It is a safe intervention, but efficacy is not well established for HIV-associated peripheral neuropathy.[33,42,43]

Several studies have investigated topical capsaicin for HIV-associated neuropathy. Capsaicin acts as an agonist for the VR1 vanilloid receptors and causes depletion of substance P. These studies demonstrated evidence of success versus placebo when the drug was applied at 8% strength and patients were followed up for 12 weeks.[33,44,45] At this higher concentration the medication is applied by a healthcare practitioner, which may be a barrier to routine usage.

Analgesics

Nonopiate analgesics

Tramadol is a weak opioid μ-receptor agonist that acts to provide pain relief. It may be less effective at rapid pain relief than stronger μ-agonists (more potent opioids such as morphine); however, less abuse potential exists. Inhibition of serotonin and norepinephrine reuptake is also associated with tramadol, and interaction with other serotonin reuptake inhibitors is a concern. Tramadol also has been shown to lower the seizure threshold and potentially cause a serotonin syndrome.[32]

Two randomized controlled trials for cannabis (in a smoked form) versus placebo have demonstrated efficacy of cannabis for HIV-associated neuropathy.[33,46,47] Intuitively, it may be difficult to truly blind the treatment group in these studies, as patients may appreciate some mood changes, mental status changes, or euphoria associated with smoking cannabis.

Opiate analgesics

Opioid medications have been utilized with FDA approval for chronic pain but not specifically chronic pain related to a peripheral neuropathy or HIV infection.[17] Opiates should be used judiciously, and recommendations exist to monitor for abuse and diversion. In particular, a higher incidence of inappropriate urine

drug test results in HIV-infected patients in a pain clinic has been documented.[48] Opioid efficacy for painful HIV-associated neuropathy has been questioned, and the observation that opioids may actually increase neuropathic pain in HIV-infected patients has been put forth. A 2005 study[33,49] demonstrated higher levels of reported pain in HIV-infected patients receiving opioids, and there is concern that opioids in the HIV-infected patient with a painful neuropathy may actually increase pain and promote painful nociception.[33]

Interventional Pain Management

Spinal cord neuromodulation (also known as dorsal column stimulation or spinal cord stimulation [SCS]) has been shown in case reports to be beneficial in patients with HIV and neuropathic pain.[50] A 20-year literature review was published in 2004 demonstrating efficacy of SCS for chronic neuropathic pain,[50,51] although a complication rate of over one-third was reported at that time. Evidence exists for the efficacy of spinal cord stimulator implantation in patients with diabetic peripheral neuropathy[50,52] as well. Limited data are available regarding SCS specifically in patients with chemotherapy neuropathy (which may be a better analogue to HIV-associated neuropathy from antiretrovirals), but some case reports have been published.[50,53,54]

In particular, longer-term studies may be beneficial to evaluate the efficacy of SCS for HIV-associated neuropathy over time; randomized controlled trials will need to be implemented as well to better support routine usage in patients with HIV-associated neuropathy. Complications were not noted in case reports specific to HIV-infected patients, but the obvious concern may be an increased risk of infection in a potentially immunocompromised patient.

Surgical Options

At this time, evidence is lacking to routinely consider any surgical interventions for HIV-associated neuropathy.

PROGNOSIS FOR PAIN AND FUNCTION

Discontinuation of any causative agent and treatment of any disease process causing neuropathies not specific to HIV are most likely to provide the best prognosis. The prognosis for pain from HIV-related neuropathies depends on an individual's response to the treatment medications. Often, a combination of nonanalgesics, analgesics, and topical treatments is required for optimal pain prognosis.

Physical therapy treatments, including tissue mobilizations, desensitization techniques, stretching, and microcurrent stimulation, have been shown to improve function and decrease pain.[55] Continued work with gait and balance training may be helpful depending on the degree of neuropathy. If the neuropathy progresses and becomes severe with lower limb weakness, ankle-foot orthosis or assistive devices may be required for ambulation. Some studies have demonstrated that physical therapy helps all types of pain related to HIV in addition to improving endurance and general functioning.[56]

A combination of medications and physical therapy treatments will lead to the best prognosis for pain and function in patients with HIV-related pain syndromes.

REFERENCES

1. Donofrio PD. Neuropathies associated with HIV infection and antiretroviral therapy. In: *Textbook of Peripheral Neuropathy*. New York: Demos Medical Publishing; 2012: 323–337.
2. Schütz SG, Robinson-Papp J. HIV-related neuropathy: current perspectives. *HIV/AIDS (Auckland, NZ)*. 2013;5: 243–251.
3. Pardo CA, McArthur JC, Griffin JW. HIV neuropathy: insights in the pathology of HIV peripheral nerve disease. *J Peripher Nerv Syst*. 2001;6:21–27.
4. Chai NC, McArthur JC. HIV and peripheral neuropathy. In: *Chronic Pain and HIV: A Practical Approach*. Chichester, UK: John Wiley & Sons, Ltd; 2016:51–62.
5. Geraci AP, Simpson DM. Neurological manifestations of HIV-1 infection in the HAART era. *Compr Ther*. 2001;27(3):232–241.
6. Kranick SM, Nath A. Neurologic complications of HIV-1 infection and its treatment in the era of antiretroviral therapy. *Continuum Lifelong Learn Neurol*. 2012;18(6 Infectious Disease):1319–1337.
7. Gabbai AA, Castelo A, Oliveira AS. HIV peripheral neuropathy. *Handb Clin Neurol*. 2013;115:515–529.
8. Simpson DM, Kitch D, Evans SR, et al. HIV neuropathy natural history cohort study: assessment measures and risk factors. *Neurology*. 2006;66(11):1679–1687.
9. Maritz J, et al. HIV neuropathy in South Africans: frequency, characteristics and risk factors. *Muscle Nerve*. 2010;41:599–606.
10. Simpson DM, Tagliati M. Nucleoside-analogue associated peripheral neuropathy in human immunodeficiency virus infection. *J Acquir Immune Defic Syndr Hum Retrovirol*. 1995;9:153–161.
11. Robinson-Papp J, et al. Substance abuse increases the risk of neuropathy in an HIV-infected cohort. *Muscle Nerve*. 2012;45:471–476.
12. Morgello S, et al. HIV-associated distal sensory polyneuropathy in the era of highly active antiretroviral therapy. *Arch Neurol*. 2004;61:546–551.
13. Robsinson-Papp J, Simpson DM. AANEM minimonograph – neuromuscular diseases associated with HIV-1 infection. *Muscle Nerve*. 2009;40:1043–1053.
14. Williams D, Geraci A, Simpson DM. AIDS and AIDS-treatment neuropathies. *Curr Neur Neurosci Rep*. 2001;I: 533–538.
15. Schaefer C, et al. Burden of illness associated with peripheral and central neuropathic pain among adults seeking treatment in the United States: a patient centered evaluation. *Pain Med*. 2014;15:2105–2119.
16. Merlin JS, et al. Pain is independently associated with impaired physical function in HIV-infected patients. *Pain Med*. 2013;14:1985–1993.
17. Scholten PM, Harden RN. Addressing and treating patients with neuropathic pain. *PM R*. 2015;7:S257–S269.
18. Hall J, et al. Does aquatic exercise relieve pain in adults with neurologic or musculoskeletal disease? A systematic review and meta-analysis of randomized controlled trials. *Arch Phys Med Rehabil*. 2008;89:873–883.
19. Rendell JW. Desensitization of the traumatized hand. In: Hunter JM, Mackin EJ, Callahan AD, eds. *Rehabilitation of the Hand: Surgery and Therapy*. 4th ed. St. Louis, MO: Mosby; 1995:693–700.
20. Merlin JS, et al. Pain self-management in HIV-infected individuals with chronic pain: a qualitative study. *Pain Med*. 2015–16;16:706–714.
21. Dorfman D, et al. Hypnosis for treatment of HIV neuropathic pain: a preliminary report. *Pain Med*. 2013;14: 1048–1056.
22. Turk DC, et al. Assessment and treatment of psychosocial comorbidities in patients with neuropathic pain. *Mayo Clin Proc*. 2010;85:S42–S50.
23. Evans S, et al. Randomized trial of cognitive behavioral therapy versus supportive psychotherapy for HIV-related peripheral neuropathic pain. *Psychosomatics*. 2003;44: 44–50.
24. Stavros K, Simpson DM. Understanding the etiology and management of HIV-associated peripheral neuropathy. *Curr HIV/AIDS Rep*. 2014;11:195–201.
25. Shlay JC, et al. Acupuncture and amitriptyline for pain due to HIV-related peripheral neuropathy. *JAMA*. 1998; 280(18):1590–1595.
26. Poduri KR, Bauernfeind M, Thakur R. PM&R Knowledge Now: Acute Herpes Zoster and Post-herpetic Neuralgia. http://www.aapmr.org/kn/.
27. Finnerup NB, Sindrup SH, Jensen TS. The evidence for pharmacological treatment of neuropathic pain. *Pain*. 2010;150:573–581.
28. Uebelacker LA, et al. Chronic pain in HIV-infected patients: relationship to depression, substance use and mental health and pain treatment. *Pain Med*. 2015;16: 1870–1881.
29. Phillips TJC, et al. Pharmacological treatment of painful HIV-associated sensory neuropathy: a systematic review and meta-analysis of randomised controlled trials. *PLoS One*. 2010;5(12):e14433.
30. Kaku M, Simpson DS. HIV neuropathy. *Curr Opin HIV AIDS*. 2014;9:521–526.

31. Krashin DL, Merrill JO, Trescot AM. Opioids in the management of HIV-related pain. *Pain Physician*. 2012;15:ES157–ES168.

32. Dworkin RH, et al. Recommendations for the pharmacological management of neuropathic pain: an overview and literature update. *May Clin Proc*. 2010;85(suppl 3):S3–S14.

33. Smith HS. Treatment considerations in painful HIV-related neuropathy. *Pain Physician*. 2011;14:E505–E524.

34. Hahn K, et al. German neuro-AIDS working group. A placebo-controlled trial of gabapentin for painful HIV-associated sensory neuropathies. *J Neurol*. 2004;251:1260–1266.

35. Simpson DM, et al. Pregabalin for painful HIV neuropathy: a randomized, double-blind, placebo-controlled trial. *Neurology*. 2010;74:413–420.

36. Walk D, Backonja M. Editorial – HIV neuropathy continues to pose a challenge. *Pain Med*. 2013;14:957–958.

37. Gilron I, Bailey M, Tu D, et al. Morphine, gabapentin, or their combination for neuropathic pain. *N Engl J Med*. 2005;352(13):1324–1334.

38. Simpson DM, et al. Lamotrigine for HIV-associated painful sensory neuropathes: a placebo-controlled trial. *Neurology*. 2003;60:1508–1514.

39. Wullf EA, Wang AK, Simpson DM. HIV-associated peripheral neuropathy. *Drugs*. 2000;59(6):1251–1260.

40. Dinat N, et al. Randomized, double-blind, crossover trial of amitriptyline for analgesia in painful HIV-associated sensory neuropathy. *PLoS One*. 2015;10(5):1–15.

41. Harrison T, et al. Experience and challenges presented by a multicenter crossover study of combination analgesic therapy for the treatment of painful HIV-associated polyneuropathies. *Pain Med*. 2013;14:1039–1047.

42. Estanislao L, et al. A randomized controlled trial of 5% lidocaine gel for HIV-associated distal symmetric polyneuropathy. *J Acquit Immune Defic Syndr*. 2004;37:1584–1586.

43. Gonzalez-Durante A, Cikurel K, Simpson DM. Managing HIV peripheral neuropathy. *Curr HIV/AIDS Rep*. 2007;4:114–118.

44. Simpson DM, Brown S, Tobias J. NGX-4010 C107 study group. controlled trial of high-concentration capsaicin patch for treatment of painful HIV neuropathy. *Neurology*. 2008;70:2305–2313.

45. Simpson DM, et al. An open-label pilot study of high-concentration capsaicin patch in painful HIV neuropathy. *J Pain Symptom Manage*. 2008;35:299–306.

46. Abrams DI, et al. Cannabis in painful HIV-associated sensory neuropathy: a randomized placebo-controlled trial. *Neurology*. 2007;68:515–521.

47. Ellis RJ, et al. Smoked medicinal cannabis for neuropathic pain in HIV: a randomized crossover clinical trial. *Neuropsychopharmacology*. 2009;34:672–680.

48. Peters J, et al. High prevalence of inappropriate urine drug tests in a pain clinic for patients with HIV. *Pain Med*. 2014;15(6):1058–1059.

49. Koeppe J, et al. Ongoing pain despite aggressive opioid pain management among persons with HIV. *Clin J Pain*. 2010;26:190–198.

50. Knezevic NN, et al. The use of spinal cord neuromodulation in the management of HIV-related polyneuropathy. *Pain Physician*. 2015;18:E643–E650.

51. Cameron T. Safety and efficacy of spinal cord stimulation for the treatment of chronic pain: a 20 year literature review. *J Neurosurg*. 2004;100:254–267.

52. Slangen R, et al. Spinal cord stimulation and pain relief in painful diabetic peripheral polyneuropathy: a prospective two center randomized controlled trial. *Diabetes Care*. 2014;37:3016–3024.

53. Cata JP, et al. Spinal cord stimulation relieves chemotherapy induced pain: a clinical case report. *J Pain Symptom Manage*. 2004;27:72–78.

54. Filho JL, Braun JM. Spinal cord stimulation in the treatment of refractory painful polyneuropathy induced by chemotherapy. *Rev Bras Anesthesiol*. 2007;57:533–538.

55. Kietrys DM, Galantino ML, Belthoff C, et al. Physical therapy interventions for individuals with HIV associated distal sensory polyneuropathy: a systematic review. *Rehabil Oncol*. 2014;32(3):52–55.

56. Pullen SD, Chigbo NN, Nwigwe EC, et al. Physiotherapy intervention as a complementary treatment for people living with HIV/AIDS. *HIV/AIDS*. 2014;6:99–107.

CHAPTER 12

Acute Herpes Zoster and Postherpetic Neuralgia

NATACHA S. FALCON, DO

INTRODUCTION

Herpes zoster (HZ) is a reactivation of the varicella zoster virus (VZV). VZV is a human α-herpes virus. Primary infection causes varicella (chickenpox), after which VZV becomes latent in the dorsal root ganglia of sensory or cranial nerves. Most cases of acute HZ are self-limited, although a variable percentage of patients may continue to experience pain for months to years after the resolution of the rash, a condition known as postherpetic neuralgia (PHN). Acute HZ is defined as infection occurring up to 30 days after rash onset, with subacute HZ occurring 30–90 days after rash onset. PHN is often defined as pain that persists for >90 days after rash onset, although some sources define it as pain that persists >6 weeks after the onset of disease. PHN is the most frequent chronic complication of HZ (shingles).[1]

PRESENTATION: HISTORICAL AND PHYSICAL FEATURES

VZV reactivates to cause HZ, characterized by a maculopapular or vesicular rash along a dermatomal distribution. The rash is characterized by severe pain, unbearable itching, aching, burning, or electric shock–like pain. The pain may precede the HZ rash. PHN is relatively common, affecting 10%–20% of those with HZ.[2,3] The most common distribution for HZ is the T3-L3 dermatomes (specifically T5 and T6) and the facial region innervated by the ophthalmic division of the trigeminal nerve. HZ preferentially afflicts the elderly and the immunosuppressed. Factors that decrease immune function such as human immunodeficiency virus (HIV) infection, chemotherapy, malignancies, and long-term steroid use may also increase the risk of developing HZ.

DEMOGRAPHICS

The incidence of PHN is 4/1000 per year. The incidence of HZ and PHN increases after 50 years of age. The incidence increases to 12/1000 among individuals aged over 80 years. Two-thirds of HZ cases occur in those aged 50 years or older, and the lifetime risk is 30%.[4] About 20% of patients with HZ develop PHN.

Advancing age and severity of acute HZ pain are the strongest risk factors for PHN. The disease usually occurs between 50 and 79 years of age, and approximately 60% of cases occur in women.[5]

COURSE

HZ arrives when VZV multiplies in sensory ganglia and advances down the affected peripheral afferent sensory nerves in the affected dermatome.[6] VZV is highly infectious, spread by respiratory droplets and direct contact with fluid from the vesicles. The disease course can be divided into four phases: prodrome, acute, subacute, and chronic.[7] The prodrome often occurs 1–5 days before the onset of the HZ rash. The prodrome period consists of hyperesthesia, paresthesias, burning dysesthesias, or pruritus along the affected dermatomes. Constitutional symptoms generally occur during the prodrome phase, consisting of fever, headaches, and malaise. The acute phase of HZ is characterized by a maculopapular or vesicular rash along a dermatomal distribution in conjunction with acute pain.

DIFFERENTIAL DIAGNOSIS

The clinical diagnosis of HZ is made if there is pain and the typical rash in a dermatomal distribution. The main consideration in the differential diagnosis is zosteriform herpes simplex (Table 12.1). Herpes simplex virus (HSV-1) causes oral herpes, also known as cold sores. Herpes simplex virus 2 (HSV-2) causes genital herpes, which usually involves the genitals, buttocks, mouth, lips, and fingers. HSV-2 most commonly affects younger adults and is not associated with chronic pain.

During the prodromal stage of HZ, the cause is not readily apparent (as the rash has not yet erupted), leading to difficulty in diagnosis. The intensity of the pain associated with HZ and PHN may lead to misdiagnosis such as renal colic, appendicitis, myocardial infarction, pleurisy, trigeminal neuralgia, acute musculoskeletal pain, or gastrointestinal or gynecologic disorders, depending on the location of symptoms. One clue may be hyperesthetic skin in the affected dermatome. The characteristic rash of HZ erupts an average of 3–5 days after the prodrome, at which point diagnosis becomes apparent.

DIAGNOSTIC TESTING

The diagnosis of HZ is usually based on clinical presentation of prodrome and rash. Laboratory confirmation

TABLE 12.1
Herpes Simplex Virus (HHV) Types

HHV1	Herpes simplex virus (HSV-1)	Oral herpes (cold sores)
HHV2	Herpes simplex virus (HSV-2)	Genital herpes
HHV3	Varicella zoster virus	Chickenpox (infected first time) Shingles (with recurrence)
HHV4	Epstein Barr virus	Mononucleosis
HHV5	Cytomegalovirus	Symptoms similar to rubella
HHV6	Roseolovirus	Roseola infantum
HHV7	Similar to HHV6	
HHV8	Kaposi sarcoma associated herpes virus	Form of cancer commonly seen in AIDS

is not usually necessary to diagnosis HZ but may be useful to differentiate HZ from herpes simplex for atypical presentations (Table 12.2). A patient may have prodromal symptoms without developing the characteristic rash (zoster sine herpete), making diagnosis difficult and requiring laboratory confirmation of VZV.[8]

If a rash is present, fluid obtained from vesicles may be evaluated with polymerase chain reaction (PCR) testing, viral culture, or direct immunofluorescent antigen staining.[8] Vesicle scrapings evaluated using immunofluorescence is the preferred method because it is rapid, specific, and very sensitive.[8,9] Standard culture is slow with a turnaround time of days and has low sensitivity. VZV DNA detection using PCR has very high sensitivity and specificity, with fast turnaround time of hours. PCR, however, is not readily available and is used only in select research laboratories.[8,9] Tzanck smears of lesions are inexpensive and can be performed at bedside. This technique is nonspecific and cannot differentiate VZV from herpes simplex virus infections.[6]

If a rash is not present, serologic (antibody) methods may be used for laboratory diagnosis of HZ. Two classes of VZV antibodies may be found in the blood: IgM and IgG. There are challenges to interpreting the results.

TREATMENT
Medication Options

Treatment of PHN includes[1] treatment of the acute viral infection,[4] treatment of the acute pain associated with HZ, and[8] prevention/treatment of PHN.

Antiviral Therapy

Antiviral therapy is the first-line treatment. Three guanosine analogues, acyclovir (Zovirax), famciclovir (Famvir), and valacyclovir (Valtrex), are approved by the US Food and Drug Administration (FDA) for the

TABLE 12.2
Laboratory Diagnostic Testing for Herpes Zoster

Test	Sensitivity	Specificity	Turnaround
Immunofluorescence	Very high (82%)	High (76%)	Hours
Culture	Low (20%)	High (99%)	Days
Polymerase chain reaction (DNA)	Very high (95%)	High (99%)	Hours
Serology	Moderate	Moderate	Weeks

Data from Schmader K. Management of herpes zoster in elderly patients. *Infect Dis Clin Pract*. 1995;4:293–299, Sauerbrei A, Eichhorn U, Schicke M, et al. Laboratory diagnosis of herpes zoster. *J Clin Virol*. 1999;14(1):31–36, and Drew WL, Mintz L. Rapid diagnosis of varicella-zoster virus infection by direct immunofluorescence. *Am J Clin Pathol*. 1980;73:699–701.

treatment of acute HZ (Table 12.3). It is recommended that treatment be initiated within 72 h after the onset of the rash. Antivirals have been shown to decease the duration of the HZ rash, reduce the formation of new lesions, reduce viral shedding, and decrease the severity of acute pain, if received within 72 h after the onset of rash and before the crusting of lesions. Studies are variable regarding the effectiveness of antivirals in preventing PHN. Treatment with antivirals is recommended for patients with an increased risk for complications with HZ, which include age >50 years of age, moderate to severe pain, severe rash, involvement of the face or eye, or immunocompromised state.[10]

In controlled clinical trials, acyclovir given within 47 h after the onset of rash shortened the mean time to last day of new lesion formation, the loss of vesicles, and full crusting compared with placebo.[11] In multiple studies, acyclovir seems to produce a moderate reduction in the development of PHN.[12] A cohort study of 419 patients with HZ found that patients receiving antiviral therapy (famciclovir vs. placebo) had a significantly lower prevalence of PHN.[13]

The choice of antiviral agent may be based on the dosing schedule and cost considerations. The most common adverse effects are nausea, headache, vomiting, abdominal pain, and dizziness.

Topical Treatments

Topical treatments may be considered for mild pain. The FDA has approved two topical medications for PHN. Lidocaine patches 5% (Lidoderm, Xylocaine), Capsaicin 0.075% cream, or Capsaicin 8% patch may be useful for pain associated with HZ. Evidence in support of their efficacy is limited. Systematic reviews suggest that topical lidocaine (5%) is beneficial for pain relief in PHN.[14,15] Capsaicin cream (Zostrix), derived from peppers, provides limited reduction in PHN and is associated with site reactions.[16]

TABLE 12.3
Antiviral Treatment for Herpes Zoster

Medication	Dosage
Acyclovir (Zovirax)	800 mg orally five times daily for 7–10 days; or 10 mg per kg intravenously every 8 h for 7–10 days
Famciclovir (Famvir)	500 mg orally three times daily for 7 days
Valacyclovir (Valtrex)	1000 mg orally three times daily for 7 days

Patches and creams should not be applied over the rash or open lesions. Topical agents are valuable treatment options in elderly and frail patients secondary to an excellent safety and tolerability profile.

See Table 12.4 for a summary of pharmacologic options for PHN.

Oral Medications
Corticosteroids

Oral corticosteroids are commonly used in the treatment of HZ. Clinical trials have shown variable results. Corticosteroids prescribed in the acute phase of HZ have been shown to be ineffective in preventing PHN in several trials and a recent review.[19]

Analgesics

First-line agents include tricyclic antidepressants (TCAs) and calcium channel α-γ ligands/anticonvulsants (gabapentin, pregabalin) for PHN. TCAs frequently used include nortriptyline (Pamelor, Aventyl), desipramine (Norpramin), amitriptyline (Vanatrip, Elavil, Endep), and imipramine (Tofranil). TCAs should be used with caution in the elderly and avoided in patients with cardiac disease, glaucoma, or a seizure disorder. Practitioners need to be knowledgeable of anticholinergic side effects, including dry mouth, urinary retention, drowsiness, blurred vision, weight gain, and constipation.

Mild to moderate pain may be relieved with acetaminophen or nonsteroidal antiinflammatories.

Tramadol, a weaker opioid medication, has also been found to be effective for neuropathic pain, including PHN.[20]

Moderate to severe pain may be treated with opioid medications (hydrocodone, oxycodone, morphine). Some clinical trials suggest that opioids (morphine and oxycodone) are effective in PHN.[21,22] A Cochrane review concluded that there was not convincing evidence supporting oxycodone in the treatment of PHN.[23]

Adjunctive therapy should be considered for pain not responding to opioids or if a patient is unable to tolerate opioids.

REHABILITATION AND PHYSICAL MEDICINE OPTIONS
Alternative Treatments

Effective treatment of PHN often requires a multimodal approach. In addition to medications, complementary and alternative medicine (CAM), transcutaneous electrical nerve stimulation (TENS), and cognitive techniques (relaxation, mind-body, hypnotism, and biofeedback) may be beneficial.

TABLE 12.4
Pharmacologic Options for Postherpetic Neuralgia

Medication	Dosage
TOPICAL AGENTS	
Capsaicin cream (Zostrix)	Apply to affected area three to five times daily
Lidocaine patch 5% (Xylocaine)	Apply patch to area of pain once daily for up to 12 h. Maximum of three patches
TRICYCLIC ANTIDEPRESSANTS	
Amitriptyline (Elavil)	Starting dosage 10–25 mg at bedtime. Usual effective dosage 75–100 mg/day. Maximum dosage 150 mg/day
Desipramine (Norpramin)	Starting dosage 25 mg at bedtime. Usual effective dosage 75–100 mg/day. Maximum dosage 150 mg/day
Nortriptyline (Pamelor)	Starting dosage 10–25 mg at bedtime. Usual effective dosage 75–100 mg/day. Maximum dosage 125 mg/day
Imipramine (Tofranil)	Starting dosage 25 mg at bedtime. Maximum dosage 150 mg/day
ANTICONVULSANTS	
Gabapentin (Neurontin)	Starting dosage 100–300 mg at bedtime. Maximum dosage of 3600 mg (divided into three doses)
Carbamazepine (Tegretol)	
Pregabalin (Lyrica)	Starting dosage 50–75 mg twice daily. Maximum dosage of 600 mg daily (divided into 2–3 doses)
Phenytoin (Dilantin)	100–300 mg at bedtime
Carbamazepine (Tegretol)	Starting 100 mg at bedtime. Increase to 200 mg three times daily
Gastroretentive (Gralise)	
OPIOID AGONISTS	
Tramadol	50 mg every 4–6 h. Maximum dose of 400 mg/day (300 mg/day in patients >75 years of age)
Oxycodone	5–15 mg every 4 h as needed
Morphine	

Data from Johnson RW, Rice AS. Clinical practice. Postherpetic neuralgia, *N Engl J Med*. 2014;371:1526–1533, Haanapaa M, Rice A, Rowbotham M. *Treating Herpes Zoster and Postherpetic Neuralgia*. International Assoc for the Study of Pain (IASP); May 2015, and Stances SJ, Dlugopolski M, Packer D. Management of herpes zoster (shingles) and postherpetic neuralgia. *Am Fam Physician*. 2000;61(8):2437–2444.

A randomized controlled trial using CAM therapies to include acupuncture, neural therapy (injection of local anesthetic), cupping and bleeding, and traditional Chinese medicinal herbs was associated with significantly reduced subacute and chronic post-HZ neuralgia pain within 3 weeks of initiating treatment. Improvements persisted for up to 2 years.[24]

Acupuncture

Acupuncture, an ancient Chinese technique, is based on the belief that when the energy force in your body (Qi) is blocked, it can create pain. With this technique, the acupuncturist inserts fine needles into your skin to help promote the flow of Qi. A trial of acupuncture did not show efficacy, as compared with placebo, for relief of PHN.[25]

Transcutaneous electrical nerve stimulation

TENS can be an important adjunct to the management of pain, especially in the elderly, when they are not able to tolerate medications. A randomized study using TENS with a biofeedback capability showed that patients treated by the true device, over the sham device, reported a statistically significant decrease in pain scores.[26] A study showed that pregabalin administration provides better results when combined with TENS therapy in reducing pain in patients with PHN.[27]

Procedural and Surgical Options

Sympathetic blockade can be performed to prevent PHN. In a retrospective study, 90% of patients were pain-free when treatment began within 2 months of zoster onset.[28]

Evidence is lacking that local anesthetic or sympathetic neurolytic blocks are beneficial in the treatment of PHN.[29]

Spinal intrathecal injections of methylprednisolone was reported to be effective in one randomized controlled trial. Concerns for safety of this intervention were raised secondary to increased risk of arachnoiditis or fungal meningitis.[30,31]

Epidural steroid injections

The PINE study assessed the effectiveness of a single epidural injection of steroids and local anesthetic for the prevention of PHN in older patients with HZ. A single epidural injection of steroids and local anesthetic in the acute phase of HZ had a modest effect in reducing zoster-associated pain for 1 month and was not effective for the prevention of long-term PHN.[32]

Intramuscular injections of methylcobalamin combined with lidocaine for acute herpetic neuralgia may be an effective therapeutic option.[4]

Botulinum toxin

Studies suggest Botox may be useful for the treatment of refractory PHN.[33,34]

Pulsed radio frequency seemed to have beneficial effects on PHN after 1 week, 1 month, and 3 months.[1]

High-frequency repetitive transcranial magnetic stimulation (rTMS) was found to be an effective and safe therapy in patients with PHN.[35] The results of this randomized controlled trial confirms that 10 daily rTMS sessions of the primary motor cortex (M1) versus sham stimulation may be effective in PHN for decreasing the intensity of pain and reducing analgesic dosages, without serious adverse events.

The International Association for the Study of Pain Neuropathic Pain Special Interest Group (NeuPSIG) evaluated systematic reviews, clinical trials & guidelines for interventional management of NP. The review concluded owing to adverse events, and low quality of evidence in support of benefit, spinal cord stimulation, deep brain stimulation, and intrathecal medication delivery is inconclusive in the treatment of PHN and should be used only as a last resort.[29]

Surgical excision of skin affected by PHN seemed be an effective treatment initially, but long-term follow-up showed this approach to be ineffective.[36]

PREVENTION OF HZ AND PHN

The only well-documented means of preventing PHN is prevention of HZ. A live attenuated VZV vaccine has been available since 2006. It was initially licensed for immunocompetent persons 60 years or older. Although the vaccine is approved for people 50 years and older, the Centers for Disease Control and Prevention does not recommend it until 60 years of age. Zostavax is the only HZ vaccine currently approved for use in the United States. Zostavax is administered as a single 0.65-mL dose subcutaneously in the deltoid region of the upper arm. Since the introduction of VZV vaccines, the rates of infection, hospitalizations, and mortality have declined. A randomized trial, including patients 60–69 years of age, found that VZV vaccines reduced the incidence of HZ by 51% and the incidence of PHN by 66%. In patients 70 years or older, the vaccine reduced the risk of HZ by 38% but had similar protection against PHN with a reduction of 67%.[37]

PROGNOSIS FOR PAIN AND FUNCTION

PHN results in suffering, reduced quality of life, and individual as well as societal healthcare costs. Patients with PHN may have sleep disorders, depression, anxiety, weight loss, and difficulty concentrating. Patients may be unable to complete activities of daily living, such as bathing, dressing, grooming, shopping, cooking, and household work. The disorder may transition an elderly person from independent living to dependent care. Patients may socialize less, resulting in reduced quality of life, physical functioning, and psychological well-being.[1,6,21]

REFERENCES

1. Johnson RW, Rice AS. Clinical practice. Postherpetic neuralgia. *N Engl J Med*. 2014;371:1526–1533.
2. Yawn BP, Saddier P, Wollan PC, St Sauver JL, Kurland MJ, Sy LS. A population-based study of the incidence and complication rates of herpes zoster before zoster vaccine introduction. *Mayo Clin Proc*. 2007;82:1341–1349.
3. Arvin A. Aging, immunity, and the varicella-zoster virus. *N Engl J Med*. 2005;352:2266–2267.
4. Kawai K, Gebremeskel BG, Acosta CJ. Systematic review of incidence and complications of herpes zoster: towards a global perspective. *BMJ Open*. 2014;4:e004833.
5. Insigna RP, Itzler RF, Pellissier JM, et al. The incidence of herpes zoster in a United States administrative database. *J Gen Intern Med*. 2005;20(8):748–753.
6. Schmader K. Management of herpes zoster in elderly patients. *Infect Dis Clin Pract*. 1995;4:293–299.
7. Volpi A, Gross G, Hercogova J, Johnson RW. Current management of herpes zoster: the European view. *Am J Clin Dermatol*. 2005;6:317–325.
8. Sauerbrei A, Eichhorn U, Schicke M, et al. Laboratory diagnosis of herpes zoster. *J Clin Virol*. 1999;14(1):31–36.

9. Drew WL, Mintz L. Rapid diagnosis of varicella-zoster virus infection by direct immunofluorescence. *Am J Clin Pathol.* 1980;73:699–701.

10. Dworkin RH, Johnson RW, Breuer J, et al. Recommendations for the management of herpes zoster. *Clin Infect Dis.* 2007;44(suppl 1):S1–S26.

11. McKendrick MW, McGill JI, White JE, Wood MJ. Oral acyclovir in acute herpes zoster. *Br Med J (Clin Res Ed).* 1986;293:1529–1532.

12. Crooks RJ, Jones DA, Fiddian AP. Zoster-associated chronic pain: an overview of clinical trials with acyclovir. *Stand J Infect Dis Suppl.* 1991;80:62–68.

13. Dworkin RH, Boon RJ, Griffin DR, Phung D. Postherpetic neuralgia: impact of famciclovir,age, rash severity, and acute pain in herpes zoster patients. *J Infect Dis.* 1998;178(suppl 1):S76–S80.

14. Derry S, Wiffen PJ, Moore RA, Quinlan J. Topical lidocaine for neuropathic pain in adults (review). *Cochrane Database Syst Rev.* 2014;7:CD010958.

15. Khaliq W, Alam S, Puri N. Topical lidocaine for the treatment of postherpetic neuralgia. *Cochrane Database Syst Rev.* 2007;(2):CD004846.

16. *Quetenza (Capsaicin) Package Insert.* Ardsley, NY: Acorda Therapeutics, Inc.; 2013.

17. Haanapaa M, Rice A, Rowbotham M. *Treating Herpes Zoster and Postherpetic Neuralgia.* International Assoc for the Study of Pain (IASP); May 2015.

18. Stances SJ, Dlugopolski M, Packer D. Management of herpes zoster (shingles) and postherpetic neuralgia. *Am Fam Physician.* 2000;61(8):2437–2444.

19. Chen N, Yang M, He L, Zhang D, Zhou M, Zhu C. Corticosteroids for preventing postherpetic neuralgia. *Cochrane Database Syst Rev.* 2010;(12):CD005582.

20. Hollingshead J, Duhmke RM, Cornblath DR. Tramadol for neuropathic pain. *Cochrane Database Syst Rec.* 2006;3:CD003726.

21. Hempenstall K, Nurmikko TJ, Johnson RW, A'Hern RP, Rice AS. Analgesic therapy in postherpetic neuralgia: a quantitative systematic review. *PLoS Med.* 2005;2(7):e164.

22. Finnerup NB, Sindrup SH, Jensen TS. The evidence of pharmacological treatment of neuropathic pain. *Pain.* 2010;150:573–581.

23. McNicol ED, Midair A, Eisenberg E. Opioids for neuropathic pain. *Cochrane Database Syst Rev.* 2013;8:CD006146.

24. Hui F, Boyle E, Vayda E, Glazier RH. A randomized controlled trial of a multifaceted integrated complementary-alternative therapy for chronic herpes zoster-related pain. *Altern Med Rev.* 2012;17(1):57–68.

25. Lewith GT, Field J, Field J, Machin D. Acupuncture compared with placebo in postherpetic pain. *Pain.* 1983;17:361–368.

26. Ing MR, Hellreich PD, Johnson DW, Chen JJ. Transcutaneous electrical nerve stimulation for chronic post-herpetic neuralgia. *Int J Dermatol.* 2015;54(4):476–480.

27. Barbarisi M, Pace MC, Passavanti MB, et al. Pregabalin and transcutaneous electrical nerve stimulation for postherpetic neuralgia treatment. *Clin J Pain.* 2010;26(7):567–572.

28. Rowbotham MC, Reinser-Keller LA, Fields H. Both intravenous lidocaine and morphine reduce the pain of postherpetic neuralgia. *Neurology.* 1991;41(7):1024–1028.

29. Dworkin RH, O'Connor AB, Kent J, et al. Interventional management of neuropathic pain: NeuPSIG recommendations. *Pain.* 2013;154:2249–2261.

30. Nelson DA, Landau WM, Lampe JB, et al. Intrathecal methylprednisolone for postherpetic neuralgia. *N Engl J Med.* 2001;344:1019–1022.

31. Kotani N, Kushikata T, Hashimoto H, et al. Intrathecal methylprednisolone for intractable postherpetic neuralgia. *N Engl J Med.* 2000;343:1514–1519.

32. van Wijck AJ, Opstelten W, Moons KG, et al. The PINE study of epidural steroids and local anesthetics to prevent postherpetic neuralgia: a randomized controlled trial. *Lancet.* 2006;367(9506):219–224.

33. Emad MR, Emad M, Taheri P. The efficacy of intradermal injection of botulinum toxin in patients with post-herpetic neuralgia. *Iranian Red Crescent Med J.* 2011;13(5):323–327.

34. Xiao L, Hui H. *Therapeutic Effect of Botulinum Toxin A in the Treatment of Postherpetic Neuralgia by Subcutaneous Injection.* AAPM; 2010. abstract 206.

35. Ma SM, Ni JX, Li XY. High-frequency repetitive transcranial magnetic stimulation reduces pain in postherpetic neuralgia. *Pain Med.* 2015;16:2162–2170.

36. Peterson KL, Rowbotham MC. Relief of post-herpetic neuralgia by surgical removal of painful skin: 5 years later. *Pain.* 2007;131:214–218.

37. Oxman MN, Levin MJ, Johnson GR, et al. A vaccine to prevent herpes zoster and postherpetic neuralgia in older adults. *N Engl J Med.* 2005;352:2271–2284.

FURTHER READING

1. Shi Y, Wu W. Treatment of neuropathic pain using pulsed radio frequency: a meta-analysis. *Pain Physician.* 2016;19:429–444.

2. Xu G, Xu S, Tang WZ, et al. Local injection of methylcobalamin combined with lidocaine for acute herpetic neuralgia. *Pain Med.* 2016;17(3):572–581.

3. Wang L, Zhu L, Zhu H. Efficacy of varicella (VZV) vaccination: an update for the clinician. *Ther Adv Vaccines.* 2016;4(1–2):20–31.

4. Finnerup NB, Attal N, Haroutounian S, et al. Pharmacotherapy for neuropathic pain in adults: a systemic review and meta-analysis. *Lancet Neurol.* 2015;14:162–173.

5. Wang SM. An integrative approach for treating postherpetic neuralgia-a case report. [abstract] *Pain Pract.* 2007;7(3):274–278.

6. Jeon YH. Herpes zoster and postherpetic neuralgia: practical consideration for prevention and treatment. *Korean J Pain.* 2015;28(3):177–184.

7. Johnson RW, Bouhassira D, Kassianos G, Leplège A, Schmader KE, Weinke T. The impact of herpes zoster and post-herpetic neuralgia on quality-of-life. *BMC Med.* 2010;8:37.
8. Gnann Jr JW, Whitley RJ. Clinical practice: herpes zoster. *N Engl J Med.* 2002;347:340–346.
9. Schmader K, Gnann Jr JW, Watson CP. The epidemiological, clinical, and pathological rationale for the herpes zoster vaccine. *J Infect Dis.* 2008;197(suppl 2):S207–S215.
10. Opstelten W, Mauritz JW, de Wit NJ, van Wijck AJ, Stalman WA, van Essen GA. Herpes zoster and postherpetic neuralgia: incidence and risk indicators using a general practice research database. *Fam Pract.* 2002;19:471–475.

CHAPTER 13

Neuropathic Pain Syndromes in Neuroborreliosis

HOUMAN DANESH, MD • ELINA ZAKIN, MD

INTRODUCTION

Lyme neuroborreliosis designates neurologic involvement during systemic infection with the spirochete *Borrelia burgdorferi*.[1] Individuals become infected with *B. burgdorferi* by the bite of an infected *Ixodes* tick.[2] Lyme disease, like syphilis (another spirochetal infection), is thought to have three stages: acute localized disease (i.e., erythema migrans), early disseminated disease, and late disseminated disease.[3] The organism can affect many organ systems, typically with the skin being the primary site of inoculation in about 80% of infected individuals. Subsequent joint involvement is also common, followed by the nervous system, which can be affected in 10%–15% of individuals infected with Lyme disease.[4] The neurologic manifestations are discussed in detail in this chapter and can range from lymphocytic meningitis to cranial neuropathies to radiculoneuritis. Additional manifestations, including post-Lyme disease syndrome and chronic Lyme disease, are also discussed in this chapter.

This chapter aims to discuss both the pharmacologic and nonpharmacologic treatment strategies for neuropathic pain secondary to neuroborreliosis. A brief discussion of antimicrobial therapy and evidence for the duration of therapy are presented later in the chapter. This is followed by a discussion of the evidence for treatment of acute neurologic manifestations of Lyme disease, followed by the treatment of late neurologic manifestations. Initial focus on antimicrobial therapy followed by a discussion of evidence for the treatment of neuropathic pain from neuroborreliosis is presented.

PATHOPHYSIOLOGY

Individuals become infected with *B. burgdorferi* by the bite of an infected *Ixodes* tick.[2] Most of the available evidence attributes the pathogenesis of Lyme neuroborreliosis to the invasion of the central and peripheral nervous system by *B. burgdorferi*. Symptoms of Lyme neuroborreliosis are due to multifocal inflammatory involvement, predominantly in the subarachnoid space and perineural tissue, with common features of a subacute course over weeks to months after initial presentation of skin lesions (i.e., erythema migrans, which occurs in about 40% of individuals)[5] (see Fig. 13.1).

NEUROLOGIC MANIFESTATIONS OF LYME DISEASE

By definition, nervous system involvement occurs only in the disseminated form of Lyme disease. Lymphocytic meningitis, cranial neuropathy (especially facial palsy), and radiculoneuritis (which may involve either sensory or motor nerves) constitute the triad of early and acute Lyme neuroborreliosis. Symptoms of a painful disseminated polyneuropathy reflect a more indolent onset and protracted time course.[6]

Central nervous system (CNS) involvement in Lyme disease most commonly presents with lymphocytic meningitis and rarely with inflammation of the actual parenchyma (an encephalomyelitis)[7] (Box 13.1). Lyme meningitis is indistinguishable from viral meningitis presenting with headache, fever, neck stiffness, and systemic symptoms. Cerebrospinal fluid analysis is critical in establishing an accurate diagnosis, with particular attention to the percentage of mononuclear cells along with clinical evidence of cranial neuropathies.[8] Lyme encephalomyelitis may present with segmental spinal cord involvement (at the level of the affected nerve root).[9] Magnetic resonance imaging of the brain and spinal cord may reveal inflammatory changes involving the brain parenchyma, and cerebrospinal fluid analysis may show an elevated total immunoglobulin level and oligoclonal bands.[10] Lyme encephalomyelitis is responsive to the appropriate antimicrobial therapy, although sequelae of neurologic injury may persist despite treatment, including neuropathic pain, intracranial hypertension, and encephalopathy.

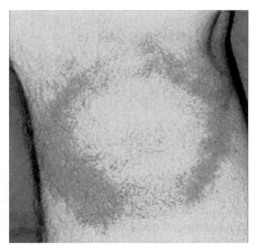

FIG. 13.1 Rash of erythema chronicum migrans on the leg in Lyme disease. (From Goering R, Dockrell H, Zuckerman M, Roitt I, Chiodini P. Vector-borne infections. In: *Mims' Medical Microbiology*, 5th ed. Elsevier Saunders; 2013; with permission.)

BOX 13.1
Summary of Central Nervous System Manifestations of Lyme Disease

Lymphocytic meningitis
Unilateral or bilateral cranial nerve palsies (most common of the facial nerve)
Radiculopathy
Peripheral neuropathy
Mononeuropathy multiplex
Cerebellar ataxia (rare)
Encephalomyelitis (rare)

Peripheral nervous system involvement in neuroborreliosis is typically a multifocal axonal inflammatory process, although the pathophysiology remains poorly understood. There are various suggested mechanisms, including a possible immunologic cross-reactivity, which may be responsible for the damage to the nerve axons.[11] No evidence of spirochetes is present on peripheral nerve analysis, with a few spirochetes identified in the dorsal root ganglia in experimental studies on monkeys.[12] Typical peripheral nervous system manifestations of Lyme disease include cranial neuropathies and radiculoneuritis, although some individuals may develop mononeuropathies, such as mononeuritis multiplex.

Cranial neuropathies occur in 8% of individuals with confirmed Lyme disease, as diagnosed with a positive anti-*B. burgdorferi* IgM antibody in the peripheral blood. They occur early in the disease course and most commonly involve the facial nerve. Other cranial nerves that can be involved include the vestibulocochlear, the lower division of the trigeminal, and the optic nerve, which can present as swelling of the optic nerve head (caused by increased intracranial pressure), inflammation of the optic nerve, or papillitis.[13] About 3% of individuals with confirmed Lyme disease may also develop radiculoneuritis, which is an inflammation of the spinal nerve or nerve roots. Pain is the most prominent presentation, often mimicking mechanical radicular pain in one or several dermatomes.[14] In addition, early in the course of neuroborreliosis, individuals may experience brachial or lumbosacral plexopathies and mononeuropathies. If the infection is left untreated, patients can develop a distal polyneuropathy clinically, which is thought to be due to a confluent mononeuropathy multiplex involving multiple smaller nerve branches.[15]

POST-LYME DISEASE SYNDROME

Some patients, despite therapy with the recommended 10–21 day course of antibiotics, may continue to have vague residual chronic symptoms, which are referred to as post-Lyme syndrome (PLS), post-Lyme disease syndrome, post-treatment chronic Lyme disease, or chronic Lyme disease. Post-Lyme disease syndrome is often used to describe nonspecific symptoms that may persist even months after antimicrobial therapy for Lyme disease, including headache, fatigue, and diffuse arthralgias.[16] According to the Infectious Diseases Society of America, criteria for the diagnosis of post-Lyme disease syndrome includes:

1. A prior history of Lyme disease treated with an accepted regimen, with subsequent resolution or stabilization of the manifestations of the disease
2. Onset of subjective symptoms (i.e., fatigue, diffuse musculoskeletal pain, or cognitive difficulties), which occur within 6 months of diagnosis of Lyme disease and are persistent for at least 6 months after completion of antimicrobial therapy.

This disease entity remains controversial, and its etiology remains unclear. The proportion of patients who develop post-Lyme disease syndrome is small.

The American Academy of Neurology (AAN) parameters present some data, although controversial, for post-Lyme disease therapy. The controversy largely lies in the question of whether PLS is a form of active infection, wherein the organism is too difficult to eradicate, or is perhaps a postinfectious or noninfectious chronic syndrome (with no active infection). In addition, the symptoms of PLS (i.e., cognitive difficulties, fatigue) are difficult to objectively evaluate with physical examination or laboratory analysis (especially if compared with those symptoms of patients with untreated Lyme disease). Data argue against persistent infection in those who have undergone curative courses of the recommended antimicrobial therapy, as there is no known antibiotic resistance to *Borrelia*, there is no correlate of persistent symptoms with any objective measures on examination or laboratory studies, and usually, there is undetectable antibody to *B. burgdorferi* (despite persistent symptoms).

OVERVIEW OF ANTIMICROBIAL THERAPY

The best available method for preventing infection with *B. burgdorferi* is to avoid exposure to vector ticks. The 2006 Infectious Disease Society of America updated guidelines for the treatment and prevention of Lyme disease state there is no recommendation for antimicrobial prophylaxis or serologic testing for the prevention of Lyme disease after a recognized tick bite. A single dose of doxycycline may be offered for adult patients and children over the age of 8 years (200 mg for adults, 4 mg/kg up to maximum 200 mg for children).[17] This regimen is contraindicated in pregnant women and children less than 8 years of age.

Depending on the stage of infection, the Infectious Disease Society has specific antimicrobial recommendations as noted in Table 13.1. Specifically, for early evidence of disease, such as erythema migrans, the recommended therapy is a 10–21 day course of doxycycline 100 mg twice per day, amoxicillin 500 mg three times per day, or cefuroxime 500 mg twice per day. The AAN published practice parameters for the treatment of CNS Lyme disease in 2007.[18] Specific recommendations for antimicrobial therapy are noted in Table 13.1. The AAN practice parameters note that evidence for antimicrobial therapy in neuroborreliosis is currently without placebo-controlled trials given the presence of residual symptoms (after therapy for erythema migrans). The initial literature in the 1980s noted that 12 patients treated with high-dose intravenous (IV) penicillin had a more rapid resolution of Lyme meningitis as compared with those who did not receive penicillin (with the untreated group later exposed to IV penicillin therapy with good recovery and fewer relapses).[19] Additional studies of antimicrobial therapy in facial nerve palsies secondary to Lyme disease did not show hastening of the palsy's resolution but did help prevent further sequelae. Studies subsequently showed comparison efficacy of various regimens presented in Table 13.1.

The AAN put forth the following recommendations in 2007:
1. Parenteral penicillin, ceftriaxone, and cefotaxime are probably safe and effective treatments for peripheral nervous system Lyme disease and CNS Lyme disease with or without parenchymal involvement.
2. Oral doxycycline is probably a safe and effective treatment for peripheral nervous system Lyme disease and for CNS Lyme disease without parenchymal involvement, with supporting data presently lacking for amoxicillin and cefuroxime as alternate therapy.

TREATMENT OF POST-LYME SYNDROME

The AAN performed three randomized, double-blind placebo-controlled trials of antibiotic therapy in PLS. Metrics evaluated included the quality of life and level of fatigue along with formal neuropsychological evaluations. Continued antimicrobial therapy was compared with placebo. The AAN concluded that PLS does not respond to prolonged courses of antibiotics. Prolonged antibiotic therapy can have detrimental effects, including infection caused by the prolonged usage of peripheral IV catheters.

PAIN IN NEUROBORRELIOSIS

The International Association for the Study of Pain defines neuropathic pain as "pain initiated or caused by a primary lesion of dysfunction in the nervous system."[20] Neuropathic pain is a manifestation of several different disorders that affect the somatosensory aspect of the nervous system, including polyneuropathies (i.e., due to diabetes, alcoholism, amyloidosis, small fiber neuropathies); hereditary neuropathies, mononeuropathies (i.e., trigeminal, glossopharyngeal, postherpetic); entrapment neuropathies, and posttraumatic nerve injuries (i.e., CRPS type II). In addition, pain syndromes can result from abnormalities in the CNS, such as a result of spinal cord injury, multiple sclerosis, or cerebrovascular events.[21]

PHARMACOLOGIC THERAPY FOR NEUROPATHIC PAIN

The current recommendation guidelines set forth by the International Association for the Study of Pain and Neuropathic Pain Special Interest Group guidelines for the treatment of neuropathic pain recommend a combination of medications over the use of monotherapy, with the recommendation to increase medication in a stepwise manner for efficacy.[22]

TABLE 13.1
Antimicrobial Therapy in Lyme Disease

Indication	Adult Regimen	Pediatric Regimen (Age < 8 years)
Erythema migrans	• PO doxycycline 100 mg BID for 14 days • PO amoxicillin 500 mg TID for 14 days • PO cefuroxime 500 mg BID for 14 days	• PO amoxicillin 50 mg/kg per day in 3 div doses (max 500 mg per dose) for 14 days • PO cefuroxime 30 mg/kg per day in 2 div doses (max 500 mg per dose) for 14 days • If < 8 yo—doxycycline 4 mg/kg per day in 2 div doses (max 100 mg per dose) for 14 days
EARLY MANIFESTATIONS (THERAPY DURATION RANGE 10–21 DAYS IN THE LITERATURE)		
Cranial neuropathy Lyme meningitis Radiculopathy	• Ceftriaxone 2 g IV daily for 14 days • Cefotaxime 2 g IV every 8 h for 14 days • Penicillin G 18–24 million U/day (div doses every 4 h) for 14 days	• Ceftriaxone 50–75 mg/kg per day IV (max 2 g per day) for 14 days • Cefotaxime 150–200 mg/kg per day in 3–4 IV doses per day (max 6 g/day) for 14 days • Penicillin G 200,000–400,000 U/kg per day in 4 div doses (max 18–24 million U/day) for 14 days
LATE MANIFESTATIONS		
Lyme arthritis without CNS manifestations	• PO doxycycline 100 mg BID for 28 days • PO amoxicillin 500 mg TID for 28 days • PO cefuroxime 500 mg BID for 28 days	• PO amoxicillin 50 mg/kg per day in 3 div doses (max 500 mg per dose) for 28 days • PO cefuroxime 30 mg/kg per day in 2 div doses (max 500 mg per dose) for 28 days • If > 8 yo, PO doxycycline 4 mg/kg per day in 2 div doses (max 100 mg per dose) for 28 days
Lyme arthritis with CNS manifestations	• Ceftriaxone 2 g IV daily for 2–4 weeks • Cefotaxime 2 g IV every 8 h for 2–4 weeks • Penicillin G 18–24 million U/day (div doses every 4 h) for 2–4 weeks	• Ceftriaxone 50–75 mg/kg per day IV (max 2 g/day) for 2–4 weeks • Cefotaxime 150–200 mg/kg per day in 3–4 IV doses per day (max 6 g/day) for 2–4 weeks • Penicillin G 200,000–400,000 U/kg per day in 4 div doses (max 18–24 million U/day) for 2–4 weeks
Peripheral neuropathy Mononeuritis multiplex	• PO doxycycline 100 mg BID for 28 days	
Encephalomyelitis Encephalopathy	• Ceftriaxone 2 g IV daily for 28 days • Cefotaxime 2 g IV every 8 h for 28 days • Penicillin G 18–24 million U/day (div doses every 4 h) for 28 days	

BID, twice daily; *CNS*, central nervous system; *IV*, intravenous; *PO*, by mouth; *TID*, three times daily.

Tricyclic Antidepressants

Based on the current guidelines, the first-line medications are the antidepressant class of medications, which have both norepinephrine and serotonin reuptake inhibition. Tricyclic antidepressants (TCAs) are cost-effective, administered once daily, and treat comorbid depression. It is advisable to initiate amitriptyline at a low dose (i.e., 10–20 mg) and increase by 25 mg every 3–7 days as tolerated. An adequate trial of amitriptyline can usually take 6–8 weeks for efficacy. Adverse side effects include the anticholinergic effects of dry mouth, orthostatic hypotension, constipation, and urinary retention. The provider should prescribe TCAs with caution to patients with cardiac disease or ventricular conduction abnormalities. It is advised that an electrocardiogram be obtained for patients over the age of 40 years and for those individuals who are receiving more than 100 mg/day.[23] Although no placebo-controlled trial exists for the use of TCAs in the management of neuropathic pain in Lyme disease, the use of amitriptyline for pain is supported by experts for the treatment of pain caused by Lyme disease.[24]

Serotonin-Norepinephrine Reuptake Inhibitors

Serotonin-norepinephrine reuptake inhibitors (SNRIs), such as duloxetine and venlafaxine, are effective in maintaining sustained pain relief for 1 year in an open-label trial in diabetic neuropathy. Duloxetine can be used as treatment of comorbid major depression and generalized anxiety disorder at a dose of 60 mg twice daily. The efficacy in the management of other neuropathic pain subtypes has not been adequately studied. Duloxetine is safe in patients with comorbid cardiac conditions but can cause nausea as an adverse side effect. Venlafaxine, another SNRI, has demonstrated efficacy at higher dosages for painful diabetic peripheral neuropathy and various polyneuropathies but not in postherpetic neuralgia.[25] Venlafaxine is available in both short- and long-acting formulations and requires 2–4 weeks to titrate to the efficacious dose. The adverse side effects have been associated with cardiac conduction blocks in patients with cardiac disease. Abruptly stopping venlafaxine can result in a withdrawal syndrome, and the drug should be tapered when discontinued.[26] There is a limited literature to support the use of SNRIs in the management of pain secondary to Lyme disease, but it is thought that SNRIs have a role in modulating central pain, which is implicated in Lyme disease.[27]

The Calcium Channel α_2-δ Ligands

Other first-line medications in the treatment of neuropathic pain are gabapentin and pregabalin, which bind to the voltage-gated calcium channels at the α_2-δ subunit and produce changes in neurotransmitter release. The presumed mechanism of action of gabapentin and pregabalin is by way of inhibiting the calcium channel activation of excitatory transmitter release and spinal sensitization. This class of drugs also activates the descending noradrenergic pain inhibitory system that is coupled to the spinal α_2 adrenoreceptors. In addition, these drugs may have an effect on proinflammatory cytokines and are effective when compared with placebo in various neuropathic pain conditions. The adverse side effects include dose-related dizziness and sedation; therefore it is recommended that these drugs be started at a low dose and titrated with caution. Gabapentin and pregabalin have few drug interactions but should be administered in reduced dosage to patients with renal insufficiency. Gabapentin is administered three times daily given the drug's complex, nonlinear pharmacokinetics (to a maximum dose of 3600 mg/day). Gabapentin may have a delayed onset to reach analgesic effect with the adequate therapeutic dose,

taking up to 2 months to reach analgesic effect, which may be difficult for some patients with neuropathic pain. Pregabalin has more predictable pharmacokinetics, with dosing starting at 150 mg/day divided in two to three doses with titration every 1–2 weeks to a maximum dose of 300 mg/day. Pregabalin has a shorter titration schedule and thus a faster onset of efficacy compared with gabapentin.

A study in Germany evaluated the effect of gabapentin monotherapy on residual pain in patients with neuroborreliosis following a course of IV ceftriaxone treatment. Ten patients with persistent neuropathic pain received doses of gabapentin, initially at 300 mg/day with titration to 500–1200 mg/day (as tolerated). Doses were escalated until pain resolved. There was a notable improvement of the subjective description of "crawling" or "burning" pain as well as a positive effect on mood at a dose of 700 mg/day. The study concluded that gabapentin monotherapy is efficacious in treating pain associated with neuroborreliosis and is associated with improved quality of life in these patients.[28]

Second-Line Agents: Opioid Analgesics and Tramadol

According to the International Meeting of the Special Interest Group on Neuropathic Pain (NeuPSIG) guidelines, second-line medications are deemed appropriate as first-line therapy in certain circumstances, such as for the treatment of acute neuropathic pain, exacerbations of severe neuropathic pain episodes, neuropathic cancer pain, or during a titration of a first-line medication when immediate pain relief is required. These second-line agents are opioid analgesics. In patients with neuropathic pain, opioid analgesics may be considered to achieve quick relief of pain while a first-line medication is being titrated to effect. However, given the current opioid epidemic, this is being done much less frequently. In addition, there are uncertain long-term data regarding the efficacy of opiate use for chronic nonmalignant pain. Opioid use could have many deleterious consequences, including opioid-associated hyperalgesia, decreased testosterone, overdose, and death. In addition, there are concerns for opioid abuse and addiction in patients who have chronic pain, thus opioids should be reserved for select cases. The use of opiates in pain secondary to Lyme disease remains controversial.

Tramadol not only is an agonist of the opioid μ-receptor but also works to inhibit the reuptake of serotonin and norepinephrine. Tramadol has 1/100th the strength of morphine on the opiate receptor; however, it is considered equianalgesic to morphine given the fact that is also affects the serotonin pathway for pain control. It is similar to other opioid analgesics, as it is effective in achieving quick analgesic efficacy and has the same recommendations by the NeuPSIG as opioids for appropriateness in treatment of neuropathic pain. The side-effect profile of tramadol is similar to other opioid analgesics. It can lower the seizure threshold and can precipitate serotonin syndrome when combined with other SNRIs and selective serotonin reuptake inhibitors. Serotonin syndrome is a potentially fatal reaction to serotonergic medications, which can result in cognitive impairment, autonomic derangements, and neuromuscular hyperactivity.[29] Dosing of tramadol can start at 50 mg once daily or twice daily, with a titration to a maximum dose of 400, or 300 mg/day in older patients.

NONPHARMACOLOGIC THERAPY FOR NEUROPATHIC PAIN

Various nonpharmacologic therapies exist for the treatment of neuropathic pain. Some strategies include meditation, acupuncture, thermos therapy, Tai Chi, transcutaneous electrical nerve stimulation, and spinal cord stimulation. These nonpharmacologic therapies have not been formally studied in the management of neuropathic pain secondary to Lyme.

Spinal cord stimulation was evaluated in a patient with bilateral foot pain following Lyme disease (for which he received a 4-week course of penicillin G IV antimicrobial therapy). The patient had a poor response to pharmacologic and physical therapy for his pain. Application of two quadrupolar electrode arrays in the dorsal epidural sac with needle placement at L2-3 and L3-4 for spinal stimulation was performed. The patient noted diminished pain duration and improved mood and sleep after stimulation. No oral pain medication was administered to the patient. After a 7-day trial, the patient reported satisfaction with pain relief; improvement persisted at 1 year after the stimulation trial. In addition, the patient discontinued all opioid medications.[30]

CONCLUSION

Neuroborreliosis can present with both acute and late manifestations. Some presentations include meningoencephalitis, cranial neuropathies, radiculopathy, and peripheral neuropathy. The entity of PLS is a controversial diagnosis. Antimicrobial therapy is first line for treatment of neuroborreliosis, with courses of therapy extending to 28 days. Limited evidence exists

for pharmacologic and nonpharmacologic therapeutic options in the management of neuropathic pain associated with CNS Lyme disease. The best evidence available is the use of gabapentin for the management of neuropathic pain secondary to Lyme disease, with notable improvements in patient quality of life. In addition, one case report revealed positive effects on the use of spinal cord stimulation for modulation of lower extremity pain in an individual patient with pain secondary to Lyme disease. Further research is needed to study the role of various pharmacologic and nonpharmacologic therapies in the management of pain secondary to Lyme disease.

REFERENCES

1. Burgdorfer W, Barbour AG, Hayes SF, Benach JL, Grunwald E, Davis JP. Lyme disease-a tick-borne spirochetosis? *Science*. 1982;216:1317–1319.
2. Fish D. Environmental risk and prevention of Lyme disease. *Am J Med*. 1995;98:S2–S8.
3. Loginian EL, Kaplan RF, Steere AC. Chronic neurologic manifestations of Lyme disease. *N Engl J Med*. 1990;323:1438–1444.
4. Gerber MA, Shapiro ED, Burke GS. Lyme disease in children in southeastern Connecticut. Pediatric Lyme disease study group. *N Engl J Med*. 1996;335:1270.
5. Ackermann R, Horstrup P, Schmidt R. Tick-borne meningopolyneuritis. *Yale J Biol Med*. 1984;57:485–490.
6. Halperin JJ. Neuroborreliosis. *Am J Med*. 1995;98:525–565.
7. Pachner AR, Steere AC. The triad of neurologic manifestations of Lyme disease: meningitis, cranial neuritis, and radiculoneuritis. *Neurology*. 1985;35:47–53.
8. Kaiser R. Neuroborreliosis. *J Neurol*. 1998;245:247–255.
9. Reik Jr L, Burgdorfer W, Donaldson JO. Neurologic abnormalities in Lyme disease without erythema chronicum migrans. *Am J Med*. 1986;81:73.
10. Halperin JJ, Volkman DJ, Wu P. Central nervous system abnormalities in Lyme neuroborreliosis. *Neurology*. 1991;41:1571.
11. Ramesh G, Bord JT, Gill A, et al. Possible role of glial cells in the onset and progression of Lyme neuroborreliosis. *J Neuroinflammation*. 2009;6:23.
12. England JD, Bohm Jr RP, Roberts ED, Philipp MT. Mononeuropathy multiplex in rhesus monkeys with chronic Lyme disease. *Ann Neurol*. 1997;41:375.
13. Halperin JJ. Lyme disease and the peripheral nervous system. *Muscle Nerve*. 2003;28:133.
14. Centers for Disease Control, Prevention (CDC). Lyme disease—United States, 2003-2005. *MMWR Morb Mortal Wkly Rep*. 2007;56:573.
15. Logigian E, Steere A. Clinical and electrophysiologic findings in chronic neuropathy of Lyme disease. *Neurology*. 1992;42:303.

16. Klempner MS, Hu LT, Evans J, et al. Two controlled trials of antibiotic treatment in patients with persistent symptoms and a history of Lyme disease. *N Engl J Med.* 2001;345:85.

17. Wormster GP, et al. The clinical assessment, treatment and prevention of Lyme disease, human granulocytic anaplasmosis, and babesiosis: clinical practice guidelines by the Infectious Diseases Society of America. *Clin Infect Dis.* 2006;43(9):1089–1134.

18. Halperin JJ, et al. Practice parameter: treatment of nervous system Lyme disease (an evidence-based review): report of the Quality Standards Subcommittee of the American Academy of Neurology. *Neurology.* 2007;69(1):91–102.

19. Steere AC, Pachner AR, Malawista SE. Neurologic abnormalities of Lyme disease: successful treatment with high-dose intravenous penicillin. *Ann Intern Med.* 1983;99:767–772.

20. Treede R, Jensen T, et al. Neuropathic pain: redefinition and a grading system for clinical and research purposes. *Neurology.* 2008;70(18):1630–1635.

21. Woolf CJ, American College of Physicians, American Physiological Society. Pain: moving from symptom control toward mechanism-specific pharmacologic management. *Ann Intern Med.* 2004;140(6):441–451.

22. Dworkin RH, et al. Recommendations for the pharmacological management of neuropathic pain: an overview and literature update. *Mayo Clin Proc.* 2010;85(3):S3–S14.

23. Kremer M, et al. Antidepressants and gabapentinoids in neuropathic pain: mechanistic insights. *Neuroscience.* 2016. pii:S0306-4522(16)30296-2.

24. Pfister HW, Rupprecht TA. Clinical aspects of neuroborreliosis and post-Lyme disease syndrome in adult patients. *Int J Med Microbiol.* 2006;296(suppl 40):11–16.

25. Fava M, et al. Emergency of adverse events following discontinuation of treatment with extended-release venlafaxine. *Am J Psychiatry.* 1997;154:1760–1762.

26. Rowbotham MC, et al. Venlafaxine extended release in the treatment of painful diabetic neuropathy: a double-blind, placebo-controlled study. *Pain.* 2004;100:697–706.

27. Dadabhoy D, Clauw DJ. Therapy insight: fibromyalgia – a different type of pain needing a different type of treatment. *Nat Clin Pract Rheumatol.* 2006;2:364–372.

28. Weissenbacher S, Ring J, Hofmann H. Gabapentin for the symptomatic treatment of chronic neuropathic pain in patients with late-stage Lyme borreliosis: a pilot study. *Dermatology.* 2005;211:123–127.

29. Gilron I, Tu D, et al. Combination of morphine with notriptyline for neuropathic pain. *Pain.* 2015;156(8):1440–1448.

30. Shui Y, et al. Spinal cord stimulation for chronic pain originating from Lyme disease: a case report. *Pain Physician.* 2012;15:511–514.

CHAPTER 14

Postmastectomy Pain Syndrome

ALLISON ZIBELLI, MD

Postmastectomy pain syndrome (PMPS) is a common, undertreated condition that affects patients who have had surgery of the breast or axilla. It was hoped that PMPS would decrease in incidence with the movement away from mastectomy and toward lumpectomy and sentinel lymph node dissection. However, it has continued to be a major complication of any breast surgery. Its causes remain poorly understood, and most patients have uncontrolled symptoms despite treatment. PMPS can lead to substantial functional impairment. Pain, sensory loss, adhesive capsulitis, or rotator cuff tendonitis can cause loss of function of the shoulder. It has been estimated that PMPS results in a billion dollars annually of lost productivity.[1]

PRESENTATION

There is no universal definition of PMPS. PMPS is often diagnosed clinically by its location in the anterior thorax or upper arm that occurs on the same side of the body as the breast surgery. The pain lasts from weeks to indefinitely and can be accompanied by phantom breast sensations, sensory loss, paresthesia, or hyperesthesia.[2] Others have defined PMPS more narrowly; Stevens defined the syndrome in 1995 as "paroxysms of sharp pain in a background of burning, aching, and constriction," which are worsened by movement, do not improve, and are not relieved by narcotics.[3] The International Association for the Study of Pain proposed a requirement that the pain has to be present at least 3 months after surgery, when normal healing presumably would have occurred.[4] Most women report that it significantly worsened their quality of life.[3] Brackstone et al. proposed a standard definition of PMPS as "pain after any type of surgery that is at least of moderate intensity and comprises neuropathic qualities, lasts longer than 6 months, is present in the ipsilateral breast/chest/arm, and is present at least half of the time."[5]

EPIDEMIOLOGY

PMPS was first described in the age of the Halstead radical mastectomy, in which the breast, skin, fat, and the major and minor pectoral muscles were removed. In the 1970s, the modified radical mastectomy surgery was developed, which leaves the pectoral muscles intact. More recently, lumpectomy (also known as partial mastectomy) became more widely used. These procedures are usually accompanied by either an axillary lymph node dissection, where multiple lymph nodes are removed and sampled, or a sentinel lymph node dissection, where one to four nodes are identified with blue dye or a radioactive tracer and removed, leaving the majority of lymph nodes intact.

It was hoped that the advent of less extensive surgeries for breast cancer would lead to a decrease in the incidence of PMPS. Unfortunately, this has not proven to be the case. Wallace et al. surveyed 282 women 1 year after breast surgery and found the highest rate of PMPS was after breast augmentation (55%), followed by mastectomy and reconstruction (49%), mastectomy alone (31%), and breast reduction (22%).[6] Fabro conducted a survey of 174 women and found an incidence of PMPS of 52%.[7] Age over 40 years or axillary lymph node dissection of more than 15 nodes conveyed a significantly higher risk. Other factors that predict for persistent postoperative pain include younger age, poorer social support, and greater preoperative anxiety.[8]

PMPS is generally regarded as being caused by damage to the intercostobrachial nerves. Paredes et al. reported on a series of patients whose intercostobrachial nerves were either sectioned or preserved.[9] The patients with sectioned nerves had anesthesia and hypoesthesia in the arm, whereas patients with intact nerves had less of both. A second study reported no difference but was limited by short follow-up and a small sample size.[10] If we accept Brackstone's proposed standard definition, then damage to a regional nerve would be implied. Damage can occur both by transection and contraction of scar tissue around the regional nerves.

PHYSICAL EXAMINATION

All patients with possible PMPS should have a thorough physical examination at baseline and periodically throughout the course of their treatment. Both arms should be measured at the widest part of the wrist, forearm, and bicep. Lymphedema is present if the measurements between the affected arm and the opposite arm differ by more than 110%. Upper body muscle strength should be assessed by testing the involved muscles against resistance. Grip strength should likewise be tested. Both arms should be tested for sensory response using pinprick and light touch. Finally, the entire arm should be palpated to assess for dysesthesia, allodynia, and hyperalgesia.[11]

COURSE

Pain from PMPS can be long lasting or even permanent. MacDonald surveyed 138 patients with a mean time after surgery of 9 years.[12] Approximately half of the patients still had pain. The majority of these patients had mastectomies, and a major risk factor was younger age. Their pain responded poorly to medical treatment.

DIFFERENTIAL DIAGNOSIS

The differential for thorax pain after breast surgery is limited. Intercostal neuroma is an underrecognized entity that is treatable. Wong reported a series of five patients who had complete relief of their pain after resection of neuroma.[13] These patients had a positive Tinel sign at one of the intercostal nerves of the lateral chest wall. This pain was relieved when the site of the Tinel sign was injected with lidocaine. All of these patients were found to have transected nerves, which were embedded in scar tissue, directly below the Tinel sign. After the neuroma was resected, the cut end was allowed to retract into the intercostal muscles. All of these patients had pain relief from 18 to 36 months after surgery. Intercostal neuromas have also been known to cause pain after breast implant placement.[14] Ultrasound-guided cryoablation is a possible treatment modality for this syndrome.[15]

Some patients may develop complex regional pain syndrome after breast surgery. This can be distinguished from PMPS by its unique symptoms. These may include autonomic changes, skin atrophy, and contraction or fibrosis of joints in the hand and arm.

Another treatable cause of postoperative pain in the axilla is axillary hematoma. This entity presents with pain and swelling of the axilla and can be mistaken for a seroma. Fluid-filled lesions are best evaluated by ultrasound. Seromas are bland, homogenous collections on ultrasound imaging. In contrast, hematomas are more complex, often with visible blood and debris.[16] Blunt et al. report a series of three cases where aspiration of

axillary hematoma resulted in substantial, long-lasting relief of pain.[17] One patient required complete resection of the hematoma cavity. They noted that pain from a hematoma may be much greater than that from a seroma of equivalent size. Aspiration of a seroma does not cure PMPS, as most seromas have resolved before the development of PMPS. The presence of a seroma is not associated with a higher risk of PMPS.[18]

Another complication of mastectomy is the axillary web syndrome. This occurs 1–6 weeks after surgery and consists of visible, painful cords in the axilla, which restrict movement. These cords cause pain with shoulder abduction. These patients can often be significantly helped by physical therapy.[19]

It is important to distinguish a compressive radiculopathy from PMPS, because the former is progressive and treatable. The pain in compressive radiculopathy is typically of gradual onset, often accompanied by numbness, severe pain, and variable weakness. The diagnostic test of choice is MRI of the cervical and thoracic spine.[20] Radiculopathy can be benign or malignant; malignant radiculopathy can be diagnosed by a mass on MRI. Malignant lesions should be treated immediately with either radiation or surgery to preserve function. Benign radiculopathy may be treated with physical therapy, nonsteroidal antiinflammatory drugs, or gabapentin.[21]

Brachial plexopathy is a rare, late sequela of radiation therapy that can occur years to decades after therapy. The mechanism is damage to blood vessels, fibrosis of connective tissue around the nerves, and direct damage to the nerves. It presents with pain, paresthesias, and inability to move the affected arm and can lead to muscular atrophy and paralysis. This entity presents late after treatment, with a median onset of 1–4 years after therapy, which helps distinguish it from PMPS.[22]

Venous thrombosis and lymphedema are easily distinguished from PMPS by the presence of erythema and edema.

DIAGNOSTIC TESTING

PMPS is a clinical diagnosis, and diagnostic testing plays a limited role. Gottrup compared patients with pain with those with no pain with sensory testing, including pinprick, thermal thresholds, and assessment of skin blood flow, during brush and pinprick stimulation.[23] He found that cutaneous blood flow measured by laser Doppler was higher on the operative side in patients with PMPS but not in patients without pain. Unfortunately, such testing is not widely available. Other, treatable causes of upper extremity pain should be excluded. In cases where edema or erythema predominates, ultrasound imaging should be performed to rule out Deep Venous Thrombosis. MRI or CT of the shoulder can be done to evaluate for symptomatic bony lesions.

TREATMENT

There is no widely accepted therapy for PMPS. A small study of pulsed high-intensity laser therapy, given three times weekly for a month, with physical therapy, showed an increase in range of movement and quality of life.[24] This study was limited by the absence of a control group. This modality continues to be used.

Psychological support can be quite helpful in helping patients cope with PMPS. Although the literature is not methodologically robust, evidence suggests that cognitive behavioral therapy can be useful for pain reduction.[25] One meta-analysis concluded that psychosocial interventions such as skills training, which helps patients conceptualize their pain differently, and educational training have a "moderate-sized" effect on pain scores.[26]

Physical therapy can be a very useful adjunct to the treatment of PMPS. Patients place a high priority on maintaining function after cancer treatment.[27] Physical therapy techniques that may be helpful include assistive devices, compensatory strategies, therapeutic exercises, and positioning.[28]

Transcutaneous electrical nerve stimulation units have been used for cancer-related pain, but the results thus far have been mixed, and few studies have been able to meet criteria for inclusion in Cochrane reviews, because of design heterogeneity and poor quality.[29] This modality, however, continues to be used because it has few side effects and can be combined with standard physical therapy. In addition, many patients prefer nonpharmacologic treatments.[28]

Myofascial release and treatment of trigger points can be helpful in patients with myofascial pain. These patients usually exhibit tenderness in the painful area, increased muscle tone, and concentrated areas of pain that are sensitive to targeted pressure.[30] Evidence is limited, but massage may provide some temporary relief for cancer-related pain.[31]

Small studies have shown the promise of autologous fat graft into surgical scars. Caviggioli treated a series of 72 patients. Fat was liposuctioned from the abdomen, centrifuged, isolated, and injected into the dermohypodermal junction of the painful surgical scars. A total of 63 patients had a significant decrease in their pain, as compared with a control group of 41 patients.[32]

A few small studies showed benefit from medical therapy. Amr randomized patients to receive placebo,

venlafaxine 37.5 mg daily, or gabapentin 300 mg daily for 10 days starting the day before surgery.[33] Both gabapentin and venlafaxine decreased immediate postoperative pain. Venlafaxine decreased the incidence and intensity of chronic pain at 6 months. Gabapentin decreased the incidence of burning pain at 6 months. An obvious limitation of this treatment is the need to start the intervention before surgery, which would require treating most patients unnecessarily. One widely cited study that claimed to show a long-term benefit of perioperative venlafaxine in decreasing the pain of PMPS was retracted because of concern about fabricated data.[34,35]

Topical capsaicin has more evidence of effectiveness. Dini et al. conducted a small open-label study of 0.025% capsaicin cream three times daily for 2 months.[36] About 70% of patients had reduction of pain. A small randomized study of topical capsaicin versus placebo resulted in 62% of patients in the experimental group having greater than 50% reduction in pain versus 10% of patients in the placebo group.[37]

CONCLUSION

Thus far, treatment for postmastectomy pain has been disappointing. Development of a standard definition of the syndrome should allow researchers to develop better medical and surgical treatments to improve the quality of life of millions of patients who develop this devastating condition every year. Rehabilitation, pharmacologic, and psychological and other modalities have been used for the treatment of PMPS, but further research is needed to find more effective therapies for these patients. PMPS can have a devastating effect on physical, social, occupational, and psychological functioning and thus deserves attention and funding proportionate to its impact. For these patients, even cure may not be enough—they want to live their lives well.

REFERENCES

1. Visnjevac O, Matson B. Postmastectomy pain syndrome: an unrecognized annual billion dollar national financial burden. *J Pain.* 2013;14(4):S33.
2. Jung BF, Ahrendt GM, Oaklander AL, Dworkin RH. Neuropathic pain following breast cancer surgery: proposed classification and research update. *Pain.* 2003;104(1-2):1-13.
3. Stevens PE, Dibble SL, Miaskowski C. Prevalence, characteristics, and impact of postmastectomy pain syndrome: an investigation of women's experiences. *Pain.* 1995;61(1):61-68.

4. Merskey HE. Classification of chronic pain: descriptions of chronic pain syndromes and definitions of pain terms. *Pain.* 1986. Suppl 3, 226.

5. Brackstone M. A review of the literature and discussion: establishing a consensus for the definition of post-mastectomy pain syndrome to provide a standardized clinical and research approach. *Can J Surg.* 2016;59(5): 294-295. http://dx.doi.org/10.1503/cjs.012016.

6. Wallace MS, Wallace AM, Lee J, Dobke MK. Pain after breast surgery: a survey of 282 women. *Pain.* 1996;66(2-3): 195-205. http://dx.doi.org/10.1016/0304-3959(96)03064-3.

7. Fabro EAN, Bergmann A, Silva BAE, et al. Post-mastectomy pain syndrome: incidence and risks. *Breast.* 2012;21(3): 321-325.

8. Kehlet H, Jensen TS, Woolf CJ. Persistent postsurgical pain: risk factors and prevention. *Lancet.* 2006;367(9522): 1618-1625.

9. Paredes JP, Puente JL, Potel J. Variations in sensitivity after sectioning the intercostobrachial nerve. *Am J Surg.* 1990;160(5):525-528. http://dx.doi.org/10.1016/S0002-9610(05)81020-7.

10. Salmon RJ, Ansquer Y, Asselain B. Preservation versus section of intercostal-brachial nerve (IBN) in axillary dissection for breast cancer – a prospective randomized trial. *Eur J Surg Oncol.* 1998;24(3):158-161. http://dx.doi.org/10.1016/S0748-7983(98)92793-7.

11. Carpenter JS, Andrykowski MA, Sloan P, et al. Postmastectomy/postlumpectomy pain in breast cancer survivors. *J Clin Epidemiol.* 1998;51(12):1285-1292.

12. Macdonald L, Bruce J, Scott N, Smith W, Chambers W. Long-term follow-up of breast cancer survivors with post-mastectomy pain syndrome. *Br J Cancer.* 2005;92(2): 225-230.

13. Wong L. Intercostal neuromas: a treatable cause of post-operative breast surgery pain. *Ann Plast Surg.* 2001;46(5): 481-484.

14. Nguyen JT, Buchanan IA, Patel PP, Aljinovic N, Lee BT. Intercostal neuroma as a source of pain after aesthetic and reconstructive breast implant surgery. *J Plast Reconstr Aesthet Surg.* 2012;65(9):1199-1203.

15. Djebbar S, Rossi IM, Adler RS. Ultrasound-guided cryo-analgesia of peripheral nerve lesions. *Semin Musculoskelet Radiol.* 2016;20(05):461-471.

16. Mohammad JA, Warnke PH, Stavraky W. Ultrasound in the diagnosis and management of fluid collection complications following abdominoplasty. *Ann Plast Surg.* 1998;41(5):498-502.

17. Blunt C, Schmiedel A. Some cases of severe post-mastectomy pain syndrome may be caused by an axillary haematoma. *Pain.* 2004;108(3):294-296.

18. Mukesh MB, Barnett G, Cumming J, et al. Association of breast tumour bed seroma with post-operative complications and late normal tissue toxicity: results from the Cambridge breast IMRT trial. *Eur J Surg Oncol.* 2012;38(10):918-924. http://dx.doi.org/10.1016/j.ejso.2012.05.008.

19. Fourie WJ, Robb KA. Physiotherapy management of axillary web syndrome following breast cancer treatment: discussing the use of soft tissue techniques. *Physiotherapy.* 2009;95(4):314-320. http://dx.doi.org/10.1016/j.physio.2009.05.001.

20. Stubblefield MD, Custodio CM. Upper-extremity pain disorders in breast cancer. *Arch Phys Med Rehabil.* 2006;87(3 suppl 1):96-99. http://dx.doi.org/10.1016/j.apmr.2005.12.017.

21. Hayes SC, Johansson K, Stout NL, et al. Upper-body morbidity after breast cancer. *Cancer.* 2012;118(S8): 2237-2249.

22. Bajrovic A, Rades D, Fehlauer F, et al. Is there a life-long risk of brachial plexopathy after radiotherapy of supraclavicular lymph nodes in breast cancer patients? *Radiother Oncol.* 2004;71(3):297-301. https://doi-org.proxy1.lib.tju.edu/10.1016/j.radonc.2004.03.005.

23. Gottrup H, Andersen J, Arendt-Nielsen L, Jensen TS. Psychophysical examination in patients with post-mastectomy pain. *Pain.* 2000;87(3):275-284.

24. Ebid AA, El-Sodany AM. Long-term effect of pulsed high-intensity laser therapy in the treatment of post-mastectomy pain syndrome: a double blind, placebo-control, randomized study. *Lasers Med Sci.* 2015;30(6):1747-1755.

25. Lossignol DAF. Psychological interventions to reduce pain in patients with cancer. *Curr Opin Oncol.* 2013;25(4):368-372. http://dx.doi.org/10.1097/CCO.0b013e3283621090.

26. Sheinfeld Gorin S, Krebs P, Badr H, et al. Meta-analysis of psychosocial interventions to reduce pain in patients with cancer. *J Clin Oncol.* 2012;30(5):539-547.

27. O'Mahony S, Goulet J, Kornblith A, et al. Desire for hastened death, cancer pain and depression: report of a longitudinal observational study. *J Pain Symptom Manage.* 2005;29(5):446-457. http://dx.doi.org/10.1016/j.jpainsymman.2004.08.010.

28. Cheville AL, Basford JR. Role of rehabilitation medicine and physical agents in the treatment of cancer-associated pain. *J Clin Oncol.* 2014;32(16):1691-1702.

29. Robb K, Oxberry SG, Bennett MI, Johnson MI, Simpson KH, Searle RD. A cochrane systematic review of transcutaneous electrical nerve stimulation for cancer pain. *J Pain Symptom Manage.* 2009;37(4):746-753. http://dx.doi.org/10.1016/j.jpainsymman.2008.03.022.

30. Gerwin R. Classification, epidemiology, and natural history of myofascial pain syndrome. *Curr Pain Headache Rep.* 2001;5(5):412-420. http://dx.doi.org/10.1007/s11916-001-0052-8.

31. Kutner JS, Smith MC, Corbin L, et al. Massage therapy versus simple touch to improve pain and mood in patients with advanced cancer: a randomized trial. (annals of internal medicine)(author abstract)(clinical report). *Ann Intern Med.* 2008;149(6):369.

32. Caviggioli F, Maione L, Forcellini D, Klinger F, Klinger M. Autologous fat graft in postmastectomy pain syndrome. *Plast Reconstr Surg.* 2011;128(2):349-352. http://dx.doi.org/10.1097/PRS.0b013e31821e70e7.

33. Amr YM, Yousef AA. Evaluation of efficacy of the perioperative administration of venlafaxine or gabapentin on acute and chronic postmastectomy pain. *Clin J Pain*. 2010;26(5):381–385. http://dx.doi.org/10.1097/AJP.0b013e3181cb406e.

34. Reuben SS, Makari-Judson G, Lurie SD. Evaluation of efficacy of the perioperative administration of venlafaxine X R in the prevention of postmastectomy pain syndrome. *J Pain Symptom Manage*. 2004;27(2):133–139. http://dx.doi.org.proxy1.lib.tju.edu/10.1016/j.jpainsymman.2003.06.004.

35. Notice of retraction. *J Pain Symptom Manage*. 2009;37(5):941. http://dx.doi.org.proxy1.lib.tju.edu/10.1016/j.jpainsymman.2009.04.001.

36. Dini D, Bertelli G, Gozza A, Forno GG. Treatment of the post-mastectomy pain syndrome with topical capsaicin. *Pain*. 1993;54(2):223–226.

37. Watson CPN, Evans RJ. The postmastectomy pain syndrome and topical capsaicin: a randomized trial. *Pain*. 1992;51(3):375–379.

CHAPTER 15

Amputation-Related Pain

STANLEY YOO, MD • MARY KESZLER, MD • ZIVA PETRIN, MD

INTRODUCTION

The prevalence of limb loss in the United States has been estimated to be approximately 1.6 million in 2005 and to increase to approximately 3.6 million by the year 2050.[1] Up to 80% of amputations in the United States are secondary to dysvascular conditions such as diabetes and peripheral vascular disease.[2] A significant number of patients with amputation have pain related to their amputation, with survey-based studies showing that up to 80% of patients have chronic pain.[3] The location of the postamputation pain can generally be divided into residual limb or residual limb pain and phantom limb pain (PLP). PLP is a unique pain syndrome, consisting of pain or painful sensations felt in the missing body part. Residual limb pain is heterogenous in origin. This chapter presents a brief review of amputation-associated nonneuropathic pain conditions important in the differential diagnosis of pain after limb amputation.

Incidence

The prevalence of pain after amputation is variable. A survey of 914 patients found that 79.9% of patients have PLP and 67.7% have residual limb pain.[4] Earlier surveys of American veteran patients with amputation show a similar prevalence of PLP in 78%[3] of patients surveyed. This correlates with a more recent study, which shows a similar prevalence of PLP (79%) in patients with peripheral vascular disease 6 months after amputation. This study also showed a 51% prevalence of residual limb pain in the same time frame.[5]

The onset of pain is variable, either appearing immediately after amputation or in the following months.[6] In approximately half the patients, the pain improves with time, with Schley et al.[6] describing improvements in phantom pain in 48.2% of patients and in residual limb pain in 47.5%.

Etiology

As it can be difficult for patients to describe the character, nature, or even the exact location of their pain, it is important to keep a broad differential diagnosis in mind. A proposed differential diagnosis can be found in Box 15.1. PLP is discussed extensively in a following section of this chapter.

Although the focus of this book is on neuropathic pain syndromes, a discussion of nonneurologic causes cannot be ignored, as they must be considered in the differential diagnosis. Identification of the etiology of pain in a patient with amputation is especially important, because along the spectrum of recovery from an amputation there may be any number of pain generators and the appropriateness of treatment approach and duration of treatment for each of those pain generators may differ.

Pain is a subjective experience, and both residual limb pain and PLP develop secondary to a variety of factors. It is unclear how many objective findings in the residual limb, such as neuromas or heterotopic ossification, contribute to the presence of PLP or how many interventions aimed at the residual limb are able to affect PLP. To further complicate matters, PLP, although not always related to prosthetic wear, may be elicited or exacerbated by poor prosthetic fit or discomfort with prosthetic wear. Although it is difficult to objectify PLP, it is generally easier to delineate many causes of residual limb pain with typical clinical and imaging findings.

RESIDUAL LIMB PAIN

Residual limb pain is heterogenous in nature, and there is no existing uniform categorization for residual limb pain, although various algorithms have been proposed.[7] Incisional and musculoskeletal pain experienced immediately after amputation, similar to that experienced in other postsurgical conditions, is typically self-limiting postsurgical pain. This is treated in the same fashion as with other surgical procedures, with antiinflammatory and narcotic medications, as warranted.

Factors that are thought to contribute to the development of postamputation pain can be divided into presurgical, surgical, and postsurgical (Box 15.2).

BOX 15.1
Differential Diagnosis of Amputation-Related Pain

- Neuropathic pain
  - Complex regional pain syndrome
  - Peripheral neuropathy
  - Radiculopathy
  - Neuroma
  - Phantom limb pain
- Musculoskeletal
  - Myofascial pain
  - Fracture
  - Osteoarthritis
  - Contractures
  - Heterotopic ossification
  - Poor prosthetic fit
- Infectious
  - Herpes zoster
  - Cellulitis
  - Septic arthritis
  - Osteomyelitis
  - Folliculitis
  - Dermatitis
- Vascular
  - Thrombus
  - Peripheral vascular disease
- Rheumatologic
  - Rheumatoid arthritis
  - Gout
- Dermatologic
  - Skin breakdown of the residual limb
  - Incisional pain
  - Choke syndrome

BOX 15.2
Factors Affecting Development of Postamputation Pain

Presurgical	Surgical	Postsurgical
Prior neuropathic pain in limb	Residual limb length	Residual limb shaping
Vasculopathy/ claudication	Nerve resection	Edema control
Infection	Bone shaping	Desensitization
Musculoskeletal pain	Incision placement	Prosthesis fit
Psychosocial	Limb shape	Wound healing
	Resection of unhealthy tissue	Psychosocial

Preexisting pain syndromes are thought to presensitize the patient to the development of postamputation pain.[8] Dysvascular limbs have higher complication rates of delayed wound healing, and chronic wounds are suggested to create a local painful structure, as well as upregulate central pain pathways.[9]

Surgical technique can also significantly affect future pain and prosthetic fit. A limb that has not been adequately amputated to resect unhealthy tissue can result in recurrence of tumor, symptomatic vascular disease with the development of ischemic or neuropathic pain, or recurrence of infection and the formation of new wounds.

A short residual limb is more difficult to fit with a prosthesis. Improper angling of the resected bone edges can create an aggressive bone edge that creates pressure points on the subcutaneous tissues. Placement of the incision within the weight-bearing point of the limb can create pain and incision breakdown.[10] Various resection techniques of peripheral nerves can possibly contribute to or reduce the formation of painful neuromas.[10-12]

Postsurgical factors that affect the development of pain include compliance with wrapping for edema control and residual limb shaping, utilization of desensitization techniques, presence of delayed wound healing, and proper prosthesis fit.

Prosthogenic pain, or pain from prosthetic wear, can occur from poor prosthetic fit and/or suspension, or the presence of skin and soft tissue adhesion, which contribute to pain with skin traction or increased focal pressure. The resulting local mechanical stress can cause a variety of disorders, such as formation of bone bruises, adventitious bursa, local callusing, pressure breakdown of the skin, or traction pain.[13] Persistent vascular disease in the residual limb can result in claudication.[14] This can be difficult to distinguish from pain caused by the prosthesis. In both cases, pain tends to worsen with increased weight-bearing activity and metabolic demand. Heterotopic ossification and aggressive bone edge can both cause local pain in the residual limb[10] and occur in a high proportion of residual limbs (up to 63% in traumatic amputees).[15] Treatment of prosthogenic pain involves identification of the offending cause (e.g., poor fit or suspension). Vascular-related pain may be treated with the combination of medications to maintain perfusion, therapy, and revascularization procedures. An in-depth discussion of diagnostic strategies for these types of pain is beyond the scope of this chapter. Critically, identifiable and sometimes reversible causes of residual limb pain should be aggressively pursued.

Neurogenic pain can occur from a local injury to a nerve, such as a neuroma, and can be sympathetically mediated, as seen in certain cases of complex regional pain syndrome (CRPS). Radiculopathy or lumbosacral plexopathy or peripheral nerve lesions can result in radiating pain. Hyperalgesia is also common postsurgically. Nociceptive pain can radiate from the spine or adjacent joints.

Diagnosis

The diagnostic approach to postamputation pain first includes differentiation of whether the pain occurs in the residual limb or in the missing body part, whether it is associated or is independent of prosthetic wear.

Detailed history and physical examination, including careful characterization of the pain, are perhaps the most helpful in delineating neurogenic from nonneurogenic causes. It should be noted that both types of pain can be experienced concurrently, and attempts to address all pain generators should be made to optimize functional progress.

Many skin findings are easily identifiable with observation and palpation. Adhesions or wounds can cause reproducible traction pain, which is typically associated with prosthetic wear. Neuromas present as a localized point of typically extreme pain with mechanical stimulation and may have a positive Tinel sign. They can frequently be palpated subcutaneously.

When the cause of pain is not so clearly identifiable, imaging modalities may be used to support or confirm a diagnosis. Plain radiography and CT scan can identify fractures, heterotopic ossification, and aggressive bony edge.[10,15] Ultrasonography has been described since 1989 as a tool for neuroma identification[16,17] and may be used for guided intervention.[18] MRI can be used to identify neuromas, adventitious bursae, bone bruising, and stress fractures from prosthetic wear, as well as identify infection and recurrence of tumor in patients with cancer.[10,13,19]

Diagnosis of PLP is clinical and is discussed in length later in this chapter. It is easily differentiated from residual limb pain as it occurs in the location of the missing body part.

Individual Diagnoses and Treatments

Treatment of postamputation pain is as heterogenous as the differential diagnosis.

The three true neuropathic syndromes in the patient with amputation include neuroma, PLP, and CRPS when its cause is neurologic.

Neuroma

Symptomatic neuromas are described to occur in 13%–32% of patients with amputation and represent the most common cause of residual limb pain.[18,20] Spindle or fusiform-shaped neuromas appear at sites of friction or local pressure, whereas terminal end nerve trauma (such as after amputation) causes terminal or end bulb neuromas, with a mass of haphazard proliferation of Schwann cells, connective tissue, and axons. Many neuromas found on imaging are asymptomatic, whereas others can be exquisitely painful, significantly limiting the quality of life and ability to tolerate prosthesis wear.

Pharmacologic interventions include anticonvulsants such as gabapentin, antidepressants such as duloxetine, and opiates.

Interventional approaches to the treatment of neuroma include guided phenol denervation,[21] pulsed radiofrequency denervation,[22] and guided steroid injection into the neuroma.[23,24] All approaches have been described with variable results. Studies are low powered and, at this time, evidence is preliminary.

Surgical approaches to treatment include resection and reimplantation into adjacent muscle,[25] reimplantation into veins,[26,27] and tibioperoneal short circuit techniques.[28] Targeted muscle reinnervation, a novel nerve transfer technique, has been extensively studied as a technique to confer more intuitive control over myoelectric prostheses. It has also been suggested to reduce reformation of neuromas by providing an intact distal scaffold for nerve regrowth.[29] These studies consist of small group sizes but have demonstrated good effects. Traction neurectomy has not been found to have favorable outcomes.[30]

Other local treatments for chronic intractable pain have been reported, primarily as case reports or small series, including transcutaneous nerve stimulation, extracorporeal shock wave therapy,[31] and peripheral neuromodulation with implantable nerve stimulators[32] with promising results.

Other general and nonspecific pain management approaches to intractable neuromas are similar to those treating phantom pain but do not have high-power evidence in the treatment of neuromas specifically. They are summarized in Table 15.1.

CRPS

Complex regional pain syndrome has been described as occurring after multiple triggering events, including amputation. Although it can occur after amputation as

TABLE 15.1
Summary of Pain Management Approaches Applicable to Phantom Limb Pain and Residual Limb Neuroma Pain

Pharmacologic	Surgical	Injection	Psychologic	Other
Opiates	Rhizotomy	Nerve block	Biofeedback	Physical therapy
NSAIDs	Dorsal column stimulation	Lumbar sympathetic block	Cognitive behavioral therapy	Occupational therapy
Anticonvulsants	Residual limb revision	Stellate ganglion block		Transcutaneous nerve stimulation
Antidepressants	Neurectomy/neuroma removal/wrapping	Trigger point injection		Mirror therapy/graded motor imagery
Partial mu agonists				Sensory discrimination training
				Multidisciplinary pain management programs

a type 1 CRPS, it is possible that it occurs as a type 2 CRPS with underlying nerve damage; the incidence of this is currently not well defined. Conversely, amputation of the affected limb has been used as a treatment for recalcitrant CRPS with some success.[33–36] However, reoccurrence of CRPS after amputation has been described in up to 24% of patients,[37] and amputation as a treatment remains controversial.

The syndrome follows a similar course in patients who develop it secondary to amputation and nonamputation patients. CRPS etiology, diagnosis, and treatment are discussed extensively in other chapters of this text.

PHANTOM LIMB PAIN

One of the most common complaints after undergoing an amputation is PLP, occurring in over 80% of patients immediately after surgery and lasting for years in up to 59%.[38] PLP is the sensation of pain in a limb that has been amputated (i.e., the perception of pain in the portion of the limb that is no longer present). Amputation has been found to be associated with neuroplastic changes in the somatosensory and motor cortices[39] in a process termed "cortical reorganization," in which neighboring somatosensory and motor representations "invade" the now deafferented cortical representation of the amputated limb.[40,41] For example, in an upper limb amputation, the somatosensory and motor representation on the face extends into the area of the cortex that previously represented the hand. For reasons that are unclear, this clinically presents itself as phantom sensation and/or pain.

When assessing a patient with pain after an amputation, the diagnosis of PLP is made clinically without any diagnostic criteria or tests. During assessment, it is important to differentiate this from phantom limb sensation, the nonpainful sensation of the presence of the amputated limb, which is experienced in most amputees and is not bothersome. Once the symptom has been confirmed as painful, the location of the pain must be verified, as patients may have a hard time differentiating pain that is in the residual limb from pain in the phantom limb. Once this has been affirmed, the patient can be diagnosed with PLP.

Those with PLP may use various words to describe the sensation, including, but not limited to, tingling, throbbing, aching, squeezing, stabbing, cramping, or feeling as if the limb is in a painful position. Over time, patients may describe that the phantom limb feels as if it is retracting into the residual limb, which is referred to as "telescoping" and is generally associated with worse PLP.[42] The symptoms can be constant or episodic, lasting for seconds to hours, and patients may notice that it is worsened by physical, psychosocial, or emotional stressors.[43] Clinicians should be cognizant that patients with PLP may be reluctant to describe their symptoms at all because of fear of being disbelieved. Promoting sensitive discussion pre- and postoperatively about PLP may be a useful technique in eliciting further clinical understanding and earlier treatment.

The incidence of PLP is independent of the patient's age, gender, history of diabetes, and etiology of amputation but is associated with residual limb pain, prosthetic use, proximal amputations, amputation of the lower limb, or bilaterality.[38,44–46] There is conflicting evidence as to the role played by preamputation pain in the development of PLP. It has been suggested by some that preamputation pain intensity is associated with an increased incidence of PLP earlier on after amputation,[7] whereas others suggest it is only predictive of more chronic PLP amputation (greater than 2 years).[8] Others yet have only found a weak association between preamputation pain and the development of PLP.[9] The duration of preamputation pain has been found not to be predicative of chronic PLP in more than one study.[7,8] Although preamputation pain intensity may be a risk factor for the development of PLP, there is little evidence to support the use of perioperative pain management to prevent PLP.[8,9,47]

Another possible risk factor for the development of PLP is depressed mood.[7,8] Multiple investigators have found an association between PLP and depressive symptoms.[4] Furthermore, it has also been suggested that coping strategies, such as catastrophizing and resting to manage pain, are predictive of the presence of PLP as well as pain intensity and lifestyle disruption.[48]

When it comes to the treatment of PLP, there are various physical and occupational therapeutic modalities that are used, with mirror therapy being the most well known. Mirror therapy is performed by placing a mirror between the amputated limb and the intact limb such that the mirror is reflecting the intact limb and the amputated limb looks whole again. The patient is then instructed to perform certain movements with the intact limb while watching the reflection and visualizing the same movements with the phantom limb. Ramachandran et al. first described mirror therapy for the treatment of PLP in 1996, with the theory being that providing visualization of the amputated limb as intact again allows the patient to have better control of the phantom limb, thereby combating the cortical reorganization of the sensory and motor homunculus that occurs after amputation.[49] Foell et al. found functional MRI (fMRI) changes before and after mirror therapy for the treatment of PLP consistent with this theory. In addition, Foell et al. found a significant reduction in pain scores after 4 weeks of training. Those patients who reported telescoping experienced less of an effect.[50] This is consistent with the notion that phantom limb telescoping is the result of advanced cortical reorganization, which may be too extensive to be corrected by mirror therapy. Chan et al. also found a significant reduction in PLP after treatment with mirror therapy as compared with those who performed sham mirror therapy or mental visualization. Moreover, eight of nine patients who crossed over to mirror therapy

from these other two groups also experienced significant pain relief.[51]

In addition to mirror therapy, mental visualization, in which patients imagine moving their phantom limb, may also be beneficial in the treatment of PLP. In a study done by MacIver et al., 13 patients with PLP were trained to meditate and use mental visualization over the course of six 1-h sessions resulting in a significant reduction in PLP intensity and unpleasantness.[52] Furthermore, those with improved symptoms demonstrated normalization of fMRI, such that it more closely resembled the imaging typical of nonamputated control subjects and subjects with amputation who did not experience PLP. Graded motor imagery is another modality in which patients are progressed in a stepwise fashion where they are first made to identify limb laterality in photographs, followed by imagined or visualized movements with the phantom limb, and then mirror therapy. In a randomized trial done by Moseley, this treatment resulted in a significant reduction of PLP.[53]

Additional nonpharmacologic therapeutic modalities are transcutaneous electrical stimulation (TENS) and sensory discrimination training. In a randomized control trail done by Finsen et al., TENS was not found to reduce PLP during the first 4 weeks post amputation as well as 1 year post amputation.[54] However, in a pilot study performed by Mulvey et al., TENS was found to significantly reduce PLP.[55] It is clear that further research needs to be done to fully evaluate this treatment modality. Another modality, sensory discrimination training, is a treatment option for those who cannot tolerate wearing a prosthesis in which behaviorally relevant stimulation is applied to the residual limb with the goal of correcting the cortical reorganization that occurs after amputation, thereby treating PLP.[42] In a small study done by Flor et al., sensory discrimination training was found to significantly reduce PLP as well as improve cortical reorganization.[56] Lastly, instructing the patient to massage their residual limb is commonly encouraged in clinical practice, although no studies have been done evaluating its effect on PLP.

As with other neuropathic pain conditions, there are numerous classes of medications that can be trialed in the treatment of PLP. One of the most commonly used classes of medications in the treatment of neuropathic pain is antiepileptic medications, especially gabapentin and pregabalin. In a Cochrane review performed by Alviar et al., although the effect of gabapentin on PLP was conflicting, the results showed a trend toward benefit.[57] In another review done by McCormick et al., there was minimal evidence to support the use of pregabalin to treat PLP.[58] Antidepressants, especially tricyclic antidepressants such as amitriptyline and nor-triptyline, are used to improve pain and sleep. In a randomized control trial done by Robinson et al., there was no improvement in PLP in the group that received amitriptyline compared with placebo.[59] This is consistent with the findings found in the Cochrane review by Alviar et al.[57] In addition, caution should be exercised when using tricyclic antidepressants in aging patients because of the potential for anticholinergic side effects.

Although opiates are frequently prescribed postoperatively, they have not been rigorously studied in the treatment of PLP. In the Cochrane review by Alviar et al., morphine was the only opiate sufficiently studied and was found to be effective in short-term relief of PLP. This class of medications should be used with caution given their significant side-effect profile and risk of tolerance and dependence. N-methyl-D-aspartate receptor antagonists are occasionally used in the treatment of neuropathic pain, and specifically ketamine and dextromethorphan may provide analgesic effect for PLP, but ketamine especially should be used with caution.[57]

If these options do not result in sufficient pain relief, multiple interventional options have been tried throughout the years, including peripheral nerve stimulation, peripheral nerve injections, and trigger point injections. In a small study done by Rauck et al., peripheral nerve stimulation with leads placed percutaneously with ultrasound guidance was found to provide significant PLP relief.[60] In a small pilot study, peripheral nerve blocks were performed in two patients, resulting in complete resolution of PLP in one patient lasting 1 year after the block, whereas the other patient had recurrence of his pain, but to a much milder extent, and only once a week, whereas before the nerve block he had continuous and severe pain.[61] There was also a case report of six patients with postamputation pain, five of whom had PLP, who underwent perineural etanercept injection. This was performed under the premise that the inflammatory cytokine, tumor necrosis factor α (TNF-α), plays a role in the development of a variety of neuropathic pain conditions. Therefore, it was proposed that local injection of a TNF-α inhibitor such as etanercept could modulate pain. Four of the five patients with PLP went on to experience improvement in PLP, one of whom had complete resolution of pain.[62] Trigger point injections were evaluated in a study performed by Reiestad et al. Patients with PLP underwent weekly myofascial trigger point injections in the residual limb with bupivacaine over the course of 5 weeks. All patients experienced an improvement in PLP after 5 weeks, with an average visual analog scale (VAS) score of nine dropping to one after treatment.[63] Although these are all promising modalities, they all need further study.

If PLP persists despite these interventions, surgical options are available, including dorsal root entry zone (DREZ) lesioning, dorsal column stimulators, motor cortex stimulator, neurectomy, and residual limb revision. In a study by Saris et al., 22 patients with postamputation pain, 16 of whom had PLP, underwent DREZ lesioning. Although it was not helpful for those who solely had residual limb pain, it was promising for those with PLP; 8 of the 16 patients with PLP had good results.[64] A small study was done to assess the benefit of motor cortex stimulators in the treatment of neuropathic pain. Of the 12 patients in the study, two had PLP, one of whom had a good outcome, whereas the other had a poor outcome.[65] Given the size of the study and the promise motor cortex stimulators have in the treatment of neuropathic pain, this needs to be further studied as a treatment option for those with PLP.

Multiple studies have been done to assess the analgesic effect of spinal cord stimulators in the case of PLP. In one of the earliest studies, six patients with PLP underwent placement of a dorsal column stimulator, five of whom had good to excellent relief.[66] However, in a study by Wester in which a dorsal column stimulator was placed in 35 patients with chronic pain from multiple etiologies (five of whom had PLP), only one patient with PLP continued to use the stimulator regularly upon follow-up. It was concluded that the stimulator provided only a weak analgesic effect in the case of PLP.[67] This finding was replicated in a study by Sanchez-Ledesma et al. in which only one of the three patients with PLP experienced a benefit from the stimulator.[68] In a more recent case series, four patients with PLP underwent spinal cord stimulator placement. In three of the patients, there was a two point decrease in PLP on the VAS, whereas the fourth patient reported the PLP was unchanged.[69] In another study by McAuley et al., 12 patients with postamputation pain, seven of whom had PLP, underwent spinal cord stimulator placement. Of these seven patients, four had sufficient relief of PLP such that it was worthwhile, but one was lost to follow-up. Of the remaining three patients, two did not experience adequate relief and the third experienced PLP relief, but not satisfactory relief of radicular pain, such that the procedure was not worthwhile.[70] Other surgical options include residual limb revision and neurectomy, but these are primarily used in the treatment of residual limb pain rather than solely PLP. Interestingly, Prantl et al. performed a prospective study of 15 transtibial amputees who underwent a surgical procedure that involved splitting the sciatic nerve and reconnecting it in a sling fashion. This was found to produce significant PLP reduction up to 1 year postoperatively.[71] Although this is a promising option for transtibial amputees, this needs to be studied further, and surgical management should generally be reserved for those cases refractory to management with more conservative measures.

Ultimately, it is very important for patients with chronic PLP to receive psychological support to learn how to cope with chronic neuropathic pain. Biofeedback techniques as well as cognitive-based therapy are commonly used in the treatment of chronic pain.

Complementary modalities, such as acupuncture may be an option. In a case report of three amputees with PLP, two patients reported resolution of their pain upon completion of a course of acupuncture.[72] However, this is a small study and randomized controlled trials may be difficult to perform with acupuncture.

Although approximately half of all patients after an amputation continue to have PLP years after surgery, there may be a reduction in pain intensity over time.[42] Up to 10% of patients have disabling PLP for years after the amputation. A prospective study done assessing employment after amputation showed higher rates of unemployment in those reporting higher levels of PLP compared with those with lower levels of PLP or no PLP. Given the prevalence of PLP and the potential debility associated with it, continued work is needed to better understand the risk factors, pathophysiology, and treatment so these patients can have improved mood and function.

CONCLUSIONS

Amputation-related pain can be neuropathic and/or nonneuropathic in etiology, although that may be clinically difficult to distinguish. Like many other types of pain, it is often multifactorial in nature. Although for many patients pain tends to improve over time, amputation-related pain may significantly diminish quality of life. In addition, this pain may limit not only participation in daily functional, vocational, and recreational activities, but also prosthetic use early on after an amputation, during a period when early incorporation of a prosthesis into mobility and/or daily activities may determine long-term prosthetic acceptance. For these reasons, proper assessment and differentiation of amputation-related pain is essential, and distinguishing neurologic versus nonneurologic causes for an individual's pain is necessary to properly guide treatment strategies. Oftentimes, multiple treatments, from therapeutic modalities to prosthetic adjustments, medications, and interventions are pursued concurrently to address all likely causes of discomfort. Further study is needed for most of these treatment modalities in these most challenging pain syndromes.

REFERENCES

1. Ziegler-Graham K, MacKenzie EJ, Ephraim PL, Travison TG, Brookmeyer R. Estimating the prevalence of limb loss in the United States: 2005 to 2050. *Arch Phys Med Rehabil.* 2008;89(3):422–429.
2. Dillingham TR, Pezzin LE, MacKenzie EJ. Limb amputation and limb deficiency: epidemiology and recent trends in the United States. *South Med J.* 2002;95(8):875–883.
3. Sherman RA, Sherman CJ, Parker L. Chronic phantom and residual limb pain among American veterans: results of a survey. *Pain.* 1984;18:83–95.
4. Ephraim PL, Wegener ST, MacKenzie EJ, Dillingham TR, Pezzin LE. Phantom pain, residual limb pain, and back pain in amputees: results of a national survey. *Arch Phys Med Rehabil.* 2005;86(10):1910–1919.
5. Richardson C, Glenn S, Nurmikko T, Horgan M. Incidence of phantom phenomena including phantom limb pain 6 months after major lower limb amputation in patients with peripheral vascular disease. *Clin J Pain.* 2006;22(4):353–358.
6. Schley MT, Wilms P, Toepfner S, et al. Painful and nonpainful phantom and residual limb sensations in acute traumatic amputees. *J Trauma.* 2008;65(4):858–864.
7. Clarke C, Lindsay D, Pyati S, Buchheit T. Residual limb pain is not a diagnosis: a proposed algorithm to classify postamputation pain. *Clin J Pain.* 2013;29(6):551–562.
8. Nikolajsen L. Postamputation pain: studies on mechanisms. *Dan Med J.* 2012;59(10):B4527.
9. Freedman G, Cean C, Duron V, Tarnovskaya A, Brem H. Pathogenesis and treatment of pain in patients with chronic wounds. *Surg Technol Int.* 2003;11:168–179.
10. Henrot P, Stines J, Walter F, Martinet N, Paysant J, Blum A. Imaging of the painful lower limb stump. *Radiographics.* 2000:S219–S235.
11. Economides JM, DeFazio MV, Attinger CE, Barbour JR. Prevention of painful neuroma and phantom limb pain after transfemoral amputations through concomitant nerve coaptation and collagen nerve wrapping. *Neurosurgery.* 2016;79(3):508–513.
12. Yüksel F, Kişlaoğlu E, Durak N, Uçar C, Karacaoğlu E. Prevention of painful neuromas by epineural ligatures, flaps and grafts. *Br J Plast Surg.* 1997;50:182–185.
13. Foisneau-Lottin A, Martinet N, Henrot P, Paysant J, Blum A, Andre J-M. Bursitis, adventitious bursa, localized soft-tissue inflammation, and bone marrow edema in tibial residual limbs: the contribution of magnetic resonance imaging to the diagnosis and management of mechanical stress complications. *Arch Phys Med Rehabil.* 2003;84.
14. Hsu E, Cohen SP. Postamputation pain: epidemiology, mechanisms, and treatment. *J Pain Res.* 2013;6:121–136.
15. Potter BK, Burns TC, Lacap AP, Granville RR, Gajewski DA. Heterotopic ossification following traumatic and combat-related amputations. Prevalence, risk factors, and preliminary results of excision. *J Bone Joint Surg Am.* 2007;89(3):476–486.
16. Provost N, Bonaldi VM, Sarazin L, Cho KH, Chem RK. Amputation residual limb neuroma: ultrasound features. *J Clin Ultrasound.* 1997;25:85–89.

17. Hurvitz EA, Ellenberg M, Lerner AM, Pope S, Wirthlin L. Ultrasound imaging of residual limbs: new use for an old technique. *Arch Phys Med Rehabil.* 1989;70:556–558.
18. O'Reilly MA, O'Reilly PM, O'Reilly HM, Sullivan J, Sheahan J. High-resolution ultrasound findings in the symptomatic residual limbs of amputees. *Mil Med.* 2013;178(12):1291–1297.
19. Boutin RD, Pathria MN, Resnick D. Disorders in the residual limbs of amputee patients: MR imaging. *AJR Am J Roentgenol.* 1998;171:497–501.
20. Pet MA, Ko JH, Friedly JL, Mourad PD, Smith DG. Does targeted nerve implantation reduce neuroma pain in amputees? *Clin Orthop Relat Res.* 2014;472(10):2991–3001.
21. Gruber H, Glodny B, Bodner G, et al. Practical experience with sonographically guided phenol instillation of residual limb neuroma: predictors of effects, success, and outcome. *AJR Am J Roentgenol.* 2008;190:1263–1269.
22. Restrepo-Garces CE, Marinov A, McHardy P, Faclier G, Avila A. Pulsed radiofrequency under ultrasound guidance for persistent residual limb-neuroma pain. *Pain Pract.* 2011;11:98–102.
23. Kesikburun S, Yaşar E, Dede I, Göktepe S, Tan AK. Ultrasound-guided steroid injection in the treatment of residual limb neuroma: pilot study. *J Back Musculoskelet Rehabil.* 2014;27(3):275–279.
24. Chen PJ, Liang HW, Chang KV, Wang TG. Ultrasound-guided injection of steroid in multiple postamputation neuromas. *J Clin Ultrasound.* 2013;41(2):122–124.
25. Ducic I, Mesbahi AN, Attinger CE, Graw K. The role of peripheral nerve surgery in the treatment of chronic pain associated with amputation residual limbs. *Plast Reconstr Surg.* 2008;121(3):908–914. Discussion 915–917.
26. Koch H, Haas F, Hubmer M, Rappl T, Scharnagl E. Treatment of painful neuroma by resection and nerve residual limb transplantation into a vein. *Ann Plast Surg.* 2003;51:45–50.
27. Mobbs RJ, Vonau M, Blum P. Treatment of painful peripheral neuroma by vein implantation. *J Clin Neurosci.* 2003;10:338–339.
28. Boroumand MR, Schulz D, Uhl E, Krishnan KG. Tibioperoneal short circuiting for residual limb neuroma pain in amputees: revival of an old technique. *World Neurosurg.* 2015;84(3):681–687.
29. Souza JM, Cheesborough JE, Ko JH, et al. Targeted muscle reinnervation: a novel approach to postamputation neuroma pain. *Clin Orthop Relat Res.* 2014;472:2984–2990.
30. Pet MA, Ko JH, Friedly JL, Smith DG. Traction neurectomy for treatment of painful residual limb neuroma in lower extremity amputee. *J Orthop Trauma.* 2015;29(9):e321–e325.
31. Jung YJ, Park WY, Jeon JH, et al. Outcomes of ultrasound-guided extracorporeal shock wave therapy for painful residual limb neuroma. *Ann Rehabil Med.* 2014;38(4):523–533.
32. Meier K, Bendtsen TF, Sørensen JC, Nikolajsen L. Peripheral neuromodulation for the treatment of postamputation neuroma pain. *A A Case Rep.* 2016. [Epub ahead of print].
33. Midbari A, Suzan E, Adler T, et al. Amputation in patients with complex regional pain syndrome. *Bone Joint J.* 2016;98-B(4):548–554.
34. Bodde MI, Dijkstra PU, den Dunnen WF, Geertzen JH. Therapy-resistant complex regional pain syndrome type I: to amputate or not? *J Bone Joint Surg Am.* 2011;93(19):1799–1805.
35. Honkamp N, Amendola A, Hurwitz S, Saltzman CL. Retrospective review of eighteen patients who underwent transtibial amputation for intractable pain. *J Bone Joint Surg Am.* 2001;83-A(10):1479–1483.
36. Kashy BK, Abd-Elsayed AA, Farag E, Yared M, Vakili R, Esa WAS. Amputation as an unusual treatment for therapy-resistant complex regional pain syndrome, type 1. *Ochsner J.* 2015;15(4):441–442.
37. Krans-Schreuder HK, Bodde MI, Schrier E, et al. Amputation for long-standing, therapy-resistant type-I complex regional pain syndrome. *J Bone Joint Surg Am.* 2012;94(24):2263–2268.
38. Frontera W, DeLisa J, Gans B, Walsh N, Robinson L, eds. *DeLisa's Physical Medicine & Rehabilitation.* 5th ed. Philadelphia: Lippincott Williams & Wilkins; 2010.
39. Flor H, Nikolajsen L, Jensen TS. Phantom limb pain: a case of maladaptive CNS plasticity? *Nat Rev Neurosci.* 2006;7:873–881.
40. Mackert B-M, Sappok T, Grusser S, Flor H, Curio G. The eloquence of silent cortex. *NeuroReport.* 2003;14:409–412.
41. Chen R, Cohen LG, Hallett M. Nervous system reorganisation following injury. *Neuroscience.* 2002;111:761–773.
42. Bakshi RR. Pain in the Amputee. 2015:243–252.
43. Bang M, Jung S. Phantom limb pain. In: Frontera WR, Silver J, Rizzo T, eds. *Frontera: Essentials of Physical Medicine and Rehabilitation.* 2nd ed. Philadelphia: Saunders; 2008:575–579.
44. Desmond DM, MacLachlan M. Prevalence and characteristics of phantom limb pain and residual limb pain in the long term after upper limb amputation. *Int J Rehabil Res.* 2010;33(3):279–282.
45. Dijkstra PU, Geertzen JH, Stewart R, van der Schans CP. Phantom pain and risk factors. *J Pain Symptom Manag.* 2002;24(6):578–585.
46. Clark RL, Bowling FL, Jepson F, Rajbhandari S. Phantom limb pain after amputation in diabetic patients does not differ from that after amputation in nondiabetic patients. *Pain.* 2013;154(5):729–732.
47. Karanikolas M, Aretha D, Tsolakis I, et al. Optimized perioperative analgesia reduces chronic phantom limb pain intensity, prevalence, and frequency: a prospective, randomized, clinical trial. *J Am Soc Anesthesiol.* 2011;114(5):1144–1154.
48. Jensen MP, Ehde DM, Hoffman AJ, Patterson DR, Czerniecki JM, Robinson LR. Cognitions, coping and social environment predict adjustment to phantom limb pain. *Pain.* 2002;95(1–2):133–142.
49. Ramachandran V, Rogers-Ramachandran D. Synaesthesia in phantom limbs induced with mirrors. *Proc R Soc Lond B.* 1996;263:377–386.

50. Foell J, Bekrater-Bodmann R, Diers M, Flor H. Mirror therapy for phantom limb pain: brain changes and the role of body representation. *Eur J Pain (United Kingdom)*. 2014;18(5):729–739.

51. Chan BL. Mirror therapy for phantom limb pain. *N Engl J Med*. 2007;357(21):2206–2207.

52. MacIver K, Lloyd DM, Kelly S, Roberts N, Nurmikko T. Phantom limb pain, cortical reorganization and the therapeutic effect of mental imagery. *Brain*. 2008;131(8): 2181–2191.

53. Moseley GL. Graded motor imagery for pathologic pain: a randomized controlled trial. *Neurology*. 2006;67(12): 2129–2134.

54. Finsen V, Persen L, Løvlien M, et al. Transcutaneous electrical nerve stimulation after major amputation. *J Bone Joint Surg Br*. 1988;70(1):109–112.

55. Mulvey MR, Radford HE, Fawkner HJ, Hirst L, Neumann V, Johnson MI. Transcutaneous electrical nerve stimulation for phantom pain and stump pain…: rehabilitation reference center. *Pain Pract*. 2013;13(4):289–296.

56. Flor H, Denke C, Schaefer M, Grüsser S. Effect of sensory discrimination training on cortical reorganisation and phantom limb pain. *Lancet*. 2001;357(9270):1763–1764.

57. Alviar M, Hale T, Dungca M. Pharmacologic interventions for treating phantom limb pain (review). *Cochrane Database Syst Rev*. 2012;(12):2011–2013.

58. McCormick Z, Chang-Chien G, Marshall B, Huang M, Harden RN. Phantom limb pain: a systematic neuroanatomical-based review of pharmacologic treatment. *Pain Med*. 2014;15(2):292–305.

59. Robinson LR, Czerniecki JM, Ehde DM, et al. Trial of amitriptyline for relief of pain in amputees: results of a randomized controlled study. *Arch Phys Med Rehabil*. 2004;85(1):1–6.

60. Rauck RL, Cohen SP, Gilmore CA, et al. Treatment of postamputation pain with peripheral nerve stimulation. *Neuromodulation*. 2014;17(2):188–196.

61. Ilfeld BM, Moeller-Bertram T, Hanling S, et al. Treating intractable phantom limb pain with ambulatory continuous peripheral nerve blocks: a pilot study. *Pain Med*. 2013;14(6):935–942.

62. Dahl E, Cohen SP. Perineural injection of etanercept as a treatment for postamputation pain. *Clin J Pain*. 2008;24(2):172–175.

63. Reiestad F, Kulkarni J. Role of myofascial trigger points in post-amputation pain: causation and management. *Prosthet Orthot Int*. 2013;37(2):120–123.

64. Saris SC, Iacono RP, Nashold BS. Dorsal root entry zone lesions for post-amputation pain. *J Neurosurg*. 1985;62(1):72–76.

65. Saitoh Y, Hirano S, Kato A, et al. Motor cortex stimulation for deafferentation pain. *Neurosurg Focus*. 2001;11(3): E1–E5.

66. Nielson K, Adams JE, Hosobuchi Y. Phantom limb pain treatment with dorsal column stimulation. *J Neurosurg*. 1975;42:301–307.

67. Wester K. Dorsal column stimulation in pain treatment. *Acta Neurol Scand*. 1987;75(2):151–155.

68. Sanchez-Ledesma M, Garcia-March G, Diaz-Cascajo P, Gomez-Moreta J, Broseta J. Spinal cord stimulation in deafferentation pain. *Stereotact Funct Neurosurg*. 1989;53:40–45.

69. Viswanathan A, Phan PC, Burton AW. Use of spinal cord stimulation in the treatment of phantom limb pain: case series and review of the literature. *Pain Pract*. 2010;10(5):479–484.

70. McAuley J, van Gröningen R, Green C. Spinal cord stimulation for intractable pain following limb amputation. *Neuromodulation*. 2013;16(6):530–536. Discussion 536.

71. Prantl L, Schreml S, Heine N, Eisenmann-Klein M, Angele P. Surgical treatment of chronic phantom limb sensation and limb pain after lower limb amputation. *Plast Reconstr Surg*. 2006;118(7):1562–1572.

72. Bradbrook D. Acupuncture treatment of phantom limb pain and phantom limb sensation in amputees. Acupuncture in medicine. *J Br Med Acupunct Soc*. 2004;22(2): 93–97.

FURTHER READING

1. Durmus D, Safaz I, Adigüzel E, et al. The relationship between prosthesis use, phantom pain and psychiatric symptoms in male traumatic limb amputees. *Compr Psychiatry*. 2015;59:45–53.

2. Hanley M, Jensen M, Smith D, Ehde D, Edwards W, Robinson L. Preamputation pain and acute pain predict chronic pain after lower extremity amputation. *J Pain*. 2007;8(2):102–109.

3. Nikolajsen L, Ilkjaer S, Christensen JH, Krøner K, Jensen TS. Randomised trial of epidural bupivacaine and morphine in prevention of stump and phantom pain in lower-limb amputation. *Lancet*. 1997;350(9088):1353–1357.

4. Nikolajsen L, Ilkjær S, Krøner K, Christensen JH, Jensen TS. The influence of preamputation pain on postamputation stump and phantom pain. *Pain*. 1997;72(3):393–405.

5. Richardson C, Glenn S, Horgan M, Nurmikko T. A prospective study of factors associated with the presence of phantom limb pain six months after major lower limb amputation in patients with peripheral vascular disease. *J Pain*. 2007;8(10):793–801.

6. Whyte A, Carroll L. A preliminary examination of the relationship between employment, pain and disability in an amputee population. *Disabil Rehabil*. 2002;24(9):462–470.

7. Ypsilantis E, Tang TY. Pre-emptive analgesia for chronic limb pain after amputation for peripheral vascular disease: a systematic review. *Ann Vasc Surg*. 2010;24(8):1139–1146.

CHAPTER 16

Postthoracotomy Pain Syndrome

YURY KHELEMSKY, MD • DAVID NECKMAN, MD

PRESENTATION: HISTORICAL AND PHYSICAL FEATURES

Postthoracotomy pain syndrome (PTPS) is a neuropathic pain syndrome that occurs in the region of a previous thoracotomy incision. It is defined by the International Association for the Study of Pain as "chronic dysesthetic burning and aching pain that recurs or persists along a thoracotomy scar at least 2 months following a surgical procedure."[1] It is thought to be related to trauma of the intercostal nerves as a result of transection, retraction, suturing, or pressure from trocar placement.[2] This is supported by the fact that patients often suffer from allodynia to touch, motion, and temperature variation along the same distribution as their pain. The ipsilateral arm can also undergo sensory and autonomic dysfunction in a complex regional pain syndrome–like fashion. The pain can restrict movement of the ipsilateral shoulder and cause significant disability and limitation to patients.[3] In addition, some patients with PTPS have a significant myofascial component that is characterized by a taut muscular band near the scapula.[4]

DEMOGRAPHICS

PTPS is a common problem for patients who undergo thoracotomy incisions. Studies over the past several decades estimate the incidence of chronic pain following thoracotomy to be anywhere from 30% to 50%, although the incidence of severe pain is much lower, approximately 5%.[5-7] Limb amputation is the only surgery that has a higher incidence of chronic postsurgical pain than thoracotomy.

The risk of developing chronic pain following surgery, in general, is increased in younger patients, female patients, and those with severe uncontrolled acute postoperative pain.[5] Although none of the abovementioned risk factors have been specifically linked to PTPS, it can be extrapolated that PTPS would behave similarly to other chronic postsurgical pain syndromes. Identification of specific preoperative risk factors for the

development of PTPS remains an important question that requires more research. The literature evaluating the risk of chronic preoperative pain as a risk factor for the development of PTPS offers no consensus. In the past, many studies that evaluated PTPS had excluded patients with preoperative chronic pain and analgesic treatment, which limits the available data. Multiple studies found no association between preoperative pain and PTPS,[8,9] whereas others have shown significant correlations between the use of preoperative analgesics and the development of PTPS.[10] More research is needed to fully elucidate this possible risk factor.

INTRAOPERATIVE FACTORS: SURGICAL TECHNIQUE

There have been attempts to decrease the incidence of PTPS via differing surgical approaches. A thoracotomy incision can be performed using four different surgical techniques: anterior, axillary, posterolateral, or muscle-sparing posterolateral (avoiding division of the latissimus dorsi muscle). There have been multiple retrospective studies evaluating these different approaches; there is a lack of convincing prospective data that favors one over another. Therefore, no consensus can be drawn on the superiority of the differing thoracotomy techniques with regard to the prevention of PTPS.[11]

Video-assisted thoracic surgery (VATS), a less invasive technique utilizing endoscopes inserted through small incisions thus avoiding the large thoracotomy incision, was expected to have a lower incidence of PTPS; however, again, the literature offers no consensus. Data from two prospective trials did not reveal a decrease in PTPS when VATS was compared with the posterolateral approach or muscle sparing posterolateral approach with classic thoracotomy incision. However, one retrospective study suggested that VATS was superior to a muscle sparing posterolateral approach for the prevention of PTPS.[12-14] The high incidence of PTPS after VATS is not surprising given that the surgical technique of placing a trocar through the intercostal space and suturing the chest wounds offer opportunities to traumatize intercostal nerves and the surrounding tissue.

Several specific surgical techniques have been successful in protecting the intercostal nerve and reducing the incidence of PTPS. These strategies include harvesting of an intercostal muscle flap, dissection and preservation of the intercostal nerve, and intracostal suturing. One review supports that these intercostal nerve protection strategies seem to decrease the incidence of PTPS, and the literature supports their use.[15]

INTRAOPERATIVE FACTORS: ANESTHETIC TECHNIQUE

Numerous anesthetic techniques have been attempted to minimize the development of PTPS with mixed results. The cornerstone of these techniques is the concept of preventative anesthesia. The goal of preventative anesthesia is to decrease the transmission of afferent pain signals arising from the surgical incision, thereby limiting central sensitization, which is thought to be instrumental in the development of chronic pain.[16] A variety of neuraxial, regional, and pharmacologic techniques have been attempted with mixed results.

Thoracic epidural anesthesia (TEA) has been used for decades in thoracic surgery, and it remains the gold standard for both acute postoperative pain and prevention of PTPS. Multiple prospective randomized controlled trials have shown that TEA both decreases the incidence of PTPS and significantly improves acute postoperative pain control when compared with intravenous opioids. In addition, significant benefit both for acute postsurgical pain and prevention of PTPS was further conferred when TEA was utilized preoperatively as opposed to postoperatively.[17,18] Although the benefit conferred by the timing of the TEA was called into question by another prospective randomized controlled trial, there is strong evidence supporting the use of TEA in the anesthetic management of patients undergoing thoracic surgery.[8]

The role of TEA has been called into question by a growing body of literature that supports the use of paravertebral blocks in lieu of TEA. Paravertebral blocks offer similar levels of analgesia for thoracotomy incisions; however, paravertebral blocks avoid the hypotension that is commonly caused by neuraxial anesthesia. In addition, paravertebral blocks have a lower incidence of common side effects following TEA, including urinary retention, nausea, and vomiting. Finally, paravertebral blocks avoid instrumenting the neuraxis, which avoids the uncommon

but catastrophic neurologic complications that can be caused by thoracic epidural placement.[19] There is some evidence supporting the use of paravertebral blocks for the prevention of chronic neuropathic pain following breast surgery. However, the use of paravertebral blocks to prevent PTPS has not been studied and requires more research.[20]

Intercostal nerve blocks and cryoanalgesia have also been studied with disappointing results. Intercostal nerve blocks show no benefit in the prevention of PTPS and were only shown to offer improved pain control during vital capacity breaths in the immediate postoperative period.[21] When compared with TEA, cryoanalgesia was actually shown to increase the incidence of allodynia and moderate to severe chronic pain that interferes with daily life following thoracotomy.[22]

Ketamine has been studied in relation to PTPS both intravenously and as an epidural adjuvant. The randomized placebo-controlled clinical trial studied the effect of a 1-mg/kg bolus of ketamine before the start of surgery, followed by an infusion of 1 mg/kg/h throughout the surgery, with a 1-mg/kg infusion over 24 h postoperatively. Although the ketamine group had improved pain control in the immediate postoperative period, there was no decrease in the development of PTPS.[23] The addition of ketamine to TEA was also studied at a low dose of 1.2 mg/h and was shown to offer no benefit for the prevention of PTPS.[24]

The effects of cyclooxygenase-2 inhibitors and acetaminophen have also been studied in postthoracotomy patients. Both drugs have been shown to improve pain control during the first 48 h after surgery when combined with TEA.[25,26] Neither drug has been studied for the prevention of PTPS and could be a target for future research.

DIAGNOSTIC CRITERIA

A diagnosis of PTPS can be made when a patient, in whom recurrent cancer and other anatomic causes of pain have been ruled out, complains of a "chronic burning and aching pain that recurs or persists along a thoracotomy scar within 2 months following a surgical procedure."[1]

DIFFERENTIAL DIAGNOSIS

There are several other causes of chronic pain in the region of a thoracotomy scar that must be ruled out before the diagnosis of PTPS can be made. These include tumor recurrence, traumatic neuroma, thoracic disc herniation, postherpetic neuralgia, and traumatic intercostal neuralgia. Tumor recurrence is the most critical diagnosis to rule out and can be difficult to distinguish given the similar nature and localization of the pain. Tumor recurrence should be suspected and investigated whenever a neuropathic PTPS-like picture occurs and the pain is recurrent after a pain-free period. However, this history does not rule out PTPS.[27] Traumatic intercostal neuroma pain is sometimes described as burning or stabbing and is often associated with a positive Tinel sign on examination, with paresthesias in the region of the patient's chronic pain elicited by percussion of the affected intercostal nerve.[28] Thoracic disc herniation can cause either unilateral or bilateral pain, can be worsened by spine flexion, and can be investigated via imaging of the spine.[29] With an acute herpes zoster infection that incidentally occurs in the region of a previous thoracotomy scar, the pain will typically be followed several days later by the characteristic dermatomal rash.[30] Postherpetic neuralgia in the region of a previous thoracotomy scar can be distinguished by history of shingles over the same area; however, if the thoracotomy was done for malignancy, then tumor recurrence should be ruled out.[31] Traumatic intercostal neuralgia can be distinguished by a history of trauma causing rib or vertebral fracture in the affected area temporally related to development of the pain, although it can also be due to surgical damage.[32]

DIAGNOSTIC TESTING

There is no specific test to diagnose PTPS, as it is a clinical diagnosis. MRI may be used to rule out a thoracic disc herniation or vertebral fracture. If suspected, ultrasound imaging can be used to evaluate for an intercostal neuroma. It is absolutely critical to rule out tumor recurrence, as the symptoms of chronic neuropathic pain and time course of tumor recurrence is easily mistaken for PTPS. Thus before a diagnosis of PTPS can be made, patients should be referred to their oncologist to obtain either chest CT or PET/CT scans to confirm that their pain is not due to tumor recurrence.[33]

REHABILITATION AND PHYSICAL MEDICINE OPTIONS AND DISCUSSION OF FUNCTION

There are no specific rehabilitation and physical medicine treatments for PTPS that have been reported in the literature. There are data supporting the use of transcutaneous electric nerve stimulation (TENS) to control acute postthoracotomy pain; however, there are no data in the literature for or against using TENS for postthoracotomy pain after 2 months. Given the

significant benefit of TENS in the acute postoperative period it would be a reasonable target for future study for the treatment of PTPS.[34,35] Other physical medicine techniques such as scar massage, desensitization techniques, biofeedback, relaxation techniques, and thoracic mobility have not been studied in the treatment of PTPS. Given the low incidence of adverse effects from physical medicine techniques, their use would be reasonable and could be a target for future research.

MEDICATION OPTIONS

Like most other neuropathic pain syndromes, PTPS can be challenging to treat. In general, opioids are less effective for neuropathic pain.[36] Tricyclic antidepressants, pregabalin, serotonin-norepinephrine reuptake inhibitors, tramadol, and lidocaine patches are useful for controlling neuropathic pain in general, although they have not been studied specifically for treating PTPS.[37] Gabapentin has shown promise as a treatment for PTPS, with limited data showing it to be safe, effective, and well tolerated in patients with PTPS.[38] Ketamine has been considered for PTPS; however, it is not widely used. There are no data to support its use for PTPS, and the literature does not support its use in chronic neuropathic pain because of its many adverse side effects and no definitive evidence for improvement in pain control.[39] Botulism toxin has been proposed as a possible treatment, and there is a case report of its successful use in a refractory case.[40] Topical 5% lidocaine medicated plaster has been shown to successfully reduce pain associated with PTPS.[41]

INTERVENTIONAL OPTIONS

The intercostal nerves offer an obvious target for interventional therapy. Intercostal nerve blocks with local anesthetics offer temporary relief for patients with PTPS. A small case series showed promising results for the use of a high concentration of local anesthetic for a controlled neurotoxic effect. Two patients with refractory PTPS received 5% tetracaine and had analgesia for up to 9 months without significant side effects.[42] Pulsed radiofrequency ablation of the affected intercostal nerves does help some patients, but retrospective data show pulsed radiofrequency ablation of the affected dorsal root ganglion to be much more effective.[43] Successful peripheral nerve field stimulation of the intercostal nerves for PTPS has also been described in a case report.[44] Although the results are promising, the support for these treatments comes from retrospective data and case reports with extremely small sample sizes, so more studies are needed to confirm the efficacy and safety of these techniques.

There are some data that epidural injections may be effective for alleviating chronic thoracic pain in general, but there are no data to support its use specifically for PTPS.[45]

For the subset of patients who are found to have a myofascial component of PTPS, trigger point injections can be beneficial. Not surprisingly, this therapy was most successful in the subset of patients found to have a trigger point present in a tight muscular band around the scapula.[4]

Spinal cord stimulation (SCS) is also an option for the subset of patients with severe PTPS that is refractory to other treatments. There have been no studies designed to evaluate the effectiveness of SCS specifically for PTPS. Two case reports in the literature showed promising results in PTPS, with both patients reporting immediate dramatic improvement in their pain and satisfaction with their treatment.[46,47] Other interventional techniques often require repeat procedures to maintain their efficacy, whereas SCS offers an effective and permanent option. When sterile technique is used correctly, infections remain rare. New advances in SCS technology, including MRI safe SCS, dorsal root ganglion (DRG) stimulation, and high-frequency SCS, are better tolerated and have fewer restrictions than traditional SCS. More studies are needed to evaluate this potentially effective treatment for patients with significant refractory PTPS.

SURGICAL OPTIONS

There are no specific surgical interventions to treat PTPS that have been reported in the literature.

COURSE/PROGNOSIS

Although pain persists for a significant number of patients, the majority of patients report mild pain. Specifically, more than 50% of patients reported that the pain interfered with their daily life, and 5% of patients reported persistent severe pain 1 year after their surgery.[48–50]

CONCLUSION

In review, PTPS is the second most common cause of chronic pain after surgery. TEA remains the gold standard for both acute postoperative pain control and prevention of chronic PTPS. Of all the procedures and medications studied in the perioperative period, only TEA has been shown to prevent the development of PTPS. Nonnarcotic pain medications are generally effective for mild to moderate pain, and interventional pain techniques such as SCS have been utilized for severe refractory cases. Although great strides have been made in the prevention and treatment of PTPS, it remains a challenging neuropathic pain syndrome that adversely affects the lives of a large percentage of patients requiring thoracic surgery. See Table 16.1 for a summary of take-home points regarding postthoracotomy pain.

TABLE 16.1 Take-Home Points of Postthoracotomy Pain	
Definition	Neuropathic pain that begins within 2 months after a thoracotomy or VATS
Diagnosis	Clinical diagnosis after other causes have been investigated. Tumor recurrence is often confused with PTPS and must be ruled out before diagnosis
Prevention	In the perioperative period, only TEA, harvesting of an intercostal muscle flap, dissection and preservation of the intercostal nerve, and intracostal suturing have been shown to lower the incidence of PTPS
Treatment	Nonopioid medications are the mainstay of treatment. Interventional techniques such as intercostal nerve blocks, peripheral nerve field stimulation, pulsed RFA, and SCS have also been used for severe cases
Prognosis	About 50% of patients with PTPS have persistent pain for over a year, 50% have pain that is severe enough to interfere with daily life, and 5% have severe pain that persists for over a year

PTPS, postthoracotomy pain syndrome; *RFA*, radiofrequency ablation; *SCS*, spinal cord stimulation; *TEA*, thoracic epidural anesthesia; *VATS*, video-assisted thoracic surgery.

REFERENCES

1. Merskey H, Bogduk N, eds. *Classification of Chronic Pain. Descriptions of Chronic Pain Syndromes and Definitions of Pain Terms.* IASP Press; 1994:i–xvi.
2. Benedetti F, Vighetti S, Ricco C, et al. Neurophysiologic assessment of nerve impairment in posterolateral and muscle-sparing thoracotomy. *J Thorac Cardiovasc Surg.* 1998;115(4):841–847.
3. d'Amours RH, Riegler FX, Little AG. Pathogenesis and management of persistent postthoracotomy pain. *Chest Surg Clin N Am.* 1998;8(3):703–722.
4. Hamada H, Moriwaki K, Shiroyama K, Tanaka H, Kawamoto M, Yuge O. Myofascial pain in patients with postthoracotomy pain syndrome. *Reg Anesth Pain Med.* 2000;25(3): 302–305.
5. Kehlet H, Jensen TS, Woolf CJ. Persistent postsurgical pain: risk factors and prevention. *Lancet.* 2006;367(9522): 1618–1625.
6. Warltier DC. Preventing and treating pain after thoracic surgery. *Anesthesiology.* 2006;(3):594–600.
7. Mongardon N, Pinton-Gonnet C, Szekely B, Michel-Cherqui M, Dreyfus JF, Fischler M. Assessment of chronic pain after thoracotomy: a 1-year prevalence study. *Clin J Pain.* 2011;27(8):677–681.
8. Ochroch EA, Gottschalk A, Augostides J, et al. Long-term pain and activity during recovery from major thoracotomy using thoracic epidural analgesia. *Anesthesiology.* 2002;97(5):1234–1244.
9. Maguire MF, Latter JA, Mahajan R, Beggs FD, Duffy JP. A study exploring the role of intercostal nerve damage in chronic pain after thoracic surgery. *Eur J Cardiothorac Surg.* 2006;29(6):873–879.
10. Keller SM, Carp NZ, Levy MN, Rosen SM. Chronic post thoracotomy pain. *J Cardiovasc Surg (Torino).* 1994;35(6 suppl 1):161–164.
11. Wildgaard K, Ravn J, Kehlet H. Chronic post-thoracotomy pain: a critical review of pathogenic mechanisms and strategies for prevention. *Eur J Cardiothorac Surg.* 2009;36(1): 170–180.
12. Kirby TJ, Mack MJ, Landreneau RJ, Rice TW. Lobectomy-video-assisted thoracic surgery versus muscle-sparing thoracotomy: a randomized trial. *J Thorac Cardiovasc Surg.* 1995;109(5):997–1002.
13. Furrer M, Rechsteiner R, Eigenmann V, Signer C, Althaus U, Ris HB. Thoracotomy and thoracoscopy: postoperative pulmonary function, pain and chest wall complaints. *Eur J Cardiothorac Surg.* 1997;12(1):82–87.
14. Landreneau RJ, Mack MJ, Hazelrigg SR, et al. Prevalence of chronic pain after pulmonary resection by thoracotomy or video-assisted thoracic surgery. *J Thorac Cardiovasc Surg.* 1994;107(4). 1079–1085-1086.
15. Visagan R, McCormack DJ, Shipolini AR, Jarral OA. Are intracostal sutures better than pericostal sutures for closing a thoracotomy? *Interact Cardiovasc Thorac Surg.* 2012;14(6):807–815.
16. Dahl JB, Kehlet H. Preventive analgesia. *Curr Opin Anaesthesiol.* 2011;24(3):331–338.
17. Senturk M, Ozcan PE, Talu GK, et al. The effects of three different analgesia techniques on long-term postthoracotomy pain. *Anesth Analg.* 2002;94(1):11–15. [table of contents].
18. Obata H, Saito S, Fujita N, Fuse Y, Ishizaki K, Goto F. Epidural block with mepivacaine before surgery reduces long-term post-thoracotomy pain. *Can J Anaesth.* 1999;46(12):1127–1132.
19. Ding X, Jin S, Niu X, Ren H, Fu S, Li Q. A comparison of the analgesia efficacy and side effects of paravertebral compared with epidural blockade for thoracotomy: an updated meta-analysis. *PLoS One.* 2014;9(5).
20. Ibarra MML, S-Carralero G-CM, Vicente GU, et al. Chronic postoperative pain after general anesthesia with or without a single-dose preincisional paravertebral nerve block in radical breast cancer surgery. *Rev Esp Anestesiol Reanim.* 2011;58(5):290–294.
21. Doyle E, Bowler GM. Pre-emptive effect of multimodal analgesia in thoracic surgery. *Br J Anaesth.* 1998;80(2):147–151.
22. Ju H, Feng Y, Yang BX, Wang J. Comparison of epidural analgesia and intercostal nerve cryoanalgesia for post-thoracotomy pain control. *Eur J Pain.* 2008;12(3): 378–384.
23. Dualé C, Sibaud F, Guastella V, et al. Perioperative ketamine does not prevent chronic pain after thoracotomy. *Eur J Pain.* 2009;13(5):497–505.
24. Ryu H-G, Lee C-J, Kim Y-T, Bahk J-H. Preemptive low-dose epidural ketamine for preventing chronic postthoracotomy pain: a prospective, double-blinded, randomized, clinical trial. *Clin J Pain.* 2011;27(4):304–308.
25. Senard M, Deflandre EP, Ledoux D, et al. Effect of celecoxib combined with thoracic epidural analgesia on pain after thoracotomy. *Br J Anaesth.* 2010;105(2):196–200.
26. Mac TB, Girard F, Chouinard P, et al. Acetaminophen decreases early post-thoracotomy ipsilateral shoulder pain in patients with thoracic epidural analgesia: a double-blind placebo-controlled study. *J Cardiothorac Vasc Anesth.* 2005;19(4):475–478.
27. Karmakar MK, Ho AMH. Postthoracotomy pain syndrome. *Thorac Surg Clin.* 2004;14(3):345–352.
28. Nguyen JT, Buchanan IA, Patel PP, Aljinovic N, Lee BT. Intercostal neuroma as a source of pain after aesthetic and reconstructive breast implant surgery. *J Plast Reconstr Aesthet Surg.* 2012;65(9):1199–1203.
29. Brown CW, Deffer PA, Akmakjian J, Donaldson DH, Brugman JL. The natural history of thoracic disc herniation. *Spine (Phila Pa 1976).* 1992;17(suppl 6):S97–S102.
30. Arvin AM. Varicella-zoster virus. *Clin Microbiol Rev.* 1996; 9(3):361–381.
31. Hadley GR, Gayle JA, Ripoll J, et al. Post-herpetic neuralgia: a review. *Curr Pain Headache Rep.* 2016;20(3):1–5.
32. Williams EH, Williams CG, Rosson GD, Heitmiller RF, Dellon AL. Neurectomy for treatment of intercostal neuralgia. *Ann Thorac Surg.* 2008;85(5):1766–1770.
33. Dane B, Grechushkin V, Plank A, Moore W, Bilfinger T. PET/CT vs. non-contrast CT alone for surveillance 1-year post lobectomy for stage I non-small-cell lung cancer. *Am J Nucl Med Mol Imaging.* 2013;3(5):408–416.

34. Ferreira FC, Issy AM, Sakata RK. Assessing the effects of transcutaneous electrical nerve stimulation (TENS) in post-thoracotomy analgesia. *Rev Bras Anestesiol.* 2011;61(5): 561–567, 308–310.

35. Freynet A, Falcoz P-E. Is transcutaneous electrical nerve stimulation effective in relieving postoperative pain after thoracotomy? *Interact Cardiovasc Thorac Surg.* 2010;10(2): 283–288.

36. Smith HS. Opioids and neuropathic pain. *Pain Physician.* 2012;15(suppl 3):ES93–ES110.

37. Dworkin RH, O'Connor AB, Audette J, et al. Recommendations for the pharmacological management of neuropathic pain: an overview and literature update. *Mayo Clin Proc.* 2010;85(suppl 3):S3–S14.

38. Solak O, Metin M, Esme H, et al. Effectiveness of gabapentin in the treatment of chronic post-thoracotomy pain. *Eur J Cardiothorac Surg.* 2007;32(1):9–12.

39. Blonk MI, Koder BG, van den Bemt PM, Huygen FJ. Use of oral ketamine in chronic pain management: a review. *Eur J Pain.* 2010;14(5):466–472.

40. Fabregat G, Asensio-Samper JM, Palmisani S, Villanueva-Perez VL, De Andres J. Subcutaneous botulinum toxin for chronic post-thoracotomy pain. *Pain Pract.* 2013;13(3): 231–234.

41. Sansone P, Passavanti MB, Fiorelli A, et al. Efficacy of the topical 5% lidocaine medicated plaster in the treatment of chronic post-thoracotomy neuropathic pain. *Pain Manag.* 2017 May;7(3):189–196.

42. Doi K, Nikai T, Sakura S, Saito Y. Intercostal nerve block with 5% tetracaine for chronic pain syndromes. *J Clin Anesth.* 2002;14(1):39–41.

43. Cohen SP, Sireci A, Wu CL, Larkin TM, Williams KA, Hurley RW. Pulsed radiofrequency of the dorsal root ganglia is superior to pharmacotherapy or pulsed radiofrequency of the intercostal nerves in the treatment of chronic postsurgical thoracic pain. *Pain Physician.* 2006;9:227–236.

44. McJunkin TL, Berardoni N, Lynch PJ, Amrani J. An innovative case report detailing the successful treatment of post-thoracotomy syndrome with peripheral nerve field stimulation. *Neuromodulation.* 2010;13(4):311–314.

45. Manchikanti L, Cash KA, McManus CD, Pampati V, Benyamin RM. A preliminary report of a randomized double-blind, active controlled trial of fluoroscopic thoracic interlaminar epidural injections in managing chronic thoracic pain. *Pain Physician.* 2010;13(6):E357–E369.

46. Graybill J, Conermann T, Kabazie AJ, Chandy S. Spinal cord stimulation for treatment of pain in a patient with post thoracotomy pain syndrome. *Pain Physician.* 2011;14(5):441–445.

47. Segal R, Stacey BR, Rudy TE, Baser S, Markham J. Spinal cord stimulation revisited. *Neurol Res.* 1998;20(5):391–396.

48. Gotoda Y, Kambara N, Sakai T, Kishi Y, Kodama K, Koyama T. The morbidity, time course and predictive factors for persistent post-thoracotomy pain. *Eur J Pain.* 2001;5(1):89–96.

49. Dajczman E, Gordon A, Kreisman H, Wolkove N. Long-term postthoracotomy pain. *Chest.* 1991;99(2):270–274.

50. Perttunen K, Tasmuth T, Kalso E. Chronic pain after thoracic surgery: a follow-up study. *Acta Anaesthesiol Scand.* 1999;43(5):563–567.

CHAPTER 17

Spinal Cord Injury–Related Neuropathic Pain

MENDEL KUPFER, MD

INTRODUCTION

Spinal cord injury is a relatively uncommon injury.[1] Spinal cord injuries are often divided as being either traumatic or nontraumatic and complete or incomplete. SCI is categorized according to the international standards for neurological classification of spinal cord 18 injury (ISNCSCI) colloquially referred to as the ASIA (American Spinal Injury Association) examination. The ASIA scale involves listing the caudal most normal level of neurologic examination in three categories—motor strength, pinprick sensation, and light touch sensation with the superior most intact level considered the overall level of the spinal cord injury. The ASIA scale further classifies the severity of the injury from A to E. A implies a complete injury, B is a sensory incomplete injury, C is a motor incomplete injury, D is a motor incomplete injury with at least half of tested muscles below the level of injury being antigravity or stronger, and E is a fully recovered spinal cord injury.[2] Spinal cord injuries are often complicated by neuropathic pain, with an estimated prevalence of approximately 50% of patients.[3–5]

Diagnostic Criteria

Patients with a spinal cord injury often present with complex multifactorial pain complaints that are difficult to describe or differentiate.[6] Multiple attempts at classifying spinal cord injury–related pain have been made. Twenty-nine systems of classification were catalogued by Hicken et al.[6–8] More recently the Spinal Cord Injury Pain Task Force of the International Association for the Study of Pain (SCIP-IASP)[9] proposed a new pain classification based on previous work by Cardenas[10] and Bryce-Ragnarsson.[11] The SCIP-IASP classification divides pain into three tiers. The first tier separates pain types into nociceptive pain, neuropathic pain, other pain, or unknown pain. Tier two then divides each of those categories into further subdivisions. Nociceptive pain is divided into musculoskeletal pain, visceral pain, and other nociceptive pain, and

then each of those categories are divided into the etiology or primary pain source in the tier 3. Neuropathic pain is divided into spinal cord injury at level pain, below level pain, and other neuropathic pain, and each one of these is divided into the contributing pain sources in tier 3. Other pain and unknown pain do not have a tier 2 subtype and are listed in tier 3 by primary pain source or pathology subtype[9] (Fig. 17.1).

Neuropathic pain has proven difficult to define and quantify, and this is particularly challenging in spinal cord injury. In 2008 the Special Interest Group on Neuropathic Pain of the IASP proposed a grading system of definite, probable, and possible neuropathic pain.[12] Definite neuropathic pain would require a pain distribution consistent with injury to the peripheral nervous system (PNS) or central nervous system (CNS) of the previous or current injury, disease affecting the PNS or CNS, and abnormal sensory signs within the body area corresponding to the injured parts of the CNS or PNS along with diagnostic tests that confirm the lesion, or disease in these structures. This definition was unsatisfactory for spinal cord–injured patients and additional criteria were proposed that include:

1. Onset of pain within 1 year following spinal cord injury.
2. No primary relation to movement, inflammation, or local tissue damage.
3. Hot, burning, tingling, pins and needles, sharp, shooting, squeezing, cold, electric, or shock-like quality of pain.[13,14]

Many additional definitions and subcategories of neuropathic pain have been proposed, including provoked and unprovoked. Multiple questionnaires have been developed in the attempt to ascertain the quality of neuropathic pain. These include the Leeds Assessment of Neuropathic Pain Scale, the Neuropathic Pain Questionnaire, and the DN4 Questionnaire. Bryce et al. have proposed a novel pain questionnaire that would be easy to administer or may even be self-administered by the patient.[15]

Tier 1: Pain type	Tier 2: Pain subtype	Tier 3: Primary pain source and/or pathology (write or type in)
☐ Nociceptive pain	☐ Musculoskeletal pain	☐ _____ e.g., glenohumeral arthritis, lateral epicondylitis, comminuted femur fracture, quadratus lumborum muscle spasm
	☐ Visceral pain	☐ _____ e.g., myocardial infarction, abdominal pain due to bowel impaction, cholecystitis
	☐ Other nociceptive pain	☐ _____ e.g., autonomic dysreflexia headache, migraine headache, surgical skin incision
☐ Neuropathic pain	☐ At level SCI pain	☐ _____ e.g., spinal cord compression, nerve root compression, cauda equina compression
	☐ Below level SCI pain	☐ _____ e.g., spinal cord ischemia, spinal cord compression
	☐ Other neuropathic pain	☐ _____ e.g., carpal tunnel syndrome, trigeminal neuralgia, diabetic polyneuropathy
☐ Other pain		☐ _____ e.g., fibromyalgia, Complex Regional Pain Syndrome type I, interstitial cystitis, irritable bowel syndrome
☐ Unknown pain		☐ _____

FIG. 17.1 International spinal cord injury pain (ISCIP) classification.[9] (From Bryce TN, Biering-Sørensen F, Finnerup NB, et al. International spinal cord injury pain classification: part I. Background and description. *Spinal Cord*. 2012;50(6):413–417. http://dx.doi.org/10.1038/sc.2011.156; with permission.)

Course

Neuropathic pain is generally reported by patients with spinal cord injury within the first 3 months to a year after injury, although it could develop over the course of the first 2 years.[16] The neuropathic pain typically does not abate, although rest, physical activity, and alcohol, as well as medication, have been found to be alleviating factors, whereas stress, anxiety, fatigue, weather changes, and cold ambient temperatures were found to be aggravating factors.[17] The severity of neuropathic pain is difficult to quantify, but the Neuropathic Pain Scale and the Neuropathic Pain Symptom Inventory have been used for this purpose.[13,18,19] Pain has been reported to be worse at night than during the day. There are conflicting reports of whether pain is worse with tetraplegia rather than paraplegia. Some of the ambiguity relates to the multifactorial nature of spinal cord injury–related pain. No correlation has been found between pain and the complete or incomplete nature of the injury.[16] Lack of pain at the initiation of acute inpatient rehabilitation has been correlated to lower long-term pain levels.[20] It has been proposed that levels of neuropathic pain can be predicted based upon sensory testing by evaluating the difference between light touch and pinprick scores on the AISA evaluation.[21]

Differential Diagnosis

Neuropathic pain as related to spinal cord injury is often difficult to differentiate from spasticity. Patients may use the term spasm when referring to a pain sensation and report pain when intending to mean spasm. The patient's complaints should be explored carefully during the acquisition of history, teasing out the nature and setting of the pain and whether spasms are actually observed versus the patient perceiving the sensation of spasm without visual confirmation of spasmodic movement. Central neuropathic pain must also be differentiated from peripheral nerve injury or lesions that may be superimposed upon the central spinal cord injury, such as peripheral compressive neuropathies and inflammatory neuropathies. Often neuropathic pain fluctuates throughout the day. However, pain that is progressively worsening or changing acutely in a previously stable patient should be concerning for a new underlying pathology, such as syrinx formation, soft tissue injury, occult fracture, heterotopic ossification (HO), or other new pathology, that may or may not be related to the spinal cord injury. Exacerbation of neuropathic pain and spasticity can also be a symptom of physiologic stress, such as infection or irritation (i.e., renal and gall bladder calculi), or psychologic stress, including somatization of mood disorders.

Diagnostic Testing

The role of diagnostic testing in the evaluation of neuropathic pain as related to spinal cord injury is limited to excluding alternative diagnoses and to confirming the underlying spinal cord pathology. Radiography is useful in the evaluation of occult fracture and HO.[22] This modality would be appropriate in the setting of exacerbation of pain with physical findings of new edema, redness, bony abnormality on palpation, or change in passive range of motion of a joint. The finding of HO lags on X-ray imaging, as the abnormal bone mineralizes and would better be diagnosed by MRI or nuclear imaging.[22] Ultrasound imaging is useful in the

evaluation of abdominal and retroperitoneal organ dysfunction, as persons with spinal cord injuries may not exhibit the typical patterns of pain associated with pathology of these organs. Calculus formation in the gall bladder and urinary system may be increased in those with spinal cord injuries.[23] Ultrasound imaging is also useful in diagnosing disorders of the circulatory system, including deep vein thrombosis[24] and vascular claudication. Computed tomography (CT) scans can be used to better visualize osseous and organ structures discussed in regards to X-ray and ultrasound imaging, albeit with an increased level of ionizing radiation. Diagnostic musculoskeletal ultrasound imaging is emerging as a useful modality in diagnosing peripheral nerve lesions in spinal cord–injured patients because electromyography and nerve conduction velocity studies are often difficult to interpret in the setting of an upper motor neuron lesion. Diagnostic musculoskeletal ultrasound imaging could also be used to evaluate musculoskeletal pathologies that mimic neuropathic pain. The role of electrodiagnostic testing is to exclude secondary diagnoses such as entrapment neuropathies and to evaluate potential comorbid disease entities such as plexopathies and peripheral polyneuropathies. Imaging of the spinal cord does not correlate with pain severity but may reveal a new diagnosis. Should syrinx be suspected, MRI is the test of choice for diagnosis.[25] CT myelogram may be used for those who cannot undergo MRI evaluation. Evidence of syrinx on CT myelogram has predictive value. However, absence of syrinx on a CT myelogram does not rule out its presence. Diagnostic testing to evaluate pain at the level of injury and below has been attempted with quantitative sensory testing. In a few controlled studies, it has been shown to be useful in predicting the treatment outcome but is not standardized nor routinely used in clinical practice.[13] Electroencephalogram and functional imaging find markers of pain by detecting a decrease in cortical activity in the frontal areas, but these tests are not in common clinical usage.[26]

Rehabilitation and Physical Medicine Options

Cognitive behavioral therapies have been postulated as being effective in the treatment of pain. A study consisting of 61 people conducted in four Dutch rehabilitation centers found that a cognitive behavioral program decreased pain intensity, pain-related disability, and anxiety in spinal cord–injured patients. However, the level of decrease in pain was less than predicted and the effect on pain-related disability was only borderline significant.[27] Roosink and Mercier[28] performed a literature review of virtual feedback for pain rehabilitation in spinal cord–injured patients. Seventeen studies were identified, and all were deemed to be of low quality. Although virtual feedback was found to have potential in improving motor function and reducing pain in spinal cord–injured patients, more research was found to be necessary in identifying appropriate patients and developing maximally effective treatment regimens. Transcranial direct current stimulation is an emerging technology that is being explored for the treatment of pain. Studies have yielded conflicting results regarding the efficacy of transcranial stimulation in the treatment of spinal cord injury–related neuropathic pain. These discrepancies may be explained by subject selection and the chronicity of the spinal cord injury in the various studies.[29,30] A small study found efficacy with exercise in the management of neuropathic pain in spinal cord–injured patients.[31] The use of transcutaneous electrical nerve stimulation (TENS) has been evaluated with inconsistent results. TENS may have improved efficacy in patients with more recent injuries. Patients should be monitored for autonomic dysreflexia if this modality is used.[32] The use of acupuncture has yielded disappointing results. A prospective study by Norrbrink and Lundeberg found a reduction in pain with a course of acupuncture; however, the results were not sustained at 2 months post study.[33] The efficacy of spinal cord stimulators and dorsal root entry zone lesioning have been studied in a very limited fashion in the setting of spinal cord injury, but the results were not encouraging.[34] A small pilot study showed promising results from having patients "virtually walk," but the sample size was small and the results were mixed.[35] As virtual reality and robotic-aided ambulation become more prevalent, their utility in treating pain will become more apparent.

MEDICATION OPTIONS
Topical Medications

Topical medications do not have a significant role in the treatment of neuropathic pain as related to spinal cord injuries because of the diffuse body areas that are usually affected. In a case series, two patients were found to respond well to topical 8% capsaicin patches applied after pretreatment with lidocaine and prilocaine.[36] Although the results were promising, it is difficult to extrapolate from a small study. The subjects in the study were ASIA classification D, which makes it further difficult to extrapolate to a broader range of patients with spinal cord injury. One must also consider the risks of autonomic dysreflexia in a patient with a spinal cord injury.

Antiepileptic Medications

Pregabalin is the only medication approved by the Federal Drug Administration for the treatment of neuropathic pain related to spinal cord injury. Pregabalin affects the voltage-gated calcium channel complexes in the presynaptic terminal. This in turn results in decreased neurotransmitter release and decreased pain sensation.[37] In a study by Carddenas et al., pregabalin was given to 108 patients with 112 placebo matched controls. Almost 80% of treated patients reported improvement of their pain.[38] A study of 137 patients with 12-week follow-up undertaken by Siddall et al. also demonstrated a significant reduction in pain levels.[39] Pregabalin is effective at 100–150 mg/day in divided doses, with a maximal dose of 600 mg/day.[39,40] Common side effects of pregabalin include somnolence (approximately 30%–40%), peripheral edema in approximately 13%, and dizziness.[40] There are a variety of less frequent, but potentially significant, adverse reactions such as weight gain, abnormalities of thought processing, and suicidal ideation.[41] Pregabalin has also been found to be effective in decreasing secondary issues related to pain, including difficulty sleeping, depression, and anxiety.[10,38,39]

Gabapentin is structurally similar to pregabalin. Gabapentin affects calcium channels at the neural bouton yielding an inhibitory effect on the neuron by diminishing calcium influx. Together with pregabalin, it is considered a first-line treatment for neuropathic pain related to spinal cord injury. A meta-analysis undertaken by Mehta, McIntyre et al. found eight studies that demonstrate significant neuropathic pain reduction with gabapentin. It is believed that there is no significant difference between the efficacies of gabapentin and pregabalin, although there is a conflicting literature to this point.[40,42]

Carbamazepine and oxcarbazepine are anticonvulsive drugs that affect voltage-gated sodium channels of the neuron. Oxcarbazepine has improved tolerance and is associated with fewer side effects than carbamazepine. Oxcarbazepine was found to be more effective than pregabalin in constant electrical, burning sensations and prickly paresthesias. In contrast, pregabalin was found to be more effective in the control of electrical shooting–like pain as well as hyperalgesia and allodynia. It has been postulated that different antiepileptic drugs may treat different subsets of the neuropathic pain.[37]

Levetiracetam is a novel antiepileptic medication. It is commonly used in posttraumatic seizure prophylaxis, but it has not been found to have meaningful efficacy in the treatment of spinal cord injury–related neuropathic pain.[43] A Cochrane review in 2014 found no evidence of efficacy of levetiracetam in the treatment of neuropathic pain.[44] Lamotrigine is an antiepileptic drug that acts upon the voltage-gated sodium channel. Lamotrigine has been found to have efficacy in the treatment of neuropathic pain, particularly in the setting of incomplete injury.[45] Valproic acid is a first-generation antiepileptic that acts upon voltage-gated sodium channels, causing a decrease in the firing frequency of neurons and also an increase in the γ-aminobutyric acid concentration of the brain. However, a double-blinded, crossover study found no significant difference in pain control between the treatment and nontreatment groups after 3 weeks.[46] Topiramate is commonly used for migraine headache prophylaxis. Its efficacy in controlling spinal cord injury–related neuropathic pain is weak, as the literature is conflicted.[47]

Antidepressant Medications

Tricyclic antidepressants act upon 5-HT2A receptors yielding an increase in serotonin-norepinephrine concentrations in the CNS. Amitriptyline has been classically used to control neuropathic pain syndromes of various etiologies. There is evidence demonstrating that amitriptyline is effective in the treatment of spinal cord injury pain in the context of depression. Of note, it has been suggested that amitriptyline may increase spasticity in spinal cord–injured patients.[48] Rantala demonstrated the efficacy of amitriptyline in a crossover study with gabapentin and an active placebo, diphenhydramine.[49] Tricyclic antidepressants are associated with anticholinergic side effects, including dry mouth, constipation, cardiac arrhythmia, glaucoma, and urinary retention. Weight gain may be significant. Other tricyclic antidepressants, such as imipramine and nortriptyline, have been found to have less adverse reactions than amitriptyline.

Trazodone is an atypical antidepressant with strong serotonin reuptake inhibition and to a lesser degree norepinephrine reuptake inhibition. In a 6-week, double-blind, placebo-controlled trial, Davidoff et al. found that trazodone was not better than placebo in controlling neuropathic pain in spinal cord–injured patients.[50] Lithium is a mood stabilizer that was studied in China for possible efficacy as a neuroregenerative agent. The study found no benefit in terms of improved function or neurologic outcome as compared with placebo, but pain was reduced with its use.[51] More research into the use of lithium is needed before a recommendation for its use can be made. Selective serotonin reuptake inhibitors are not found to have efficacy in controlling neuropathic pain. Selective serotonin norepinephrine reuptake inhibitors (SSNRIs) are found to have efficacy in the treatment of neuropathic pain, particularly in the setting of concomitant depression. In a study conducted by Vranken, 48 patients received escalating doses of duloxetine or placebo to a maximal dose of 120 mg/day and found a statistically significant decrease in dynamic pain and cold allodynia; however, tactile and pressure pain thresholds did not improve. Only one domain in an SF36 survey (a patient-reported survey of patient health) showed improvement. The Pain Disability Index survey did not show any significant improvement with the addition of duloxetine. The study's conclusion was to withhold judgment on the efficacy of this medication on central neuropathic pain.[52]

Opioid Medications

Opioid medications are commonly used to treat pain of many etiologies. Although there is controversy regarding the use of opioids in non-cancer-related chronic pain, opioids are commonly used in the treatment of spinal cord injury–related neuropathic pain. In a study of 7447 male veterans with spinal cord injury, 70% were noted to have received opioid medications.[53] A survey study by Cardenas found that 58% of responding patients had a therapeutic trial on opioid medications and that, as a medication class, opioids provided more relief from pain than any other class of oral medication.[54] A study conducted in Spain showed significant benefit in terms of neuropathic pain reduction by opioid medications in spinal cord–injured patients.[55] This finding is consistent with previous research on the role of opioid medications for the treatment of neuropathic pain.[56] The misuse of opioids in the spinal cord–injured population was found to be consistent with that in the general population with chronic pain.[57]

Recommendations for responsible opioid prescribing include the use of "opioid contracts," obtaining informed consent from the patient, performing random urine drug screens and pill counts, monitoring for aberrant behaviors, consulting with state data banks to minimize the risk of multiple providers prescribing opioids, using abuse deterrent formulations when appropriate, and setting treatment goals based upon functional outcomes.[58,59] Many of these measures, however, are more difficult to perform with persons with spinal cord injuries. For example, patients performing bladder routines may need catheter kits and nursing assistance to provide a urine drug screen. This patient population may find it difficult to bring in medications for review because of poor dexterity and a fear of theft that they cannot prevent. Often these patients have a reliance on others to dispense medications, which complicates their responsibility for safe storage of medications. Aberrant behaviors and substance abuse may have been the etiology of the spinal cord injury but it does not negate the validity of the new pain syndromes suffered.[60] Patients with spinal cord injuries may travel to distant medical centers, including crossing state lines, for specialized care, a behavior that may be suspicious in other patient populations. Individuals with dysphagia may not be able to use certain sustained-release formulations or abuse deterrent formulations. A variety of screening tools and surveys have been developed with the goal of identifying misuse of opioid medications in the population with chronic pain[61,62]; however, they are not well studied in the population with spinal cord injury.

Patients receiving opioid medications should also be monitored for medical side effects, including urinary retention, constipation, somnolence, respiratory depression, depressed testosterone levels, pruritis, mood disorders, and hyperalgesic syndrome. Caution should be exercised when prescribing opioid medications concurrent with benzodiazepine medications, commonly prescribed for the treatment of spasticity.

Tramadol

Tramadol is a unique medication in that it is a weak µ-opioid agonist with weak monoamine reuptake inhibition. Tramadol has been found to be effective in improving at level and below level neuropathic pain in a crossover study performed by Norbrink and Lundeberg.[63]

Cannabinoids

There is an emerging availability and interest in cannabinoid medications for the treatment of pain and spasticity. The body of the literature for the use of cannabinoids in spinal cord injury–related pain is scant, although a small study found no efficacy with the use of dronabinol as compared with active control.[64] Limitations of that study include a small sample size; it also only tested a specific extract of marijuana. There is a growing body of evidence that cannabis has efficacy in the treatment of neuropathic pain and spasticity as related to multiple sclerosis, particularly in its vaporized form.[65,66] Following the multiple sclerosis literature, further research into the application of cannabis to spinal cord injury patients is warranted.

Miscellaneous Medications

Nonsteroidal antiinflammatory drugs are ineffective in the treatment of neuropathic pain.[67] Their use in the acute phase of spinal cord injury may be contraindicated in the context of recent spine surgery and possible effects on bone healing. Acetaminophen does not have a significant efficacy in neuropathic pain[68]; however, it is often used to potentiate opioid medications.[69]

INTERVENTIONAL OPTIONS

Botulinum Toxin Injections

Early evidence indicates that subcutaneous injections of botulinum toxin are effective in treating spinal cord injury–related neuropathic pain. In one study, 40 patients were given a one-time dose of 200 units of botulinum toxin subcutaneously at the level of pain, with the finding of a significant reduction on the visual analog pain scale.[70] Similarly, supportive findings were found in other neuropathic pain syndromes, although the best route of delivery and specific indications have not been established.[71]

Intravenous Medications

Several intravenous medications have been trialed in the treatment of spinal cord injury–related pain. Pain may improve with lidocaine infusions and intravenous ketamine acting as a sodium channel and N-methyl-D-aspartate receptor antagonist, respectively. Although the ketamine and high-dose lidocaine were found to have efficacy in lessening neuropathic pain, they are not thought of as practical medications because of difficulty of administration and the risk of adverse reactions and toxicity.[72]

Intrathecal Medicine

Intrathecal baclofen is commonly used in the treatment of spasticity as related to spinal cord injury but has not been found to significantly reduce neuropathic pain related to spinal cord injury.[73] Intrathecal baclofen pumps may also be used to administer other medications to the intrathecal space. The use of this modality for the treatment of spinal cord injury–related neuropathic pain has not been well studied.[74] A small study by Siddall et al. consisting of 15 patients revealed that patients enjoyed significant benefit from intrathecal morphine and clonidine.[75] Intrathecal morphine or clonidine separately was not found to have better efficacy than placebo, but in combination, there was significant pain reduction. A limitation of the Siddall study is that patients underwent only a short course of intrathecal morphine and clonidine and long-term sequelae and efficacy were not characterized. Loubser et al. found that a single dose of intrathecal lidocaine yielded significant pain reduction for a mean duration of 2 hours.[76] The effects of a continuous infusion were not investigated. A case report found that the combination of intrathecal ziconotide and hydromorphone provided significant pain relief in a single patient.[77] It should be noted that in both the case series of intrathecal morphine and baclofen and the case report of intrathecal hydromorphone and ziconotide, the at-level pain preferentially improved, whereas the below-level pain persisted.

Surgical Options

A range of neurosurgical techniques have been explored in the treatment of spinal cord injury–related neuropathic pain. Neuromodulation by means of spinal cord stimulation has been studied in a limited fashion without impressive results.[34] Aggressive procedures, such as intrathecal phenol, thalamotomies, anterior spinal cord decompression commissurotomy, and surgical sympathectomy have also not yielded satisfying results.[3] The use of dorsal root entry zone (DREZ) lesions and cordotomies has been found to have efficacy in certain spinal cord–injured patients with intractable severe neuropathic pain.[3] A modified surgical DREZotomy procedure has been claimed to have improved outcomes in a small single-site study.[78] One potential application for aggressive surgical procedures may be in parts of the world were access to close medical care and medications are not possible.[79]

Prognosis

A rational approach to the treatment of neuropathic pain in the spinal cord–injured patient would be to first understand the specific functional impairments that are limited because the patient is having pain. Second, function-based goals and realistic expectations for analgesia should be set. Third, comorbid ailments should be treated, provocative factors mitigated, and exacerbating conditions addressed. Fourth, noninvasive medicine-sparing modalities should be trialed. Fifth, medications should be added in a stepwise fashion from the least invasive and best tolerated to the most invasive with more serious potential side effects, all with concurrent monitoring for adverse reactions. Gabapentin or pregabalin remain the first-line medications for this pain syndrome; however, patients should be monitored for side effects, including dizziness, sedation, and edema. Antidepressant medications such as tricyclic antidepressants or SSNRIs may be used in place of, or in conjunction with, an antiepileptic drug, particularly in the context of pain with depression. If the patient has difficulty sleeping, urinary incontinence, or difficulty with secretion management, the anticholinergic effects of a

tricyclic antidepressant may be desirable. Judicious use of opioids may also be indicated in the treatment of neuropathic pain. The patient should be monitored for compliance and aberrant behaviors, as well as for medical side effects of chronic opioid use. Pharmacologic treatments may be augmented by complementary treatments such as cognitive behavioral therapy. If pain is confined to an isolated body part, topical medications, such as capsaicin, may be of benefit. Future directions to be investigated include the use of subcutaneous botulinum toxins, cortical stimulation, and cannabis. The role for aggressive interventional procedures is limited. Intrathecal medications may be considered in recalcitrant cases.

REFERENCES

1. Spinal cord injury (SCI) 2016 facts and figures at a glance. *J Spinal Cord Med.* 2016;39(4):493–494. http://dx.doi.org/10.1080/10790268.2016.1210925.
2. Marino RJ, Barros T, Biering-Sorensen F, et al. International standards for neurological classification of spinal cord injury. *J Spinal Cord Med.* 2003;26 (suppl 1):S50–S56. http://www.pubmedcentral.nih.gov/articlerender.fcgi?artid=4066420&tool=pmcentrez&rendertype=abstract%5Cnhttp://www.ncbi.nlm.nih.gov/pubmed/16296564.
3. Siddall PJ, Loeser JD. Pain following spinal cord injury. *Spinal Cord.* 2001;39(2):63–73. http://www.ncbi.nlm.nih.gov/pubmed/11402361.
4. Siddall PJ, McClelland JM, Rutkowski SB, Cousins MJ. A longitudinal study of the prevalence and characteristics of pain in the first 5 years following spinal cord injury. *Pain.* 2003;103(3):249–257. http://dx.doi.org/10.1016/S0304-3959(02)00452-9.
5. Burke D, Fullen BM, Stokes D, Lennon O. Neuropathic pain prevalence following spinal cord injury: a systematic review and meta-analysis. *Eur J Pain.* 2017;21(1):29–44. http://dx.doi.org/10.1002/ejp.905.
6. Putzke JD, Richards JS, Hicken BL, Ness TJ, Kezar L, DeVivo M. Pain classification following spinal cord injury: the utility of verbal descriptors. *Spinal Cord.* 2002;40(3):118–127. http://0.180.245.238.
7. Calmels P, Mick G, Perrouin-Verbe B, Ventura M. Neuropathic pain in spinal cord injury: identification, classification, evaluation. *Ann Phys Rehabil Med.* 2009;52(2):83–102. http://dx.doi.org/10.1016/j.rehab.2008.12.012.
8. Hicken BL, Putzke JDRJ. Classification of pain following spinal cord injury: literature review and future directions. In: Burchiel K, Yezierski RP, ed. *Spinal Cord Injury Pain: Assessment, Mechanisms, Management.* vol. 23. Seattle, WA: International Association for the Study of Pain; 2002:25–38.
9. Bryce TN, Biering-Sørensen F, Finnerup NB, et al. International spinal cord injury pain classification: part I. Background and description. *Spinal Cord.* 2012;50(6):413–417. http://dx.doi.org/10.1038/sc.2011.156.

10. Cardenas DD, Emir B, Parsons B. Examining the time to therapeutic effect of pregabalin in spinal cord injury patients with neuropathic pain. *Clin Ther*. 2015;37(5):1081–1090. http://dx.doi.org/10.1016/j.clinthera.2015.02.028.

11. Bryce TN, Dijkers MPJM, Ragnarsson KT, Stein AB, Chen B. Reliability of the Bryce/Ragnarsson spinal cord injury pain taxonomy. *J Spinal Cord Med*. 2006;29(2):118–132.

12. Saulino M. Spinal cord injury pain. *Phys Med Rehabil Clin N Am*. 2014;25(2):397–410.

13. Felix ER. Chronic neuropathic pain in SCI: evaluation and treatment. *Phys Med Rehabil Clin N Am*. 2014;25(3):545–571. http://dx.doi.org/10.1016/j.pmr.2014.04.007.

14. Finnerup NB, Baastrup C. Spinal cord injury pain: mechanisms and management. *Curr Pain Headache Rep*. 2012;16(3):207–216. http://dx.doi.org/10.1007/s11916-012-0259-x.

15. Bryce TN, Richards JS, Bombardier CH, et al. Screening for neuropathic pain after spinal cord injury with the spinal cord injury pain instrument (SCIPI): a preliminary validation study. *Spinal Cord*. 2014;52(5):407–412. http://dx.doi.org/10.1038/sc.2014.21%5Cn. http://www.ncbi.nlm.nih.gov/pubmed/24614856.

16. Celik EC, Erhan B, Lakse E. The clinical characteristics of neuropathic pain in patients with spinal cord injury. *Spinal Cord*. 2012;50(8):585–589. http://dx.doi.org/10.1038/sc.2012.26.

17. Finnerup NB, Johannesen IL, Sindrup SH, Bach FW, Jensen TS. Pain and dysesthesia in patients with spinal cord injury: a postal survey. *Spinal Cord*. 2001;39(5):256–262.

18. Galer BS, Jensen MP. Development and preliminary validation of a pain measure specific to neuropathic pain the Neuropathic Pain Scale. *Neurology*. 1997;48(2):332–338. http://www.neurology.org/content/48/2/332%5Cnhttp://www.ncbi.nlm.nih.gov/pubmed/9040716%5Cnhttp://www.neurology.org.libproxy.ucl.ac.uk/content/48/2/332.

19. Bouhassira D, Attal N, Fermanian J, et al. Development and validation of the neuropathic pain symptom inventory. *Pain*. 2004;108(3):248–257.

20. Zanca JM, Dijkers MP, Hammond FM, Horn SD. Pain and its impact on inpatient rehabilitation for acute traumatic spinal cord injury: analysis of observational data collected in the SCIRehab study. *Arch Phys Med Rehabil*. 2013;94(4 suppl).

21. Levitan Y, Zeilig G, Bondi M, Ringler E, Defrin R. Predicting the risk for central pain using the sensory components of the international standards for neurological classification of spinal cord injury. *J Neurotrauma*. 2015;32(21):1684–1692. http://online.liebertpub.com/doi/10.1089/neu.2015.3947%5Cn. http://www.ncbi.nlm.nih.gov/pubmed/26244708.

22. Sautter-Bihl ML, Hültenschmidt B, Liebermeister E, et al. Heterotopic ossification following traumatic brain injury and spinal cord injury. *J Am Acad Orthop Surg*. 2009;17(11):689–697. http://dx.doi.org/10.1371/journal.pone.0016632.

23. Moonka R, Stiens SA, Resnick WJ, et al. The prevalence and natural history of gallstones in spinal cord injured patients. *J Am Coll Surg*. 1999;189(99):274–281. http://dx.doi.org/10.1016/S1072-7515(99)00143-X.

24. Kelly BM, Yoder BM, Tang C-T, Wakefield TW. Venous thromboembolic events in the rehabilitation setting. *PM R*. 2010;2(7):647–663. http://dx.doi.org/10.1016/j.pmrj.2010.03.029.

25. Le Chapelain L, Perrouin-Verbe B, Fattal C. Chronic neuropathic pain in spinal cord injury patients: what relevant additional clinical exams should be performed? *Ann Phys Rehabil Med*. 2009;52(2):103–110.

26. Pascoal-Faria P, Yalcin N, Fregni F. Neural markers of neuropathic pain associated with maladaptive plasticity in spinal cord injury. *Pain Pract*. 2015;15(4):371–377. http://dx.doi.org/10.1111/papr.12237.

27. Heutink M, Post MWM, Bongers-Janssen HMH, et al. The CONECSI trial: results of a randomized controlled trial of a multidisciplinary cognitive behavioral program for coping with chronic neuropathic pain after spinal cord injury. *Pain*. 2012;153(1):120–128. http://dx.doi.org/10.1016/j.pain.2011.09.029.

28. Roosink M, Mercier C. Virtual feedback for motor and pain rehabilitation after spinal cord injury. *Spinal Cord*. 2014;52(12):860–866. http://dx.doi.org/10.1038/sc.2014.160.

29. Wrigley PJ, Gustin SM, McIndoe LN, Chakiath RJ, Henderson LA, Siddall PJ. Longstanding neuropathic pain after spinal cord injury is refractory to transcranial direct current stimulation: a randomized controlled trial. *Pain*. 2013;154(10):2178–2184. http://dx.doi.org/10.1016/j.pain.2013.06.045.

30. Ngernyam N, Jensen MP, Arayawichanon P, et al. The effects of transcranial direct current stimulation in patients with neuropathic pain from spinal cord injury. *Clin Neurophysiol*. 2015;126(2):382–390. http://dx.doi.org/10.1016/j.clinph.2014.05.034.

31. Norrbrink C, Lindberg T, Wahman K, Bjerkefors A. Effects of an exercise programme on musculoskeletal and neuropathic pain after spinal cord injury—results from a seated double-poling ergometer study. *Spinal Cord*. 2012;50(6):457–461. http://dx.doi.org/10.1038/sc.2011.160.

32. Felix ER. Chronic neuropathic pain in SCI. Evaluation and treatment. *Phys Med Rehabil Clin N Am*. 2014;25(3):545–571.

33. Norrbrink C, Lundeberg T. Acupuncture and massage therapy for neuropathic pain following spinal cord injury: an exploratory study. *Acupunct Med*. 2011;29:108–115. http://dx.doi.org/10.1136/aim.2010.003269.

34. Dworkin RH, O'Connor AB, Kent J, et al. Interventional management of neuropathic pain: NeuPSIG recommendations. *Pain*. 2013;154(11):2249–2261. http://dx.doi.org/10.1016/j.pain.2013.06.004.

35. Jordan M, Pain N. Effects of virtual walking treatment on spinal cord injury related neuropathic pain: pilot results and trends related to location of pain and at-level neuronal hypersensitivity. *Am J Phys Med Rehabil*. 2016;95(5):390–396. http://dx.doi.org/10.1097/PHM.0000000000000417.

36. Trbovich M, Yang H. Capsaicin 8% patch for central and peripheral neuropathic pain of persons with incomplete spinal cord injury: two case reports. *Am J Phys Med Rehabil/Assoc Acad Physiatr.* 2015;94(8):e66–72. http://dx.doi.org/10.1097/PHM.0000000000000301.

37. Min K, Oh Y, Lee S-H, Ryu JS. Symptom-based treatment of neuropathic pain in spinal cord-injured patients. *Am J Phys Med Rehabil.* 2016;95(5):330–338. http://dx.doi.org/10.1097/PHM.0000000000000382.

38. Cardenas DD, Nieshoff EC, Suda K, et al. A randomized trial of pregabalin in patients with neuropathic pain due to spinal cord injury. *Neurology.* 2013;80(6):533–539. http://dx.doi.org/10.1212/WNL.0b013e318281546b.

39. Siddall PJ, Cousins MJ, Otte A, Griesing T, Chambers R, Murphy TK. Pregabalin in central neuropathic pain associated with spinal cord injury: a placebo-controlled trial. *Neurology.* 2006;67(10):1792–1800.

40. Mehta S, McIntyre A, Dijkers M, Loh E, Teasell RW, Teasell M. Gabapentinoids are effective in decreasing neuropathic pain and other secondary outcomes after spinal cord injury: a meta-analysis. *Arch Phys Med Rehabil.* 2014;95(11):2180–2186. http://dx.doi.org/10.1016/j.apmr.2014.06.010.

41. Lyrica Package Insert, https://www.accessdata.fda.gov/drugsatfda_docs/label/2011/021446s026,022488s005lbl.pdf Accessed 9/7/17

42. Pérez C, Navarro A, Saldaña MT, Masramón X, Rejas J. Pregabalin and gabapentin in matched patients with peripheral neuropathic pain in routine medical practice in a primary care setting: findings from a cost-consequences analysis in a nested case-control study. *Clin Ther.* 2010;32(7):1357–1370. http://dx.doi.org/10.1016/j.clinthera.2010.07.014.

43. Finnerup NB, Grydehøj J, Bing J, et al. Levetiracetam in spinal cord injury pain: a randomized controlled trial. *Spinal Cord.* 2009;47(12):861–867. http://dx.doi.org/10.1038/sc.2009.55.

44. Wiffen PJ, Derry S, Moore RA, Lunn MP. Levetiracetam for neuropathic pain in adults. In: Derry S, ed. *Cochrane Database of Systematic Reviews.* Chichester, UK: John Wiley & Sons, Ltd; 2014. http://dx.doi.org/10.1002/14651858.CD010943.pub2.

45. Finnerup NB, Sindrup SH, Bach FW, Johannesen ILJT. Lamotrigine in spinal cord injury pain: a randomized controlled trial. *Pain.* 2002;96(3):375–383.

46. Drewes AM, Andreasen A, Poulsen LH. Valproate for treatment of chronic central pain after spinal cord injury. A double-blind cross-over study. *Paraplegia.* 1994;32(8):565–569. http://dx.doi.org/10.1038/sc.1994.89.

47. Dinoff BL, Richards JSNT. Use of topiramate for spinal cord injury-related pain. *J Spinal Cord Med.* 2003;26(4):401–403.

48. Teasell RW, Mehta S, Aubut J-AL, et al. A systematic review of pharmacologic treatments of pain after spinal cord injury. *Arch Phys Med Rehabil.* 2010;91(5):816–831. http://dx.doi.org/10.1016/j.apmr.2010.01.022.

49. Rintala DH, Holmes SA, Courtade D, Fiess RN, Tastard LV, Loubser PG. Comparison of effectiveness of amitriptyline and gabapentin on chronic neuropathic pain in persons with spinal cord injury. *Arch Phys Med Rehabil.* 2007;88(12):1547–1560.

50. Davidoff G, Guarracini M, Roth E, Sliwa J, Yarkony G. Trazodone hydrochloride in the treatment of dysesthetic pain in traumatic myelopathy: a randomized, double-blind, placebo-controlled study. *Pain.* 1987;29(2):151–161. http://www.ncbi.nlm.nih.gov/pubmed/3302841.

51. Yang ML, Li JJ, So KF, et al. Efficacy and safety of lithium carbonate treatment of chronic spinal cord injuries: a double-blind, randomized, placebo-controlled clinical trial. *Spinal Cord.* 2012;50(2):141–146. http://dx.doi.org/10.1038/sc.2011.126.

52. Vranken JH, Hollmann MW, van der Vegt MH, et al. Duloxetine in patients with central neuropathic pain caused by spinal cord injury or stroke: a randomized, double-blind, placebo-controlled trial. *Pain.* 2011;152(2):267–273. http://dx.doi.org/10.1016/j.pain.2010.09.005.

53. Carbone LD, Chin AS, Burns SP, et al. Morbidity following lower extremity fractures in men with spinal cord injury. *Osteoporos Int.* 2013;24(8):2261–2267. http://dx.doi.org/10.1007/s00198-013-2295-8.

54. Cardenas DD, Jensen MP. Treatments for chronic pain in persons with spinal cord injury: a survey study. *J Spinal Cord Med.* 2006;29(2):109–117.

55. Barrera-Chacon JM, Mendez-Suarez JL, Jáuregui-Abrisqueta ML, Palazon R, Barbara-Bataller E, García-Obrero I. Oxycodone improves pain control and quality of life in anticonvulsant- pretreated spinal cord-injured patients with neuropathic pain. *Spinal Cord.* 2011;49(1):36–42. http://www.scopus.com/inward/record.url?eid.=2-s2.0-78651286587&partnerID=40&md5=e2694748ea649d55bcfa67599cc829d6.

56. Finnerup NB, Otto M, McQuay HJ, Jensen TS, Sindrup SH. Algorithm for neuropathic pain treatment: an evidence based proposal. *Pain.* 2005;118(3):289–305.

57. Krause JS, Clark JMR, Saunders LL. Pain medication misuse among participants with spinal cord injury. *Spinal Cord.* 2015;53(8):630–635. http://dx.doi.org/10.1038/sc.2015.42.

58. Peppin JF, Passik SD, Couto JE, et al. Recommendations for urine drug monitoring as a component of opioid therapy in the treatment of chronic pain. *Pain Med.* 2012;13:886–896.

59. Pain N, Practices PB, Cone EJ, et al. Risks and responsibilities in prescribing opioids risks and responsibilities in prescribing opioids for chronic noncancer pain, part 2: best practices. 2017;5481(May). http://dx.doi.org/10.3810/pgm.2014.11.2841.

60. Passik SD. Challenges in using opioids to treat pain in persons with substance use disorders. *Addict Sci Clin Pract.* 2008;(2):4–25.

61. Jones T, Moore T, Levy JL, et al. original article A comparison of various risk screening methods in predicting discharge from opioid treatment. *Clin J Pain.* 2012;28(2):93–100.

62. Soapp-r CPP, Butler SF, Budman SH, Fernandez KC, Fanciullo GJ, Jamison RN. Cross-validation of a screener to predict opioid misuse in chronic pain patients. *J Addict Med.* 2009;3(2):66–73.

63. Norrbrink C, Lundeberg T. Tramadol in neuropathic pain after spinal cord injury. *Clin J Pain*. 2009;25(3):177–184. http://dx.doi.org/10.1097/AJP.0b013e31818a744d.

64. Rintala DH, Fiess RN, Tan G, Holmes SA, Bruel BM. Effect of dronabinol on central neuropathic pain after spinal cord injury. *Am J Phys Med Rehabil*. 2010;89(10):840–848. http://dx.doi.org/10.1097/PHM.0b013e3181f1c4ec.

65. Schrot RJ, Hubbard JR. Cannabinoids: medical implications. *Ann Med*. 2016;48(3):128–141. http://dx.doi.org/10.3109/07853890.2016.1145794.

66. Leung L. Cannabis and its derivatives: review of medical use. *J Am Board Fam Med*. 2011;24(4):452–462. http://dx.doi.org/10.3122/jabfm.2011.04.100280.

67. Moore RA, Chi C-C, Wiffen PJ, Derry S, Rice ASC. Oral nonsteroidal anti-inflammatory drugs for neuropathic pain. In: Moore RA, ed. *Cochrane Database of Systematic Reviews*. Chichester, UK: John Wiley & Sons, Ltd; 2015. http://dx.doi.org/10.1002/14651858.CD010902.pub2.

68. Wiffen PJ, Knaggs R, Derry S, Cole P, Phillips T, Moore RA. Paracetamol (acetaminophen) with or without codeine or dihydrocodeine for neuropathic pain in adults. In: Moore RA, ed. *Cochrane Database of Systematic Reviews*. Chichester, UK: John Wiley & Sons, Ltd; 2016. http://dx.doi.org/10.1002/14651858.CD012227.pub2.

69. Shinozaki T, Yamada T, Nonaka T, Yamamoto T. Acetaminophen and non-steroidal anti-inflammatory drugs interact with morphine and tramadol analgesia for the treatment of neuropathic pain in rats. *J Anesth*. 2015;29(3):386–395. http://dx.doi.org/10.1007/s00540-014-1953-0.

70. Han Z-A, Song DH, Oh H-M, Chung ME. Botulinum toxin type A for neuropathic pain in patients with spinal cord injury. *Ann Neurol*. 2016;79(4):569–578. http://dx.doi.org/10.1002/ana.24605.

71. Francisco GE, Tan H, Green M. Do botulinum toxins have a role in the management of neuropathic pain? *Am J Phys Med Rehabil*. 2012;91(10):899–909. http://dx.doi.org/10.1097/PHM.0b013e31825a134b.

72. Attal N, Mazaltarine G, Perrouin-Verbe B, Albert T. Chronic neuropathic pain management in spinal cord injury patients. What is the efficacy of pharmacological treatments with a general mode of administration? (oral, transdermal, intravenous). *Ann Phys Rehabil Med*. 2009;52(2):124–141.

73. Loubser PG, Akman NM. Effects of intrathecal baclofen on chronic spinal cord injury pain. *J Pain Symptom Manage*. 1996;12(4):241–247.

74. Bensmail D, Ecoffey C, Ventura M, Albert T. Chronic neuropathic pain in patients with spinal cord injury. What is the efficacy of regional interventions? Sympathetic blocks, nerve blocks and intrathecal drugs. *Ann Phys Rehabil Med*. 2009;52(2):142–148. http://dx.doi.org/10.1016/j.rehab.2008.12.004.

75. Siddall PJ, Molloy AR, Walker S, Mather LE, Rutkowski SB, Cousins MJ. The efficacy of intrathecal morphine and clonidine in the treatment of pain after spinal cord injury. *Anesth Analg*. 2000;91(6):1493–1498. http://dx.doi.org/10.1097/00000539-200012000-00037.

76. Loubser PG, Donovan WH. Diagnostic spinal anaesthesia in chronic spinal cord injury pain. *Paraplegia*. 1991;29(1):25–36. http://dx.doi.org/10.1038/sc.1991.4.

77. Saulino M. Successful reduction of neuropathic pain associated with spinal cord injury via of a combination of intrathecal hydromorphone and ziconotide: a case report. *Spinal Cord*. 2007;45(11):749–752. http://dx.doi.org/10.1038/sj.sc.3102027.

78. Chun H-J, Kim YS, Yi H-J. A modified microsurgical DREZotomy procedure for refractory neuropathic pain. *World Neurosurg*. 2011;75(3–4):551–557. http://dx.doi.org/10.1016/j.wneu.2010.12.005.

79. Taira T. Ablative neurosurgical procedure for pain after spinal cord injury. *World Neurosurg*. 2011;75(3–4):449–450. http://dx.doi.org/10.1016/j.wneu.2010.12.049.

CHAPTER 18

Pain Syndromes Associated With Traumatic Brain Injury

BRIAN T. KUCER, MD

Traumatic brain injuries (TBIs) are a worldwide significant cause of mortality and morbidity. There are approximately 1.4 million TBIs each year in the United States seen by healthcare providers and an estimated 1–3 million more mild injuries that do not seek medical attention.[1] The overall prevalence rate for TBI survivors experiencing disability in the United States is estimated at 3–5 million.[2] Chronic pain syndromes are common after TBI, estimated to affect approximately 50%–80% of TBI survivors, the majority of whom suffer from chronic headache and back pain.[3–6] There may be a negative correlation between pain reporting and injury severity, with mild TBI survivors reporting more pain than moderate to severe TBI survivors.[7] This difference can be attributed to a variety of factors including attentional, insight, and awareness impairments in moderate to severe TBI survivors versus increased activity and cognitive strain in the mild TBI population. Pain that persists beyond the initial phase (3 months) of healing[8] is considered a chronic pain syndrome, although the time frame when acute becomes chronic has been clinically defined and may be more arbitrary. Concurrent posttraumatic stress disorder, especially among veterans, is common.[9]

Management of chronic pain syndromes after TBI clinically requires understanding of the incidence, physiology, and pathophysiology of central nervous system (CNS) injuries and their effect on pain perception and modulation, relevant anatomic considerations, and a thorough understanding of nonorganic factors that contribute to ongoing reporting of pain. Key tenets of good physiatric management of patients with centrally mediated pain include taking a thorough history from the patient and possibly their caretakers, a comprehensive physical examination, evaluation of objective testing, and then developing a plan of care that allows for treatment of the whole patient, with an emphasis on improving function and quality of life.

DEFINITIONS OF PAIN

The definition of pain is widely accepted as: An unpleasant sensory and emotional experience associated with actual or potential tissue damage, or described in terms of such damage.[10] The pain pathways can involve an external stimulus, peripheral sensory nociceptors, subcortical structures, and cortical pathways. In addition, individual psychological factors contribute to pain in the acute and chronic phases and may predominate in these later stages.[11] Assessment of chronic pain involves consideration of factors in each of these areas. Localized tissue damage, the activation of cytokine mediated pathways, and changes in regional blood flow and metabolism have all been associated with physiologic changes after TBI. In regards to anatomic differences, acute painful stimuli generally activate somatosensory, insular, and cingulate cortical regions, whereas spontaneous pain and allodynia activate the prefrontal cortex and limbic regions.[12]

Chronic pain is common after TBI and can be grouped into a few main subtypes: somatic and musculoskeletal injuries, peripheral nociceptive pain, and central and peripheral neuropathic pain syndromes. Nociceptive pain is pain generated from peripheral damaged tissues, whereas neuropathic pain is pain with a generator from either a peripheral nerve or from an aberrant signal from the CNS. The incidence of the peripheral nerve injuries in patients with concomitant TBI is estimated at 34%.[13] Traumatic neuropathies most commonly affect the brachial plexus, followed by the radial, ulnar, and peroneal nerves. About 50% of patients with peripheral nerve lesions experienced neuropathic pain, and patients with traumatic peripheral neuropathies had significantly decreased quality of life reporting.[14] Somatic and musculoskeletal injuries are vast and can include the spectrum of soft tissue injuries (including tendinous, ligamentous, and capsular injuries and joint instability), fractures (both clinically acute and late-diagnosed fractures), heterotopic ossification, and visceral injuries with referred pain. Centrally mediated neuropathic pain can present as either a headache syndrome or more peripheral pain syndromes and is described in more detail in the following sections (Table 18.1[15]).

POSTTRAUMATIC HEADACHES

By far, the most common centrally mediated pain syndrome after TBI is posttraumatic headache. The incidence of posttraumatic headache varies; the most widely accepted definition is from the International Classification of Headache disorders (ICHD). The ICHD-Beta 3 defines posttraumatic headache as occurring within 7 days of trauma or the ability to sense and report headache after trauma. It is usually classified as tension-type headache or migraine.[16] The 7-day cutoff may underestimate the number of TBI survivors who experience headaches, which has been reported as up to 71% in the first year.[17] The anatomy of headache involves modulation of a complex series of excitatory and inhibitory neuronal networks, involving changes in afferent input to the trigeminocervical nucleus as well as changes in modulation of nociceptive inputs as excellently summarized by Bogduk.[18]

Diagnostic criteria for posttraumatic headaches rely exclusively on patient reporting, and thus the clinician should document the location, duration, onset, radiation, associated symptoms, and ameliorating and exacerbating factors with each visit. Pain-related behaviors and the consistency of those behaviors should also be observed and documented. In addition, headache logs and standardized questionnaires are more likely to be used in specialty headache centers as part of the evaluation process.[19] Serial administration of standardized headache questionnaires such as the Migraine Disability Assessment score can be useful in determining the impact on quality of life.[20] Factors associated with prolonged headaches include history of prior headaches, less severe injury, female gender, and history of psychiatric disorder.[16] This comprehensive assessment helps to document changes in headache character over time and also aids in the detection of inconsistencies, which may represent manifestations of secondary gain.

Although these approaches can be helpful in treating mild TBI survivors, unique challenges exist for patients with moderate to severe injuries. Difficulty with alertness, attention, verbal expression, insight/awareness, and agitation may make it difficult to

TABLE 18.1
Potential Etiologies of Pain in Traumatic Brain Injuries

Pain Syndrome	Causes	Manifestations	Treatment
Peripheral nociceptive pain syndrome	Damage to tissues: Crush injuries, Visceral injuries, Fractures, Sprains, Strains, Hematoma, Abrasions, Wounds, Burns, Heterotopic ossification	Typically occurs at or near the site of injury	Reduction of inflammation, Relative rest, Stretching, Myofascial release, Modalities including ice and heat, Immobilization or mobility to improve healing
Peripheral neuropathic pain syndrome	Damage (trauma or autoimmune/disease process specific to the peripheral nervous system	Typically follows a more distal to proximal progression (length-dependent process)	Rule out chronic impingement requiring surgical intervention, Medication, Desensitization techniques, Modalities
Central neuropathic pain syndrome	Damage to central nervous system, usually thalamus	More distal than proximal, may occur focally or globally, does not follow dermatomal distribution	Medications, Desensitization, Cortical stimulation, Complementary and alternative medicine

Data from International Classification of Headaches, Beta-3. Available at: https://www.ichd-3.org/.

understand for certain whether a patient is in pain as well as make it difficult to understand the specific characteristics of the painful condition, such as subtleties of any ameliorating or exacerbating factors.[21] Observation of pain-related behaviors, correlation between physical movements and worsening agitation, fluctuations in vital signs, and any asymmetry on physical examination can be a clue to the clinician to pursue further diagnostic studies.

International Classification of Headaches (ICHD-Beta 3) taxonomy delineates a few different headache syndromes. The first is acute headache attributable to moderate or severe injury to the head and must include one of the following: (1) loss of consciousness for >30 min; (2) Glasgow Coma Scale score <13; (3) posttraumatic amnesia lasting >24 h; (4) alteration in the level of awareness for >24 h; (5) imaging evidence of a traumatic head injury, such as intracranial hemorrhage and/or brain contusion.[22] Acute headache caused by mild TBI involves lack of inclusion into the moderate or severe category, plus one of the following: (1) transient confusion, disorientation, or impaired consciousness; (2) loss of memory for events immediately before or after the head injury (anterograde or retrograde amnesia); (3) two or more other symptoms suggestive of mild TBI: nausea, vomiting, visual disturbances, dizziness and/or vertigo, impaired memory and/or concentration.[23] Chronic headache is defined as symptom duration lasting more than 3 months.[24]

The awareness of the morbidity of blast-related injury after military deployment has led to more research into the prevalence of headache in this population. Military veterans with history of deployment-related TBI report more frequent, persistent headaches than age-matched controls.[25]

Differential diagnosis of posttraumatic headache involves probing into contributing and potential external factors. The presence of intracranial bleeding or mass lesion is typically ruled out with CT scan of the head in the initial management of TBI. The presence of an intracranial lesion should prompt neurosurgical consultation. Typically, a negative CT scan with persistent symptoms is followed by MRI to rule out any other mass or demyelinating process.

The presence of cervicogenic headache due to instability and/or pain from the cervical joints and associated ligaments, as well as the potential for trigger-point associated referred pain patterns, should be considered. Palpation of the posterior cervical musculature should also be assessed, as it can contribute to headache reporting, and patients with chronic tension-type headaches have lower pain thresholds for trigger points

than patients without chronic headache.[26] Orthopedic spinal injuries affecting spinal stability should be evaluated, as these injuries can contribute to chronic headache symptoms via referred pain pathways.[27]

Assessment of the patient's psychological milieu is imperative. Often traumatic events are associated with attributing premorbid symptoms to the event. Teasing out the presence or absence of symptoms before the TBI is an important clinical strategy. Malingering and other forms of secondary gain constitute a minority of cases of chronic headache; there is some evidence to suggest that societal factors influence persistent symptom reporting.[28]

The course of posttraumatic headache is variable and unpredictable, although the overall prognosis is generally good. The most common presentation resembles tension-type headache and/or migraine or a mixture of headache syndromes and is most commonly reported in the temporal region[29] (see Table 18.2). Eighty percent of patients improve over time; however, the duration of improvement can vary widely up to 6 months.[30] Approximately 20% of patients report infrequent headaches at 1 year after their injury, with 5% of patients reporting persistent daily headache.[17]

TABLE 18.2
Common Primary Headaches

Common Types of Primary Headache	Clinical Manifestations
Migraine headache	May or may not be accompanied by aura or prodrome Female predominance Deep pulsating pain or throbbing Sound/light sensitivity Nausea and vomiting are common
Tension-type headache	Typically described as bitemporal, dull ache Female predominance Nausea and vomiting are rare Not associated with aura May last several days
Cluster headache (the most common of the trigeminal autonomic cephalgias)	Unilateral, stabbing pain, usually around the eye Sudden onset Male predominance Nausea and vomiting are rare

Clinical worsening of headache presentation may be attributable to changes in environmental factors, including referred pain from musculoskeletal disorders, an increase in activity, increased depression, frustration or negative impact related to changes in social participation and fulfillment of societal roles, or medication overuse headaches.

The current clinical guidelines for treatment recommend identification of the most closely associated headache type and treatment of headaches based on the headache type. Posttraumatic tension-type headaches should be treated according to clinical practice guidelines for tension-type headaches in the non-TBI population, whereas migraine-type posttraumatic headaches should be treated according to clinical practice guidelines for migraine-type headaches in the non-TBI population.[31] The medications recommended by the Ontario Neurotrauma Foundation Guidelines for mild TBI and persistent symptoms are given in Table 18.3.[31]

In addition to oral therapies, botulinum toxin is an effective treatment[32] for chronic migraine and tension-type headaches. It may be a useful agent in patients with medication noncompliance.[33] Botox should be considered when first- or second-line medications are unable to effectively manage chronic migraine headaches. The US Food and Drug Administration indications for botulinum treatment are for patients experiencing more than 15 days of headaches per month for more than 4 h per day.[34] It has been shown to have long-lasting and reproducible long-term effectiveness with repeat treatments, typically 155 units injected over 31 areas.[35] Other future treatment options may include antibodies to neuropeptide calcitonin gene-related peptide, which are currently being studied in animal models[36] and Phase II clinical trials.[33,37–39]

Medication overuse headaches should be considered in those headaches that persist. Medication overuse headaches are defined as headaches occurring more than 15 days per month with use of simple analgesics more than 15 days/month or a combination analgesic more than 10 days per month for 3 months or more.[40] If this diagnosis is made, withdrawal of medication is the recommended treatment. However, there are no evidence-based clinical practices that have been shown to be more effective than others.[41] Special considerations regarding TBI include safety of nonsteroidal antiinflammatory drugs or triptans in the setting of any recent intracranial hemorrhage.

Several nonmedication modalities have been shown to be effective for the treatment of posttraumatic headache. Mindfulness therapy is a meditative therapy with emphasis on focusing on individual aspects of body function

TABLE 18.3
Medication Treatment Options in Headaches

Headache Type	First-Line Therapy	Second-Line Therapy	Third-Line Therapy
Tension type Unclassified type	Amitriptyline or nortriptyline 10 mg PO QHS, increasing 10 mg every 1–2 weeks as necessary/tolerated to a dose of 50–100 mg PO QHS. Choose amitriptyline if concomitant sleep issues	Gabapentin 100–300 mg PO QHS, increasing by 100–300 mg every 5 days as needed to a maximum of 600 mg PO TID	
Migraine type	Amitriptyline or nortriptyline 10 mg PO QHS, increasing 10 mg every 1–2 weeks as necessary/tolerated to dose of 50–100 mg PO QHS Or Nadolol 20 mg PO BID and increasing by 20 mg every 5 days as necessary/tolerated to 30–80 mg PO BID or Propranolol 20 mg PO TID and increasing by 20 mg every 5 days as necessary/tolerated to a maximum of 80 mg PO TID	Topiramate starting at 12.5 mg PO QHS and increasing by 12.5 mg PO QHS weekly as necessary/tolerated to a maximum of 100 mg PO QHS Or Gabapentin 100–300 mg PO QHS and increasing by 100–300 mg every 5 days as necessary/tolerated on a TID schedule to a maximum of 600 mg PO TID	Verapamil 40 mg PO TID and titrating to 80 mg PO TID as necessary/tolerated Or Pizotifen 0/5 mg PO QHS and increasing by 0.5 mg every week to a maximum dose of 3.0 mg PO QHS Or Flunarizine 5 mg PO QHS and increasing to 10 mg PO QHS after 10–14 days

Data from Ontario Neurotrauma Foundation. Guidelines for mild traumatic brain injury and persistent symptoms. *Development*. 2011:1–156. papers2://publication/uuid/E0B125F9-5DC8-40D8-AB0F-1F3601245329.

while blocking out distracting thoughts. It was studied in chronic episodic migraineurs and led to a statistically insignificant reduction in headaches compared with standard therapy.[42] Another small study in tension-type headaches showed a benefit of mindfulness therapy.[43]

Group-based acceptance and commitment therapy, a form of psychotherapy that recognizes the current difficult situation at hand and attempts to move forward toward a desired goal, significantly reduced disability and anxiety, in a mix of patients with chronic tension-type and migraine-type headaches. In addition, yoga has been shown to be of benefit in the reduction of symptoms of chronic migraine in addition to conventional therapies.[44,45]

Transcranial magnetic stimulation treatments were observed to reduce chronic migraine headache-related frequency and intensity as efficaciously as Botox, although the effect was reduced after 8 weeks, whereas the Botox-related effect persisted for about 12 weeks.[46] Acupuncture has been generally accepted as an effective treatment for chronic headache and has been shown to decrease headache intensity.[47] Overall, the use of complementary and alternative medicine (CAM) in the setting of chronic migraine has been shown to reduce moderate mental distress in women with chronic headache but not in men.[48] The use of CAM is higher in the population with chronic headache than in the general population[42,49] and is growing, and it is estimated to have been utilized in approximately 30% of the general population in the last 12 months.[50]

Overall, a multidisciplinary and holistic approach to posttraumatic headache offers patients the best possible prognosis. Patients should be counseled regarding sleep hygiene, adequate hydration, environmental modulation, and stress management as a foundation for using other therapeutic interventions. In general, this prognosis is very good. Most patients with TBI with posttraumatic headaches see resolution or a significant reduction of their headaches within 6 months.[51] The management of persistent, chronic headache is best achieved with a calculated, comprehensive approach that involves the identification of medical, musculoskeletal, psychiatric, and environmental factors that may be contributing to the persistence of posttraumatic headaches and then targeting therapies to help reduce symptom burden, with a focus on improving functional status.

CENTRAL NEUROPATHIC PAIN SYNDROMES AFTER TBI

Rare cases of centrally mediated neuropathic pain disorders after TBI have been reported,[52] typically involving direct thalamic injuries or injuries to the spinothalamic pathways, with patients exhibiting impaired thermal sensation.[53] Onset has typically been reported with a delay of 1–9 months.[53–55]

Theoretical constructs for centrally mediated pain involve a reduction in the activity of inhibitory neurons in the thalamus and projections from the thalamus into the pre- and post-central gyri, which lead to an increase in peripheral sensation from primary afferents.[56] Functional MRI studies of patients with mild TBI versus controls have shown that patients with mild TBI exhibited less activity in the thalamus, pons, anterior cingulate cortex, insula, dorsolateral prefrontal cortex, and medial prefrontal cortices than the healthy control group.[57] Ongoing hyperesthesia, hyperalgesia, or allodynia, with continued dysmodulation of inhibitory central systems, may lead to the development of spontaneous pain. This is usually not restricted to a certain peripheral nerve distribution or dermatome. It may affect a large region of the body or be localized to one specific area. It is most commonly described as a burning pain and, when present, most often affects the distal extremities.[58]

Diagnosis and treatment should evaluate for the possibility that fractures, soft tissue injuries, and visceral injuries may have been missed during the acute traumatic management of the patient. In addition to these occult injuries, the effects of sequelae of traumatic brain injury should also be considered, i.e. spasticity, contracture, or heterotopic ossification.

Treatment of centrally mediated pain syndrome can be divided into rehabilitative, pharmacologic, and surgical approaches. Rehabilitative approaches include regular stretching, strengthening, use of modalities to reduce inflammation and pain, desensitization techniques such as rubbing with progressively rougher surfaces, and documenting the progressive trajectory of function. Proper ergonomic principles should be applied to prevent misalignments or joint subluxation.

Medication trials have been sparse and are generally informed from the treatment of central pain syndromes in the non-TBI population. Specific caveats in the TBI population when applying medications are to minimize the use of medications with cognitive side effects and "start low and go slow" in regards to titration of medication.[21,55,59] Gabapentin[60] or pregabalin is considered first-line therapy in central pain syndrome and in combination with other agents such as opioids or topical agents may have an additive effect in the treatment of neuropathic pain syndromes.[61]

The most commonly prescribed medication for centrally mediated pain syndrome is gabapentin, a central γ-aminobutyric acid agonist. Gabapentin has been shown to be an effective pharmacological agent in primary headache disorders, including chronic daily headache.[62] Other antiepileptic medications, such as valproic acid or topiramate, have also been shown to reduce headaches.[31] Individual approaches to medication management include titration of the medication up to the highest tolerated dose before switching agents and medication holidays after effective treatment to assess the need for ongoing pain medication versus improvements related to spontaneous recovery.

Intramuscular botulinum toxin injection has been shown to be effective in reducing pain caused by cervical dystonia. However, its results have been mixed for the treatment of other painful head and neck conditions.[63] Botulinum toxin has been shown to be effective in reducing chronic migraine headache and should be considered in patients who have failed multiple agents or who may be sensitive to systemic medication in regards to side-effect profiles.[35] Continued Botox injections may reduce the need for prophylactic or breakthrough medications for patients with chronic migraine.[35]

Surgical treatment approaches have been directed at minimizing restrictions in range of motion and correcting any skeletal or muscular deformities that may be contributing to an ongoing chronic pain syndrome. These can include surgical treatment of heterotopic ossification, repair of muscular injuries (i.e., rotator cuff repair), surgical release of joint contracture to reduce spasticity and improve passive positioning (thereby reducing exacerbations of pain), or spinal surgeries meant to improve spinal alignment and prevent peripheral nerve impingement.

A case report of a patient with a central neuropathic pain syndrome revealed that implantation of a motor cortex stimulator led to a subsequent 70%–80% reduction in pain.[54] The motor cortex stimulation increased ventrolateral thalamic blood flow in a combined PET study but did not alter somatosensory potentials.[64] Deep brain stimulation has had variable success with pain reduction.[65,66] As functional neurosurgery approaches become more widespread, cortical stimulation may be a future target of surgical treatment for central neuropathic pain syndrome.

PERIPHERAL PAIN SYNDROMES AFTER TRAUMATIC BRAIN INJURY

One-third of TBIs are associated with peripheral nerve and soft tissue injuries.[13] The presence of more than one peripheral lesion is a risk factor for ongoing functional disability.[67] In addition, the presence of peripheral injuries affects central neuroinflammation and may contribute to persistent functional deficits after TBI.[68] Complex regional pain syndrome (CRPS) develops in 12% of TBI survivors who report that they have chronic pain.[69] Treatment would mimic current treatment of CRPS. Modulation of treatment plans would revolve around the individual TBI survivor's ability to tolerate the generally unpleasant desensitization techniques (contrast baths, rubbing of progressively rougher surfaces on affected skin) that are a hallmark of treatment.

LUMBAR PAIN SYNDROMES AFTER TRAUMATIC BRAIN INJURY

Chronic lower back pain is approximately as common as posttraumatic headache in TBI survivors.[6] Factors that may contribute to low back pain include the mechanism of injury with associated strain or sprain of the lumbar spine. Premorbid osteoarthritis or spinal instability may be exacerbated during the traumatic event.

Spasticity or postural changes as a result of the TBI, including positioning in wheelchair or in bed, should be evaluated frequently. The loss or change in ability to ambulate and transfer may place additional stress on patients with back pain. Changes in cognitive abilities, including the ability to tolerate or ignore a painful stimulus, also play a role in how the patient perceives or is able to manage the pain. This is secondary to the reduction in the supraspinal inhibitory pathways that modulate the threshold and intensity at which we experience pain.

Treatment of low back pain in individuals with TBI should follow standard practice guidelines with special considerations for the TBI population. Supraspinal factors affect the perception of low back pain[70] and can be influenced by pain medications, especially those with cognitive and arousal based side effects. These medications should also be evaluated for the risk of potential for drug-drug interactions with concurrent antiepileptic or antispasticity medications. Modified pain scales such as the Wong-Baker FACES[71] as well as input from caregivers help quantify pain in the cognitively impaired patient.

In patients with moderate to severe TBI who are undergoing rehabilitation, the ability to participate meaningfully in therapy and activities of daily living should improve. As brain injury survivors recover, they can better articulate the exact nature, character, location, and presence of ameliorating and exacerbating factors to their medical team. It is important to prevent worsening or development of lower back pain during the rehabilitation process through close monitoring of the patients' individual wheelchair positioning needs and modifications to the chair.

Exercise prescription is an important component to any rehabilitative treatment plan.[51] The definition of any amount of activity that can be performed without exacerbation of symptoms is important, and a shift in a patient's expectations regarding what is meaningful may be required, especially in patients who were very active before their injury.[59] Structuring activity into the treatment program helps brain injury survivors who benefit from a structured activity pattern.

SUMMARY/DISCUSSION

Chronic pain is common after TBI. Neuropathic pain may involve structures from the peripheral afferents to more central pathways that modulate the nociceptive pathways. Overall the prognosis is good for treatment of pain disorders after TBI, with central neuropathic pain the most difficult subtype to manage. Pain management must be an important part of physiatric treatment regardless of the initial severity of the injury, as there is a wide variability of outcomes within each severity subgroup that makes it difficult to prognosticate outcomes. A patient-centered, multidisciplinary approach to the diagnosis and management of patients with TBI with chronic pain is paramount, with particular emphasis on maximizing function and quality of life.

REFERENCES

1. CDC TBI Statistics. No Title. CDC Website. https://www.cdc.gov/TraumaticBrainInjury/data/index.html.
2. Frieden TR, Houry D, Baldwin G. Traumatic brain injury in the United States: epidemiology and rehabilitation. In: *CDC NIH Rep to Congr*; 2015:1–74. http://dx.doi.org/10.3171/2009.10.JNS091500.
3. Nampiaparampil DE. CLINICIAN'S CORNER prevalence of chronic pain. *JAMA*. 2009. http://dx.doi.org/10.1001/jama.300.6.711.
4. Lahz S, Bryant RA. Incidence of chronic pain following traumatic brain injury. *Arch Phys Med Rehabil*. 1996;77(9):889–891.
5. Lew HL, Otis JD, Tun C, Kerns RD, Clark ME, Cifu DX. Prevalence of chronic pain, posttraumatic stress disorder, and persistent postconcussive symptoms in OIF/OEF veterans: polytrauma clinical triad. *J Rehabil Res Dev*. 2009;46(6):697–702.
6. Bosco MA, Murphy JL, Clark ME. Chronic pain and traumatic brain injury in OEF/OIF service members and veterans. *Headache*. 2013:1518–1522. http://dx.doi.org/10.1111/head.12172.
7. Uomoto JM. PCE. Traumatic brain injury and chronic pain: differential types and rates by head injury severity. *Arch Phys Med Rehabil*. 1993;74(1):61–64.
8. Carmon A. Classification of Chronic Pain 1994.
9. Gauntlett-Gilbert J, Wilson S. Veterans and chronic pain. *Br J Pain*. 2013;7(2):79–84. http://dx.doi.org/10.1177/2049463713482082.
10. International Association for the Study of Pain. http://www.iasp-pain.org/Taxonomy.
11. Karzmark P, Hall K, Englander K. Late-onset post-concussion symptoms after mild traumatic brain injury: the role of premorbid, injury-related, environmental, and personality factors. *Brain Inj*. 1995;9(1):21–26.
12. Akparian AV. The brain in chronic pain: clinical implications. *Pain Manag*. 2012;1(6):577–586. http://dx.doi.org/10.2217/pmt.11.53.The.
13. Stone L, Keenan MA. Peripheral nerve injuries in the adult with traumatic brain injury. *Clin Orthop Relat Res*. 1988;233:136–144.
14. Brown EA, Kenardy JA, Dow BL. PTSD perpetuates pain in children with traumatic brain injury. *J Pediatr Psychol*. 2014. http://dx.doi.org/10.1093/jpepsy/jsu014.
15. International Classification of Headaches, Beta-3. https://www.ichd-3.org/.
16. International Classification of Headache Disorders. https://www.ichd-3.org/5-headache-attributed-to-trauma-or-injury-to-the-head-andor-neck/.
17. Hoffman JM, Lucas S, Dikmen S, et al. Natural history of headache after traumatic brain injury. *J Neurotrauma*. 2011;1725(September):1719–1725. http://dx.doi.org/10.1089/neu.2011.1914.
18. Bogduk N. Anatomy and physiology of headache. *Biomed Pharmacother*. 1995;49(10):435–445. http://dx.doi.org/10.1016/0753-3322(96)82687-4.
19. Brown AW, Watanabe TK, Hoffman JM, Bell KR, Lucas S, Dikmen S. Headache after traumatic brain injury: a national survey of clinical practices and treatment approaches. *PM R*. 2015;7(1):3–8. http://dx.doi.org/10.1016/j.pmrj.2014.06.016.
20. Tamburin S, Paolucci S, Magrinelli F, Musicco M, Sandrini G. The Italian Consensus Conference on Pain in Neurorehabilitation: rationale and methodology. *J Pain Res*. 2016;9(6):311–318. http://dx.doi.org/10.2147/JPR.S84646.
21. Sherman KB, Goldberg M, Bell KR. Traumatic brain injury and pain. *Phys Med Rehabil Clin N Am*. 2006;17:473–490. http://dx.doi.org/10.1016/j.pmr.2005.11.007.
22. Acute Headache Attributable to Moderate to Severe Injury to the Head. https://www.ichd-3.org/5-headache-attributed-to-trauma-or-injury-to-the-head-andor-neck/5-1-acute-headache-attributed-to-traumatic-injury-to-the-head/5-1-1-acute-headache-attributed-to-moderate-or-severe-traumatic-injury-to-the-head/.
23. Acute Headache due to Mild Traumatic Brain Injury. https://www.ichd-3.org/5-headache-attributed-to-trauma-or-injury-to-the-head-andor-neck/5-1-acute-headache-attributed-to-traumatic-injury-to-the-head/5-1-2-acute-headache-attributed-to-mild-traumatic-injury-to-the-head/.

24. Persistent Headache Definition. https://www.ichd-3.org/5-headache-attributed-to-trauma-or-injury-to-the-head-andor-neck/5-2-persistent-headache-attributed-to-traumaticinjury-to-the-head/.

25. Couch JR, Stewart KE. Headache prevalence at 4-11 years after deployment-related traumatic brain injury in veterans of Iraq and Afghanistan wars and comparison to controls: a matched case-controlled study. *Headache*. 2016;56(6):1004–1021. http://dx.doi.org/10.1111/head.12837.

26. Palacios-Cena M, Wang K, Castaldo M, et al. Trigger points are associated with widespread pressure pain sensitivity in people with tension-type headache. *Cephalalgia*. 2016;0(0):1–9. http://dx.doi.org/10.1177/0333102416679965.

27. Travell J, Simons DSL. *Myofascial Pain and Dysfunction: The Trigger Point Manual*. 2nd ed. Lippincott, Williams & Wilkins; 1999.

28. Evans RW. *Headache Currents Persistent Post-traumatic Headache, Postconcussion Syndrome, and Whiplash Injuries: The Evidence for a Non-traumatic Basis with an Historical Review*; 1866:716–724.

29. Defrin R. Chronic post-traumatic headache: clinical findings and possible mechanisms. *J Man Manip Ther*. 2014;22. http://dx.doi.org/10.1179/2042618613Y.0000000053.

30. Keidel M, Diener HC. Der posttraumatische Kopfschmerz. *Nervenarzt*. 1997;68(10):769–777. http://dx.doi.org/10.1007/s001150050193.

31. Ontario Neurotrauma Foundation. Guidelines for mild traumatic brain injury and persistent symptoms. *Development*. 2011:1–156. papers2://publication/uuid/E0B125F9-5DC8-40D8-AB0F-1F3601245329.

32. Göbel H. Botulinum toxin in migraine prophylaxis. *J Neurol*. 2004;(251 suppl 1):I8–I11. http://dx.doi.org/10.1007/s00415-004-1103-y.

33. Sun H, Dodick DW, Silberstein S, et al. Safety and efficacy of AMG 334 for prevention of episodic migraine: a randomised, double-blind, placebo-controlled, phase 2 trial. *Lancet Neurol*. 2016;15(4):382–390. http://dx.doi.org/10.1016/S1474-4422(16)00019-3.

34. Allergan. *Botox Package Insert*. vol. 50. 2016.

35. Aicua-Rapun I, Martínez-Velasco E, Rojo A, et al. Real-life data in 115 chronic migraine patients treated with onabotulinumtoxin A during more than one year. *J Headache Pain*. 2016;17(1):112. http://dx.doi.org/10.1186/s10194-016-0702-1.

36. Bree D, Levy D. Development of CGRP-dependent pain and headache related behaviours in a rat model of concussion: implications for mechanisms of post-traumatic headache. *Cephalalgia*. 2016;0(0):1–13. http://dx.doi.org/10.1177/0333102416681571.

37. Bigal ME, Edvinsson L, Rapoport AM, et al. Safety, tolerability, and efficacy of TEV-48125 for preventive treatment of chronic migraine: a multicentre, randomised, double-blind, placebo-controlled, phase 2b study. *Lancet Neurol*. 2015;14(11):1091–1100. http://dx.doi.org/10.1016/S1474-4422(15)00245-8.

38. Pascual J. CGRP antibodies: the Holy Grail for migraine prevention? *Lancet Neurol*. 2015;14(11):1066–1067. http://dx.doi.org/10.1016/S1474-4422(15)00244-6.

39. Ramos ML, Pascual J. AMG 334 CGRP antibody for migraine: time to celebrate? *Lancet Neurol*. 2016;15(4):347–349. http://dx.doi.org/10.1016/S1474-4422(16)00040-5.

40. Medication Overuse Headaches. https://www.ichd-3.org/8-headache-attributed-to-a-substance-or-its-withdrawal/8-2-medication-overuse-headache-moh/.

41. de Goffau MJ, Klaver ARE, Willemsen MG, Bindels PJE, Verhagen AP. The effectiveness of treatments for patients with medication overuse headache; a systematic review and meta-analysis. *J Pain*. 2016. http://dx.doi.org/10.1016/j.jpain.2016.12.005.

42. Wells RE, Burch R, Paulsen RH, Wayne PM, Houle TT, Loder E. Meditation for migraines: a pilot randomized controlled trial. *Headache*. 2014;54(9):1484–1495. http://dx.doi.org/10.1111/head.12420.

43. Cathcart S, Galatis N, Immink M, Proeve M, Petkov J. Brief mindfulness-based therapy for chronic tension-type headache: a randomized controlled pilot study. *Behav Cogn Psychother*. 2013:1–15. http://dx.doi.org/10.1017/S1352465813000234.

44. Kisan R, Sujan M, Adoor M, et al. Effect of yoga on migraine: a comprehensive study using clinical profile and cardiac autonomic functions. *Int J Yoga*. 2014;7(2):126–132. http://dx.doi.org/10.4103/0973-6131.133891.

45. John PJ, Sharma N, Sharma CM, Kankane A. Effectiveness of yoga therapy in the treatment of migraine without aura: a randomized controlled trial. *Headache*. 2007;47(5):654–661. http://dx.doi.org/10.1111/j.1526-4610.2007.00789.x.

46. Shehata HS, Esmail EH, Abdelalim A, et al. Repetitive transcranial magnetic stimulation versus botulinum toxin injection in chronic migraine prophylaxis: a pilot randomized trial. *J Pain Res*. 2016;9:771–777. http://dx.doi.org/10.2147/JPR.S116671.

47. Zhao L, Guo Y, Wang W, Yan L. Systematic review on randomized controlled clinical trials of acupuncture therapy for neurovascular headache. *Chin J Integr Med*. 2011;17(8):580–586. http://dx.doi.org/10.1007/s11655-011-0709-z.

48. Rhee TG, Harris IM. Gender differences in the use of complementary and alternative medicine and their association with moderate mental distress in U.S. adults with migraines/severe headaches. *Headache J Head Face Pain*. 2016. http://dx.doi.org/10.1111/head.12986. [Cdc].

49. Wells RE, Bertisch SM, Buettner C, Phillips RS, McCarthy EP. Complementary and alternative medicine use among adults with migraines/severe headaches. *Headache*. 2011;51(7):1087–1097. http://dx.doi.org/10.1111/j.1526-4610.2011.01917.x.

50. Zhang Y, Leach MJ, Hall H, et al. Differences between male and female consumers of complementary and alternative medicine in a national US population: a secondary analysis of 2012 NIHS data. *Evid Based Complement Altern Med*. 2015;2015. http://dx.doi.org/10.1155/2015/413173.

51. Gironda RJ, Clark ME, Ruff RL, et al. Traumatic brain injury, polytrauma, and pain: challenges and treatment strategies for the polytrauma rehabilitation. *Rehabil Psychol.* 2009;54(3):247–258. http://dx.doi.org/10.1037/a0016906.

52. Donnellan CP. Acupuncture for central pain affecting the ribcage following traumatic brain injury and rib fractures–a case report. *Acupunct Med.* 2006;24(3):129–133.

53. Ofek H, Defrin R. The characteristics of chronic central pain after traumatic brain injury. *Pain.* 2007;131:330–340. http://dx.doi.org/10.1016/j.pain.2007.06.015.

54. Son BC, Won S, Seok E, Hoon J, Hong JT. Motor cortex stimulation for central pain following a traumatic brain injury. *Pain.* 2006;123:210–216. http://dx.doi.org/10.1016/j.pain.2006.02.028.

55. Ivanhoe CB, Hartman ET. Clinical caveats on medical assessment and treatment of pain after TBI. *J Head Trauma Rehabil.* 2004;19(1):29–39.

56. White JC, Sweet WH. *Pain: Its Mechanisms and Neurosurgical Control*; 1955.

57. Leung A, Shukla S, Yang E, et al. Diminished supraspinal pain modulation in patients with mild traumatic brain injury. *Mol Pain.* 2016. http://dx.doi.org/10.1177/1744806916662661.

58. NIH Central Pain Syndrome Information. https://www.ninds.nih.gov/Disorders/All-Disorders/Central-Pain-Syndrome-Information-Page.

59. Young JA. Pain and traumatic brain injury. *Phys Med Rehabil Clin.* 2007;18:145–163. http://dx.doi.org/10.1016/j.pmr.2006.11.008.

60. Hesami O, Beladimoghadam N, Assarzadegan F. The efficacy of gabapentin in patients with central post-stroke pain. *Iran J Pharm Res.* 2015;14(suppl):95–101.

61. Vorobeychik Y, Gordin V, Mao J, Chen L. Combination therapy for neuropathic pain a review of current evidence. *CNS Drugs.* 2011;25(12):1023–1034.

62. Perloff MD, Berlin RK, Gillette M, Petersile MJ, Kurowski D. Gabapentin in headache disorders: what is the evidence? *Pain Med.* 2016;17(1):162–171. http://dx.doi.org/10.1111/pme.12931.

63. Sycha T, Kranz G, Auff E, Schnider P. Botulinum toxin in the treatment of rare head and neck pain syndromes: a systematic review of the literature. *J Neurol.* 2004;251(1):i19–i30. http://dx.doi.org/10.1007/s00415-004-1106-8.

64. Peyron R, Mertens P, Gregoire MC, Lavenne F, Le Bars D. Electrical stimulation of motor cortex for pain control: a combined PET-scan and electrophysiological study. *Pain.* 1999;83.

65. Kumar K, Toth C, Nath RK. Deep brain stimulation for intractable pain: a 15-year experience. *Neurosurgery.* 1997;40(4):736–737.

66. Rasche D, Rinaldi PC, Young RF, Tronnier VM. Deep brain stimulation for the treatment of various chronic pain syndromes. *Neurosurg Focus.* 2006;21(6):E8.

67. Groswasser Z, Cohen M, Blankstein E. Polytrauma associated with traumatic brain injury: incidence, nature and impact on rehabilitation outcome. *Brain Inj.* 1990;4(2):161–166.

68. Mcdonald SJ, Sun M, Agoston DV, Shultz SR. The effect of concomitant peripheral injury on traumatic brain injury pathobiology and outcome. *J Neuroinflammation.* 2016. http://dx.doi.org/10.1186/s12974-016-0555-1.

69. Gellman H, Keenan MA, Stone L, Hardy SE, Waters RL, Stewart C. Reflex sympathetic dystrophy in brain-injured patients. *Pain.* 1992;51(3):307–311. http://www.ncbi.nlm.nih.gov/pubmed/1491858.

70. Perlepe V, Haenecour L, Duprez T, Omoumi P, Berg BC, Lecouvet FE. Lumbar pain with intracranial origin. *Acta Radiol.* 2013;54(3):324–326. http://dx.doi.org/10.1177/0284185112471794.

71. Jensen M. Wong-Baker FACES pain rating scale. In: Wittink C, Carr D, eds. *Evidence, Outcomes, and Quality of Life in Pain Treatment.* 2003:2–3. http://dx.doi.org/10.1037/t05330-000.

CHAPTER 19

Pain Syndromes Associated With Cerebrovascular Accidents

MARY KESZLER, MD • TULASI GUDE, MD • KIMBERLY HECKERT, MD

Cerebrovascular events are one of the most common causes of morbidity and mortality in the United States, with nearly 800,000 new strokes yearly and a prevalence of 6.6 million in people 20 years or older.[1] In addition to associated neurologic deficits, stroke survivors may have various pain conditions, some of which are unique to this patient population. Although there are many potential causes of chronic pain after stroke, this chapter focuses on four of the more common pain conditions that can have neuropathic etiologies: central poststroke pain (CPSP), shoulder hand syndrome, poststroke headache, and hemiplegic shoulder pain (HSP).

CENTRAL POSTSTROKE PAIN

CPSP, previously known as Dejerine-Roussy syndrome and thalamic pain syndrome, is a feared complication of cerebrovascular accidents and has been described by Tasker as "among the most spectacular, distressing, and intractable of pain syndromes."[2] It affects approximately 8% of patients after a stroke but is more common after strokes that involve the lateral medulla and inferior-lateral thalamus, with a prevalence of 25% and 17%–18%, respectively.[3,4]

Patients primarily complain of pain within the distribution of the body affected by the stroke. The majority of patients, approximately 67%, have allodynia and may also endorse dysesthesia, hypoesthesia, or hyperpathia, whereas 40% of patients may experience hypoalgesia.[5,6] The pain typically fluctuates in intensity as well as distribution throughout the day.[7] In addition to the pain complaint, patients may present with hemiplegia as a result of the stroke, although approximately 52% do not have any weakness.[8] They generally present with other sensory findings besides painful symptoms, such as astereognosis and altered temperature perception.[3,9] Of note, the affected body area is generally objectively cooler, especially as the pain worsens.[5] The majority of patients also have ataxia, found in up to 62%.[8] Although a patient's neurologic deficits as a result of the stroke are evident immediately, CPSP can present days to months after the stroke. Less than 40% of patients with CPSP are reported to develop the painful symptoms at the time of the stroke.[5] The majority of patients have onset of symptoms within a month of the stroke, whereas 18% develop symptoms within the first 6 months and the remaining 18% develop symptoms after 6 months.[4] Most patients have pain constantly, whereas the remaining 15% have pain daily.[9]

In addition to the sensory and motor changes previously mentioned, on physical examination the patient has impaired pinprick, temperature, and touch sensation, as well as notable coolness of the affected area.[3,5] Vibration and proprioception sensation are intact. The lowered skin temperature is attributed to autonomic instability in the area affected by the stroke.[5] CPSP is the result of dysfunction of the spino-thalamocortical tract as it courses from the spinal cord through the brainstem and thalamus to the sensory cortex.[4,10]

The diagnosis of CPSP is made solely based upon the history and physical examination. Imaging can be done to rule out other diagnoses and to confirm the history of a stroke. To diagnose a patient with CPSP, the patient must have a history of a stroke or stroke-like event if no imaging has been done, pain in a neuroanatomically plausible distribution based upon the location of the stroke, and pain and temperature sensory deficits.[8] The presence of allodynia is pathognomonic but is not required for a diagnosis of CPSP. In addition, paradoxic burning or burning pain induced with cold stimulation increases the possibility of the symptoms being attributable to CPSP but is not diagnostic.[5]

Differential diagnosis is broad, as there are many conditions with overlapping symptoms. Depending on the location and distribution of the pain, the physician has to consider a diagnosis of multiple sclerosis, syringomyelia, peripheral neuropathy, complex regional pain syndrome (CRPS), poststroke headache, spasticity, HSP, frozen shoulder, rotator cuff tendinopathy or tear, herpes zoster, and deep venous thrombosis.[3]

Upon evaluation of patients in whom CPSP is suspected, desensitization with various tactile stimuli is initiated, as it is commonly a first-line treatment in clinical practice. When treating these patients, there are few evidence-based nonpharmacologic and noninterventional options. A small study of 15 patients was done to examine the effects of transcutaneous electrical nerve stimulation (TENS) on CPSP. After receiving treatment, four patients had pain relief, five had a transient increase in pain, and six reported no change in their pain.[8] In addition to this weak evidence, the painful area tends to be quite extensive to which it would be difficult, if not impossible, to adequately apply TENS pads to provide sufficient electrical stimulation. An emerging therapeutic option for CPSP is transcranial magnetic stimulation (TMS). In a prospective study of 14 patients who underwent five sessions of TMS, there was a modest improvement in pain 4 weeks after treatment with $P = .018$.[11]

Pharmacologic therapeutic options include several classes of medications. The most extensively studied class is the tricyclic antidepressants, specifically amitriptyline. As amitriptyline inhibits norepinephrine and serotonin reuptake, this modulates thalamic burst firing activity, one of the proposed theories for the development of CPSP, thereby reducing pain.[12] The side-effect profile should be considered, especially in the elderly patient with stroke, in which case adverse effects may be experienced before therapeutic benefit. Other tricyclic antidepressants such as nortriptyline, desipramine, imipramine, and doxepin have been studied less extensively. Other antidepressants that can be used are trazodone, venlafaxine, and maprotiline.[3] Although fluvoxamine can also be tried, selective serotonin reuptake inhibitor (SSRI) antidepressants are generally ineffective.[3,5]

Anticonvulsants, specifically lamotrigine, gabapentin, pregabalin, carbamazepine, and phenytoin, may be used, although supporting evidence is based primarily on case reports, therefore not placing them as first-line treatment. As with other chronic pain conditions, opioids can be trialed; however, there is no evidence demonstrating their effectiveness in CPSP and associated potential for adverse effects should be considered, especially in the elderly. Various cardiac medications have also been recommended as possible treatment options, specifically clonidine, mexiletine, and β-blockers.[9,13]

More experimental pharmacologic treatments include propofol, intrathecal baclofen, ketamine, and intravenous lidocaine.[5] A small, double-blind study consisting of six patients with CPSP receiving intravenous lidocaine showed reduction of pain for 45 min after the injection, with resumption of pain thereafter.[8] In a double-blind randomized controlled trial studying naloxone, 3 of the 20 patients in the study had transient relief with naloxone, whereas 4 had relief with saline and an additional 4 had relief with both.[14] If pharmacologic or therapeutic modalities are ineffective at managing the patient's symptoms, patients may undergo a sympathetic blockade, which may provide initial pain relief that generally recurs.[9]

Surgical options include thalamotomy or mesencephalic tractotomy in which abnormal reticulothalamic neuronal pools, a proposed source of pain, are removed. As a result, it is less likely that these pain sources are reactivated. These procedures are better at ameliorating allodynia and hyperpathia than burning pain.[15] Dorsal root entry zone (DREZ) lesioning can also be done, but for chronic pain conditions in general, the recurrence rate 2 years after DREZ lesioning ranges from 60% to 80%.[16] Less permanent procedures include implanted spinal cord, deep brain, and motor cortex stimulators. In a prospective study of 30 patients who underwent spinal cord stimulator trials for CPSP, 30% had good pain relief and 20% had fair pain relief, whereas the remaining 50% had poor pain relief. Ultimately, 10 of the original 30 patients underwent spinal cord stimulator placement, 9 of whom had long-term pain relief, lasting for 28 months on average.[17] The results from studies examining the effects of deep brain stimulators on CPSP are conflicting and in limited cases have shown improvement in allodynia and improved sensory discrimination.[8] For motor cortex stimulators, a retrospective study examined 14 patients with various diagnoses, 7 of whom had CPSP.[18] There was evidence that the best long-term results were seen in those with CPSP as two subjects had excellent long-term results and three had satisfactory results, but the magnitude of relief waned over time.

Limited success with pharmacologic, interventional, and surgical options has resulted in having many patients explore complimentary modalities, such as acupuncture and massage. There are no studies that have examined the effects of acupuncture on CPSP, but there have been case reports of favorable results. Interestingly, there are two cases of subjects with CPSP who experienced instantaneous and sustained pain relief after vestibular caloric stimulation.[19] Ramachandran theorizes that cold water vestibular caloric irrigation activates the posterior insula, which in turn inhibits the generation of pain in the anterior cingulate. Although this technique needs further study, if further evidence supports it, it would provide a safe pain-relief alternative for patients. Ultimately, what is most important for these patients is to learn coping and relaxation techniques as the pain is generally lifelong and can lead to depression and be aggravated by stress.[5]

The overall course and prognosis for these patients is poor. Pain is often the most limiting symptom after their stroke.[3] The most favorable prognostic factor is early initiation of treatment after onset of symptoms.[7] Even if treatment is started quickly, patients may still have lifelong pain. In one survey, practitioners reported that 50% of patients experienced pain relief with medication.[7] Like other chronic pain conditions, CPSP negatively affects the patient's quality of life, ability to participate in rehabilitation, and quality of sleep. Given the high prevalence of stroke, the aging population, the frequency of CPSP, and the associated disability, treatments for this condition that lead to adequate analgesia are important to treat many people for years to come.

SHOULDER-HAND SYNDROME

CRPS is a chronic neuropathic pain condition that can develop after various musculoskeletal injuries or surgeries or as a result of injuries to the peripheral or central nervous system. In patients who had stroke, the most common form of CRPS is shoulder-hand syndrome (SHS), with an incidence ranging from 1.5% to 50%.[20,21] Patients with SHS frequently report pain in the shoulder but may describe pain in the hand or both.[21] Although the disease course can be difficult to predict, the prognosis has been found to correlate with the patient's motor deficit, spasticity, vibratory sensory deficits, and initial coma.[22]

To make a diagnosis of SHS, a patient must meet diagnostic criteria for CRPS of the upper limb with a history of a stroke. What complicates the diagnosis in clinical practice is that the physician must be able to tease out the findings and symptoms that are attributable to the stroke itself rather than a separate diagnosis of SHS. As stated by the Budapest Criteria, for patients to be diagnosed with CRPS, they must have pain and vasomotor, sudomotor, and motor or trophic changes.[23] Patients with SHS may experience allodynia, hyperalgesia, hyperpathia, or thermal hyperesthesia or allodynia. There may also be vasomotor or sudomotor changes, such as temperature dysregulation, skin color change, or edema, as a result of the stroke and disuse. In regards to motor changes, it is not uncommon for patients to a have upper limb weakness after a stroke depending on the site of the lesion. In the case of SHS, the limb is weaker than expected compared with the other stroke deficits and the patient generally has a decreased range

TABLE 19.1 Differential Diagnosis for Shoulder-Hand Syndrome
Differential Diagnosis
• Other poststroke pain conditions
• CPSP
• Hemiplegic shoulder pain
• Musculoskeletal
• Myofascial pain
• Rotator cuff pathology
• Tendonitis
• Fracture
• Subluxation
• Osteoarthritis
• Neurologic
• CRPS type 1 or 2[a]
• Peripheral polyneuropathy
• Peripheral mononeuropathy
• Radiculopathy
• Infectious
• Herpes zoster
• Cellulitis
• Septic arthritis
• Osteomyelitis
• Vascular
• Thrombus
• Peripheral vascular disease
• Lymphedema
• Rheumatologic
• Rheumatoid arthritis
• Gout

CPSP, central poststroke pain; *CRPS*, complex regional pain syndrome.
[a]See Chapter 6 for definition.

of motion and poor muscle coordination, and approximately 50% have a tremor.[21] Just as those with CRPS, those with SHS may have trophic findings, such as nail or hair growth changes. It is also common for these patients, just like other patients with chronic pain, to have anxiety or depression as a result of the pain.[21] The symptoms of SHS overlap with many other conditions, some of which are unique to the stroke population. A possible differential diagnosis is listed in Table 19.1.

Although the diagnosis is made clinically, there is some testing to assist in confirming the diagnosis. Traditional three-phase bone scintigraphy has been studied as a diagnostic tool for CRPS with variable sensitivity and specificity, but one study done by Park et al. showed that quantitative three-phase bone scintigraphy had a sensitivity of 80.8% and specificity of 100%

for diagnosing very acute stage CRPS.[24] In a study done by Kumar et al., dual-energy X-ray absorptiometry scan was shown to correlate with the duration and severity of SHS.[25] There is a lack of good evidence to support the use of electromyography as a diagnostic tool to predict the development of SHS, as presence of spontaneous activity in muscles of the effected limb is correlated with the development of SHS in 65% of paretic patients, whereas only 4% of patients without spontaneous activity developed SHS.[26] Other tests, including nuclear magnetic resonance and thermography may show abnormalities, such as bone and subcutaneous edema or reduced skin temperature, respectively, but these are not diagnostic of CRPS or SHS. Furthermore, normal findings on thermography do not rule out SHS. Stellate ganglion blocks may also be tried as a diagnostic and therapeutic tool; however, lack of improvement does not rule out SHS, as not all patients with CRPS have sympathetically mediated pain.[21]

Rehabilitation options available for SHS help with symptom management. Although keeping the affected limb elevated can help reduce the swelling, there is no evidence to support a combination of kinesiotherapy and manual lymphatic drainage to control the edema. Desensitization is commonly used to treat CRPS and is therefore used in SHS to manage allodynia.[21] Cacchio et al. also found that mirror therapy can lead to significant improvement in pain and motor function after 4 weeks and 6 months compared with controls.[27] In addition to modalities that assist with cortical remapping, restricting arm movement has also been shown to be helpful. Kondo et al. found a significant reduction in the development of SHS when passive movement of the upper limb affected by the stroke was restricted.[28] Also, Hartwig et al. showed that a shoulder joint functional orthosis reduced SHS symptoms compared with the control group.[29]

In addition to therapeutic modalities, multiple classes of medications can be used to manage the painful symptoms. Nonsteroidal antiinflammatory medications may be of most use in the early phase of SHS; however, the efficacy is low. Tricyclic antidepressants are also used, as they can reduce neuropathic pain and improve mood and sleep. These medications must be used with caution in the elderly population given the anticholinergic side-effect profiles. Unfortunately, other classes of antidepressants, specifically SSRIs, have not been found to be efficacious in treating neuropathic pain. Antiepileptics, specifically gabapentin, have been used to treat various sources of neuropathic pain and may be useful in the treatment of SHS; however, this has not been studied. Although topical medications have moderate efficacy in treating CRPS, they are not often used for SHS. Capsaicin, lidocaine, and dimethylsulfoxide cream may be used, especially if oral medications prove ineffective or cannot be tolerated. Opioids are the last pharmacologic option in the treatment of SHS, as they have not been studied as a treatment for CRPS, let alone SHS, and are associated with other side effects and concerns. There are currently preliminary studies examining the effects of botulinum toxin and thalidomide, as well as a case reporting the benefit of bisphosphonates in the treatment of SHS.[21,30] These treatment options require further study.

If pain persists despite these treatments, a sympathetic or somatic block can be performed. A sympathetic block is generally attempted first, but it generally reduces pain only if the pain is sympathetically mediated. As previously stated, not all patients with CRPS have sympathetically mediated pain; therefore such a block may not be effective. If a sympathetic block is successful, the patient should immediately start physical and occupational therapy. If there is no relief after a sympathetic block, a somatic block can be performed. This can be done either at the brachial plexus or as an epidural. Unfortunately, the literature in support of these interventions is scarce and primarily anecdotal. Spinal cord stimulators and intrathecal analgesia with opioids, ziconitide, or clonidine have also been used in the treatment of CRPS and SHS and may be an option for patients who have uncontrollable pain.[21]

There are few surgical options for patients with intractable SHS. Sympathectomies can be performed surgically, chemically, or via radiofrequency ablation. Although these may provide pain relief initially, it is rarely permanent and patients may develop new pain syndromes that prove to be just as difficult to control. As a result, this procedure is generally avoided. A Cochrane review of sympathectomies in the treatment of SHS showed sympathectomies are not effective for neuropathic pain relief overall and can lead to significant complications.[31] If all else fails and if a patient is properly counseled, some patients choose to have the affected limb amputated. Patients must understand that only a small percentage experience pain relief and that new pain syndromes and problems may arise as a result of the amputation.[21]

Just as in CPSP, what is critical for these patients is proper psychological support, including counseling and relaxation, and biofeedback techniques to manage the chronic pain as well as depression that can develop as a result of chronic pain and stroke.

POSTSTROKE HEADACHE

Both headaches and strokes are individually quite prevalent, and headaches that occur at the onset of stroke have been well studied and occur in 27%–31%.[32] What is less clear is the prevalence and disease course of poststroke headache. This is described as a headache that is associated with the stroke and persists after completion of the stroke. This type of headache has a reported incidence ranging from 10.8% to 23.3%, although most studies report a range between 10% and 12%. The headaches are primarily tension type but may present as migraine type or a combination of both. Patients with poststroke headache most often describe the pain as a pressing sensation and generally deny change in headache with movement or associated photophobia, phonophobia, nausea, or vomiting. Those with poststroke headache may have daily headaches or headaches a few times a month, and the headaches can range in duration from less than an hour to constant pain. The pain can also range in severity but is generally reported as moderate to severe. Although there are no distinct diagnostic criteria for poststroke headache, the onset of the headache at onset of stroke is the most distinguishing factor between stroke-attributed and non-stroke-attributed headaches.[33]

Patients are more likely to develop poststroke headache if the stroke is in the right hemisphere, specifically in the temporal lobe. A history of headaches before stroke also increases the risk of developing poststroke headache with a rate of 17.3% compared with 4.1% in patients without a history of headaches. Interestingly, there is no increased risk of developing headache after a hemorrhagic versus ischemic stroke.[33] At this time, the overall course and prognosis is not well described; however, a headache at stroke onset is predictive of poststroke headache 6 months after the stroke.[34]

When assessing a patient who had a stroke and is complaining of headache, the differential diagnosis is quite broad, some of which are included in Table 19.2. Interestingly, medication overuse headache was found to be the cause of headache in 11.5% of patients with stroke in a study done by Hansen et al.[33]

Diagnosis is made clinically. Advanced imaging, such as computed tomography or magnetic resonance imaging, may be useful in ruling out other potential causes of headache in this patient population. Although no medications have been specifically studied in the treatment of poststroke headache, medications typically used to treat the more common types of headaches are applied in clinical practice. These include, but are not limited to, analgesic medications such as acetaminophen and nonsteroidal antiinflammatories, migraine

TABLE 19.2
Differential Diagnosis for Post-Stroke Headache

Differential Diagnosis

- Neurologic
  - Subdural or subarachnoid hemorrhage
  - Increased intracranial pressure due to cerebral edema or hemorrhage
  - Migraine
  - Tension-type headache
  - Cluster headache
  - Cervicogenic headache
  - Trigeminal neuralgia
  - Occipital neuralgia

- Vascular
  - Temporal arteritis

- Infectious
  - Meningitis
  - Herpes zoster
  - Dental carries

- Iatrogenic
  - Medication side effect
  - Medication overuse

medication, botulinum toxin injections, and tricyclic antidepressants or membrane stabilizers such as gabapentin or topiramate. Unfortunately, these medications are among the few treatment options available, as rehabilitation modalities and other interventions have not been formally investigated to date.

HEMIPLEGIC SHOULDER PAIN

A commonly described poststroke pain syndrome is HSP, with an incidence commonly reported as approximately 70%.[35] As the name implies, HSP is a term that encompasses a number of conditions in stroke survivors in which pain develops in the shoulder of the paretic upper limb. There are a multitude of potential etiologies, including, but not limited to, spasticity, glenohumeral subluxation, rotator cuff impingement or tear, and neuropathic syndromes such as the previously described shoulder hand syndrome and CRPS. Diagnosis is clinical and relies primarily on history and physical examination, which vary depending on the underlying etiology of pain. History of preexisting shoulder pain should be noted. A thorough musculoskeletal and neurologic examination of the affected limb is warranted, including active and passive range of motion, palpation of the shoulder girdle muscles, biceps tendons, and acromioclavicular joint, sensory testing, reflexes, strength, and

TABLE 19.3
Statistical Analysis of Combined Clinical Tests in the Diagnosis of Hemiplegic Shoulder Pain

Clinical Tests	Sensitivity	Specificity	Positive Predictive Value	Negative Predictive Value
• Positive Neer test • Hand-behind-neck numerical rating scale ≥5 • Passive external rotation >10° difference compared to unaffected side	96.7%	99.0%	96.7%	99.0%

tone. Rajaratnam and colleagues found that HSP could be successfully diagnosed by using specific clinical tests, as listed in Table 19.3.[36]

Poststroke patients are at the greatest risk of injury that leads to the development of HSP during the early stages of poststroke recovery, as the affected arm is typically more flaccid and the patients rely more heavily on caregivers to assist with transfers and positioning. Risk factors for developing HSP within the first 6 months after stroke are impaired voluntary motor control, diminished perception, tactile extinction, and impaired sensation. Other risk factors include spasticity of elbow flexors, restricted range of motion of shoulder abduction and external rotation, trophic changes, and type 2 diabetes.[37]

HSP may have a presentation similar to various other conditions, and a broad differential must be considered. Differential diagnosis is listed in Table 19.4. Glenohumeral subluxation, spasticity, acute rotator cuff injury, acute long head biceps tendinopathy, adhesive capsulitis, and myofascial pain are not included in the differential diagnosis, as they are in fact different components that make up HSP rather than separate entities.

In addition to the history and physical examination, there are various diagnostic tools that can be used to assist with the diagnosis and further characterization of HSP, thereby providing guidance in the development of a treatment plan. A tool that is rarely used, but considered gold standard in the diagnosis of rotator cuff tears, is X-ray arthrography. In a study performed by Lo and colleagues of 32 poststroke patients with HSP, 50% of patients had X-ray arthrographic evidence of adhesive capsulitis in the affected shoulder, 44% had glenohumeral subluxation, 22% had rotator cuff tears, and 16% had CRPS type I.[38] With such a high frequency of adhesive capsulitis in HSP, magnetic resonance arthrography (MRA) can also be useful in diagnosing this pain contributor, as it is a better tool for diagnosis of soft tissue abnormalities than X-ray arthrography. In a study done by Távora and colleagues, stroke survivors

TABLE 19.4
Differential Diagnosis for Hemiplegic Shoulder Pain

Differential Diagnosis

- Other poststroke pain conditions
  - CPSP
  - SHS
- Musculoskeletal
  - Rotator cuff pathology
  - Long head biceps tendinopathy
  - Humeral or clavicular fracture
  - Glenohumeral or acromioclavicular joint osteoarthritis
  - Myofascial pain
  - Shoulder subluxation
  - Soft tissue contracture
- Neurologic
  - CRPS
  - Peripheral mononeuropathy, e.g., axillary or suprascapular
  - Brachial plexopathy
  - Radiculopathy
  - Spasticity
- Infectious
  - Herpes zoster
  - Cellulitis
  - Septic arthritis
  - Osteomyelitis
- Vascular
  - Thrombus
  - Lymphedema
- Rheumatologic
  - Rheumatoid arthritis
  - Gout

CPSP, central poststroke pain; *CRPS*, complex regional pain syndrome; *SHS*, shoulder-hand syndrome.

with and without shoulder pain underwent MRA of the hemiplegic shoulder. Although both groups had findings consistent with adhesive capsulitis, including synovial capsule thickening and enhancement, and enhancement in the rotator cuff interval, these changes were more pronounced in patients with shoulder pain. The study also revealed no significant differences in shoulder joint effusion, subacromial bursal fluid, acromioclavicular capsular hypertrophy, rotator cuff tendinopathy, or muscle atrophy, supporting the lower rates of these findings in the study by Lo et al.[39]

For patients who are unable to undergo an MRA, ultrasonography may also be a useful tool and has the added benefit of being a dynamic study. Lee and colleagues performed ultrasound imaging on the affected shoulder of 71 patients with HSP and found that the most common abnormality was subacromial-subdeltoid bursal effusion, followed by supraspinatus tendinosis, supraspinatus tendon partial-thickness tear, and supraspinatus tendon full-thickness tear.[40] They found no ultrasound evidence consistent with adhesive capsulitis. Interestingly, in the study performed by Kim and colleagues analyzing the physical examination, shoulder X-ray, and shoulder ultrasound image of 94 patients with HSP, they found that adhesive capsulitis, shoulder subluxation, and long head of biceps tendon effusion had the highest prevalence at 1 month post stroke; however, by 3 and 6 months, these were less common and supraspinatus pathology had the highest prevalence.[41] One must consider the relative strengths and weaknesses of the various diagnostic imaging modalities in working through the differential keeping in mind that the etiology may be multifactorial.

Despite the underlying pathology, there are modalities and treatments that can be universally applied to all patients with HSP. From stroke onset, prevention of shoulder injury through proper positioning and handling is key. All caretakers must be educated to reduce the risk of injury. Although there are no studies supporting one position versus another, it is commonly suggested that the shoulder be kept abducted, externally rotated, and flexed, a position opposite of the posturing commonly seen in spastic hemiparesis after a stroke. When a patient is supine in bed, it is generally recommended that the shoulder be protracted with the arm forward, wrist neutral to slightly supinated, and the fingers extended.[35]

Strapping or taping may also be used to maintain the shoulder in an anatomic position; however, the evidence is mixed as to its effectiveness in reducing pain. Although Griffin and colleagues found that strapping led to a statistically significant increase in pain-free days compared with placebo and control groups, Hanger

and colleagues found no significant difference in pain, range of motion, or functional outcomes.[42,43] Slings may be helpful in reducing the gravitational pull on the hemiplegic arm; however, positioning with a standard sling keeps the shoulder adducted and internally rotated and may lead to decreased range of motion in the shoulder or contracture. Therefore use of a sling is recommended only when a patient with flaccid hemiparesis is upright to protect the limb. An alternative to the traditional sling is the GivMohr sling, which maintains the flaccid limb in an appropriate position while also supporting the shoulder joint. In a study by Dieruf et al., the GivMohr sling was found to reduce shoulder subluxation when compared with a humeral cuff sling, so it may be more useful in patients with HSP.[44] When a patient is sitting, an arm trough or lap tray may be used to ensure that the arm does not get caught behind the wheel as well as to promote shoulder abduction and limit excessive internal and external rotation.[35]

With the help of physical or occupational therapists, patients and their caregivers can be taught how to passively range the shoulder to help maintain the range of motion without injuring the rotator cuff. Pain-free passive range of motion is also important for these patients, as it has been found to reduce the reports of shoulder pain by 43%.[45] It is important that these gentle stretches be done manually and not with the use of an overhead pulley, as it may cause impingement and rotator cuff injury, especially as these patients generally have impaired sensation in the affected limb.[46] Heat and cold packs may also be used, keeping in mind that patients with impaired sensation should be monitored closely. TENS, which is another commonly used modality in physical and occupational therapy, may be beneficial for patients with HSP, specifically high intensity compared with low intensity.[47]

In addition to TENS, other forms of electrical stimulation have been found to be beneficial for patients with HSP. Functional and intramuscular electrical stimulation are two forms that result in muscle contractions; therefore they may be helpful for patients who are not able to voluntarily activate certain muscles. Functional electrical stimulation (FES) is generally directed at the supraspinatus and posterior deltoid for patients with HSP. Although some individual studies have shown improvement in shoulder pain after receiving FES, a Cochrane review done by Price and colleagues found that patients with HSP benefited with improved pain-free passive external rotation of the shoulder and reduced glenohumeral subluxation, but there was no overall improvement in resting pain or motor impairments.[48] Intramuscular electrical stimulation provides more direct and targeted stimulation, as the electrodes are placed intramuscularly, unlike FES. Chae and colleagues found that patients treated with intramuscular electrical stimulation had a significant reduction in pain 1 year after treatment compared with those treated with slings.[49] In a series of eight case reports, Chae and colleagues further reported that placement of a single percutaneous peripheral nerve stimulator in the deltoid resulting in axillary nerve stimulation resulted in 70% reduction of pain at the end of 3 weeks of treatment and 61% reduction in pain 4 weeks later.[50]

Like other musculoskeletal or neuropathic pain conditions, HSP persists if untreated. In a study performed by Lo and colleagues, patients who had HSP attributable to adhesive capsulitis had a worsening of their symptoms the longer it went untreated. Therefore it is important to initiate treatment early.[38] When considering pharmacologic treatment, it is generally recommended to start with acetaminophen or nonsteroidal antiinflammatory drugs. Although there are no studies analyzing these medications in the treatment of this specific patient population, they are generally well tolerated.[35] Topical medications, such as lidocaine or capsaicin, may also be used; however, there are no studies to support or refute their use at this time. As in neuropathic pain conditions, antiepileptics such as gabapentin or pregabalin, tricyclic antidepressants such as amitriptyline and nortriptyline, or SSRIs and serotonin–norepinephrine reuptake inhibitors such as fluoxetine may be tried. Antispasmodics may also help patients better participate and tolerate therapies by controlling excess tone.

The impact of complementary therapeutic modalities for HSP is being explored. A systematic review of seven randomized controlled trials that studied acupuncture in the treatment of HSP found that when acupuncture is combined with therapeutic exercise, patients experience better relief than with either modality alone.[51] Shin and Lee performed a study examining the benefits of combining aromatherapy and acupressure and found that those who received acupressure alone or acupressure combined with aromatherapy experienced a significant reduction in pain but those who received both experienced significant improvement compared with those who received acupressure alone.[52] As these treatments have little to no adverse effects and do not interact with medications, they are great adjunctive options for patients who are interested in alternative medicine.

If conservative measures fail in controlling a patient's pain, a few interventional options may be offered. Trigger point injections may be tried when myofascial etiology is a suspected contribution. Chemodenervation with botulinum toxin can be considered when spasticity contributes to pain and restricted motion. In a small study done by Kong and colleagues, patients experienced improved range of motion and reduced pain after receiving a botulinum toxin compared with those who received placebo.[53] Unfortunately, these findings were not replicated in a randomized controlled trial performed by Marciniak and colleagues. In this study, 21 patients were randomized to receive botulinum toxin in the pectoralis major with or without treatment of the teres major versus a placebo injection. It was found that both groups experienced reduced pain without a significant difference. Yet, those who received botulinum toxin showed a significant improvement in hygiene score for the Disability Assessment Score.[54] Beyond the traditional intramuscular botulinum toxin injection, Castiglione and colleagues performed a small pilot study analyzing the pain effects of intraarticular botulinum toxin injections and found that there was a reduction in pain, but this treatment needs further study.[55]

If patients are experiencing symptoms most consistent with neuropathic pain and CRPS, a stellate ganglion block can be tried with the added benefit of being both diagnostic and therapeutic. However, if a patient has symptoms more consistent with adhesive capsulitis, glenohumeral or acromioclavicular joint arthritis, rotator cuff impingement, or tendinopathy of the long head of the biceps, a corticosteroid injection can be considered. There are multiple studies showing that corticosteroid injections lead to reduced pain.[56–58] Lakse and others showed that a subacromial or intraarticular corticosteroid injection when combined with physical therapy led to significantly reduced pain and increased range of motion compared with physical therapy alone.[59] Corticosteroids can also be used in a suprascapular nerve block. In a randomized controlled trial of 64 patients with stroke randomized to suprascapular nerve block and physical therapy or placebo injection with physical therapy, the treatment group had a statistically significant reduction in pain after treatment as well as 12 weeks later.[60] As there is no sensory component to the suprascapular nerve, a phenol block can also be used in the case of difficult-to-manage spasticity for a more lasting response. This should be weighed against the potential for motor recovery in the innervated muscles.

Surgical intervention may be necessary pending structural integrity and response to conservative management. Procedures include muscle contracture release, fracture or rotator cuff repair, and scapular or glenoid capsular mobilization. Braun and colleagues performed a small study of 25 patients with HSP and muscle contractures; 13 underwent surgical release of these contractures, whereas the remaining 12 were in the control group. They found that 10 of the patients who underwent surgery experienced pain relief 2 months postoperatively, whereas the entire control group continued to report pain up to 6 months later.[61] There is little evidence to support surgical rotator cuff repair in patients with HSP, and it is generally limited to those who experience an acute tear sometime after the stroke.[35] A newer surgical option is a fully implanted peripheral nerve stimulator specifically targeting the axillary nerve. In a case study, the patient experienced sustained pain relief and increased pain-free range of motion once the device was implanted.[62]

As previously mentioned, if HSP goes untreated, it will likely worsen over time and develop into a chronic condition. As is the case for CPSP, SHS, and poststroke headache, further investigation is necessary to better understand and treat these pain syndromes.

REFERENCES

1. Mozaffarian D, Benjamin EJ, Go AS, et al. Heart disease and stroke statistics-2016 update a report from the American Heart Association. *Circulation*. 2016;133. http://dx.doi.org/10.1161/CIR.0000000000000350.
2. Henry JL, Lalloo C, Yashpal K. Central poststroke pain: an abstruse outcome. *Pain Res Manag*. 2008;13(1):41–49. https://www.ncbi.nlm.nih.gov/pubmed/18301815.
3. Frontera WR, Silver JK, Rizzo TD. *Essentials of Physical Medicine and Rehabilitation: Musculoskeletal Disorders, Pain, and Rehabilitation*. Elsevier Health Sciences; 2015.
4. Flaster M, Meresh E, Rao M, Biller J. Central poststroke pain: current diagnosis and treatment. *Top Stroke Rehabil*. 2013;20(2):116–123. https://www.ncbi.nlm.nih.gov/pubmed/23611852.
5. Bowsher D. Central post-stroke ('thalamic syndrome') and other central pains. *Am J Hosp Palliat Med*. 1999;16(4):593–597.
6. Backonja MM, Serra J. Pharmacologic management part 2: lesser-studied neuropathic pain diseases. *Pain Med*. 2004;5(suppl 1):48–59. http://dx.doi.org/10.1111/j.1526-4637.2004.04021.x.
7. Bowsher D. The management of central post-stroke pain. *Postgrad Med J*. 1995;71(840):598–604.
8. Harvey RL. *Central Post-stroke Pain Syndrome*. 2014;378–383.e2.
9. DeLisa JA, Gans BM, Walsh NE, et al. *DeLisa's Physical Medicine & Rehabilitation: Principles and Practice*. Philadelphia: Lippincott Williams & Wilkins; 2005.
10. Hansson P. Post-stroke pain case study: clinical characteristics, therapeutic options and long-term follow-up. *Eur J Neurol*. 2004;11(suppl 1):22–30. https://www.ncbi.nlm.nih.gov/pubmed/15061821.
11. Hasan M, Whiteley J, Bresnahan R, et al. Somatosensory change and pain relief induced by repetitive transcranial magnetic stimulation in patients with central poststroke pain. *Neuromodulation*. 2014;17(8):731–736. Discussion 736. https://www.ncbi.nlm.nih.gov/pubmed/24934719.
12. Jensen TS, Lenz FA. Central post-stroke pain: a challenge for the scientist and the clinician. *Pain*. 1995;61(2):161–164.
13. Awerbuch GI, Sandyk R. Mexiletine for thalamic pain syndrome. *Int J Neurosci*. 1990;55(2–4):129–133. http://dx.doi.org/10.3109/00207459008985960.
14. Bainton T, Fox M, Bowsher D, Wells C. A double-blind trial of naloxone in central post-stroke pain. *Pain*. 1992;48(2):159–162.
15. Segatore M. Understanding central post-stroke pain. *J Neurosci Nurs*. 1996;28(1):28–35.
16. Nicholson BD. Evaluation and treatment of central pain syndromes. *Neurology*. 2004;62(5). http://dx.doi.org/10.1212/wnl.62.5_suppl_2.s30.
17. Aly MM, Saitoh Y, Hosomi K, Oshino S, Kishima H, Yoshimine T. Spinal cord stimulation for central poststroke pain. *Neurosurgery*. 2010;67(3):ons206-12; discussion ons212. https://www.ncbi.nlm.nih.gov/pubmed/20679928.
18. Sokal P, Harat M, Zielinski P, Furtak J, Paczkowski D, Rusinek M. Motor cortex stimulation in patients with chronic central pain. *Adv Clin Exp Med*. 2015;24(2):289–296. https://www.ncbi.nlm.nih.gov/pubmed/25931362.
19. Ramachandran VS, McGeoch PD, Williams L. Can vestibular caloric stimulation be used to treat Dejerine-Roussy syndrome? *Med Hypotheses*. 2007;69(3):486–488. https://www.ncbi.nlm.nih.gov/pubmed/17321064.
20. Chae J. Poststroke complex regional pain syndrome. *Top Stroke Rehabil*. 2010;17(3):151–162. https://www.ncbi.nlm.nih.gov/pubmed/20797958.
21. Pertoldi S, Di Benedetto P. Shoulder-hand syndrome after stroke. A complex regional pain syndrome. *Eura Medicophys*. 2005;41(4):283–292. https://www.ncbi.nlm.nih.gov/pubmed/16474282.
22. Daviet JC, Preux PM, Salle JY, et al. Clinical factors in the prognosis of complex regional pain syndrome type I after stroke. *Am J Phys Med Rehabil*. 2002;81(1):34–39.
23. Harden RN, Bruehl S, Perez RS. Validation of proposed diagnostic criteria (the "Budapest criteria") for complex regional pain syndrome. *Pain*. 2010;150(2):268–274. http://dx.doi.org/10.1016/j.pain.2010.04.030.
24. Park SG, Hyun JK, Lee SJ, Jeon JY. Quantitative evaluation of very acute stage of complex regional pain syndrome after stroke using three-phase bone scintigraphy. *Nucl Med Commun*. 2007;28(10):766–770. http://dx.doi.org/10.1097/MNM.0b013e32828e513f.
25. Kumar V. A study of bone densitometry in patients with complex regional pain syndrome after stroke. *Postgrad Med J*. 2001;77(910):519–522.

26. Cheng PT, Hong CZ. Prediction of reflex sympathetic dystrophy in hemiplegic patients by electromyographic study. *Stroke*. 1995;26(12):2277–2280.

27. Cacchio A, De Blasis E, De Blasis V, Santilli V, Spacca G. Mirror therapy in complex regional pain syndrome type 1 of the upper limb in stroke patients. *Neurorehabil Neural Repair*. 2009;23(8): 792–799 8pp. http://dx.doi.org/10.1177/1545968309335977.

28. Kondo I, Hosokawa K, Soma M, Iwata M, Maltais D. Protocol to prevent shoulder-hand syndrome after stroke. *Arch Phys Med Rehabil*. 2001;82(11):1619–1623.

29. Hartwig M, Gelbrich G, Griewing B. Functional orthosis in shoulder joint subluxation after ischaemic brain stroke to avoid post-hemiplegic shoulder-hand syndrome: a randomized clinical trial. *Clin Rehabil*. 2012;26(9):807–816. http://dx.doi.org/10.1177/0269215511432355.

30. Santamato A, Ranieri M, Panza F, et al. Role of biphosphonates and lymphatic drainage type Leduc in the complex regional pain syndrome (shoulder-hand syndrome). *Pain Med*. 2009;10(1):179–185. https://www.ncbi.nlm.nih.gov/pubmed/19222778.

31. Mailis-Gagnon A, Furlan A. Sympathectomy for neuropathic pain. *Cochrane Database Syst Rev*. 2003;(2):CD002918. http://dx.doi.org/10.1002/14651858.CD002918.

32. Hansen AP, Marcussen NS, Klit H, Andersen G, Finnerup NB, Jensen TS. Pain following stroke: a prospective study. *Eur J Pain*. 2012;16(8):1128–1136. https://www.ncbi.nlm.nih.gov/pubmed/22407963.

33. Hansen AP, Marcussen NS, Klit H, Kasch H, Jensen TS, Finnerup NB. Development of persistent headache following stroke: a 3-year follow-up. *Cephalalgia*. 2015;35(5):399–409. https://www.ncbi.nlm.nih.gov/pubmed/25164919.

34. Harrison RA, Field TS. Post stroke pain: identification, assessment, and therapy. *Cerebrovasc Dis*. 2015;39(3–4):190–201. http://dx.doi.org/10.1159/000375397.

35. Vasudevan JM, Browne BJ. Hemiplegic shoulder pain: an approach to diagnosis and management. *Phys Med Rehabil Clin N Am*. 2014;25(2):411–437. internal-pdf://213.2.7.238/HSP-browne.pdf.

36. Rajaratnam BS, Venketasubramanian N, Kumar PV, Goh JC, Chan YH. Predictability of simple clinical tests to identify shoulder pain after stroke. *Arch Phys Med Rehabil*. 2007;88(8):1016–1021. http://dx.doi.org/10.1016/j.apmr.2007.05.001.

37. Roosink M, Renzenbrink GJ, Buitenweg JR, Van Dongen RT, Geurts AC, Ijzerman MJ. Persistent shoulder pain in the first 6 months after stroke: results of a prospective cohort study. *Arch Phys Med Rehabil*. 2011;92(7):1139–1145. http://dx.doi.org/10.1016/j.apmr.2011.02.016.

38. Lo SF, Chen SY, Lin HC, Jim YF, Meng NH, Kao MJ. Arthrographic and clinical findings in patients with hemiplegic shoulder pain. *Arch Phys Med Rehabil*. 2003;84(12):1786–1791. internal-pdf://0980201408/arthrogram.pdf.

39. Távora DGF, Gama RL, Bomfim RC, Nakayama M, Silva CEP. MRI findings in the painful hemiplegic shoulder. *Clin Radiol*. 2010;65(10):789–794. http://dx.doi.org/10.1016/j.crad.2010.06.001.

40. Lee IS, Yong BS, Moon TY, Yeon JJ, Jong WS, Dong HK. Sonography of patients with hemiplegic shoulder pain after stroke: correlation with motor recovery stage. *Am J Roentgenol*. 2009;192(2):40–44. http://dx.doi.org/10.2214/AJR.07.3978.

41. Kim YH, Jung SJ, Yang EJ, Paik NJ. Clinical and sonographic risk factors for hemiplegic shoulder pain: a longitudinal observational study. *J Rehabil Med*. 2014;46(1):81–87. internal-pdf://84.158.49.224/longitudinal study.pdf.

42. Griffin A, Bernhardt J. Strapping the hemiplegic shoulder prevents development of pain during rehabilitation: a randomized controlled trial. *Clin Rehabil*. 2006;20(4):287–295. internal-pdf://231.74.35.126/strapping 1.pdf.

43. Hanger HC, Whitewood P, Brown G, et al. A randomized controlled trial of strapping to prevent post-stroke shoulder pain. *Clin Rehabil*. 2000;14(4):370–380. http://dx.doi.org/10.1191/0269215500cr339oa.

44. Dieruf K, Poole JL, Gregory C, Rodriguez EJ, Spizman C. Comparative effectiveness of the GivMohr sling in subjects with flaccid upper limbs on subluxation through radiologic analysis. *Arch Phys Med Rehabil*. 2005;86(12):2324–2329. http://dx.doi.org/10.1016/j.apmr.2005.07.291.

45. Caldwell CB, Wilson DJ, Braun RM. Evaluation and treatment of the upper extremity in the hemiplegic stroke patient. *Clin Orthop Relat Res*. 1969;63:69–93. http://www.scopus.com/inward/record.url?eid=2-s2.0-0014487496&partnerID=40&md5=03f95db62c095264bdf2a412bd3a719c.

46. Kumar R, Metter EJ, Mehta AJ, Chew T. Shoulder pain in hemiplegia. The role of exercise. *Am J Phys Med Rehabil*. 1990;69(4):205–208. http://dx.doi.org/10.1097/00002060-199008000-00007.

47. Leandri M, Parodi CI, Corrieri N, Rigardo S. Comparison of TENS treatments in hemiplegic shoulder pain. *Scand J Rehabil Med*. 1990;22(2):69–72.

48. Price CIM, Pandyan AD. Electrical stimulation for preventing and treating post-stroke shoulder pain: a systematic Cochrane review. *Clin Rehabil*. 2001;15(1):5–19. http://dx.doi.org/10.1191/026921501670667822.

49. Chae J, Yu DT, Walker ME, et al. Intramuscular electrical stimulation for hemiplegic shoulder pain. *Am J Phys Med Rehabil*. 2005;84(11):832–842. http://dx.doi.org/10.1097/01.phm.0000184154.01880.72.

50. Chae J, Wilson RD, Bennett ME, Lechman TE, Stager KW. Single-lead percutaneous peripheral nerve stimulation for the treatment of hemiplegic shoulder pain: a case series. *Pain Pract*. 2013;13(1):59–67. internal-pdf://98.198.130.147/nerve stimulation.pdf.

51. Lee JA, Park SW, Hwang PW, et al. Acupuncture for shoulder pain after stroke: a systematic review. *J Altern Complement Med*. 2012;18(9):818–823. http://dx.doi.org/10.1089/acm.2011.0457.

52. Shin BC, Lee MS. Effects of aromatherapy acupressure on hemiplegic shoulder pain and motor power in stroke patients: a pilot study. *J Altern Complement Med*. 2007;13(2):247–251. internal-pdf://1.64.244.215/accupressure.pdf.

53. Kong KH, Neo JJ, Chua KSG. A randomized controlled study of botulinum toxin A in the treatment of hemiplegic shoulder pain associated with spasticity. *Clin Rehabil.* 2007;21(1):28–35. http://ovidsp.ovid.com/ovidweb.cgi?T=JS&CSC=Y&NEWS=N&PAGE=fulltext&D=emed8&AN=2007056615%5Cnhttp://lib.exeter.ac.uk:4556-/resserv?sid=OVID:embase&id=pmid:&id=doi:10.1177%2F0269215506072082&issn=0269-2155&isbn=&volume=21&issue=1&spage=28&pages=28-35&date=20.

54. Marciniak CM, Harvey RL, Gagnon CM, et al. Does botulinum toxin type a decrease pain and lessen disability in hemiplegic survivors of stroke with shoulder pain and spasticity? *Am J Phys Med Rehabil.* 2012;91. http://dx.doi.org/10.1097/PHM.0b013e31826ecb02.

55. Castiglione A, Bagnato S, Boccagni C, Romano MC, Galardi G. Efficacy of intra-articular injection of botulinum toxin type A in refractory hemiplegic shoulder pain. *Arch Phys Med Rehabil.* 2011;92(7):1034–1037. internal-pdf://69.145.130.75/intraarticular botox.pdf.

56. Snels IA, Beckerman H, Twisk JW, et al. Effect of triamcinolone acetonide injections on hemiplegic shoulder pain: a randomized clinical trial. *Stroke.* 2000;31(10):2396–2401. internal-pdf://197.203.149.52/steroid rct.pdf.

57. Dekker JHM, Wagenaar RC, Lankhorst GJ, de Jong BA. The painful hemiplegic shoulder: effects of intra-articular triamsinolone acetonide. *Am J Phys Med Rehabil.* 1997;76:43–48. internal-pdf://61.139.169.97/intraarticular steroids.pdf.

58. Rah UW, Yoon SH, Moon DJ, et al. Subacromial corticosteroid injection on poststroke hemiplegic shoulder pain: a randomized, triple-blind, placebo-controlled trial. *Arch Phys Med Rehabil.* 2012;93(6):949–956. http://dx.doi.org/10.1016/j.apmr.2012.02.002.

59. Lakse E, Gunduz B, Erhan B, Celik EC. The effect of local injections in hemiplegic shoulder pain: a prospective, randomized, controlled study. *Am J Phys Med Rehabil.* 2009;88(10):805–811. http://dx.doi.org/10.1097/PHM.0b013e3181b71c65.

60. Adey-Wakeling Z, Crotty M, Shanahan EM. Suprascapular nerve block for shoulder pain in the first year after stroke: a randomized controlled trial. *Stroke.* 2013;44(11):3136–3141. internal-pdf://111.25.236.193/nerve block.pdf.

61. Braun RM, West F, Mooney V, Nickel VL, Roper B, Caldwell C. Surgical treatment of the painful shoulder contracture in the stroke patient. *J Bone Joint Surg Am.* 1971;53(7):1307–1312.

62. Yu DT, Friedman AS, Rosenfeld EL. Electrical stimulation for treating chronic poststroke shoulder pain using a fully implanted microstimulator with internal battery. *Am J Phys Med Rehabil.* 2010;89(5):423–428. http://dx.doi.org/10.1097/PHM.0b013e3181d8d06f.

CHAPTER 20

Multiple Sclerosis Pain

MICHAEL SAULINO, MD, PHD

INTRODUCTION

Multiple sclerosis (MS) results in a number of serious impairments including paralysis, sensory loss, spasticity, cognitive impairment, and neurogenic bowel/bladder dysfunction, but perhaps no MS-associated condition is more vexing to the treating clinician than chronic pain. Although some of these MS-related impairments can be accommodated with compensatory strategies, neuropathic pain associated with MS often remains quite recalcitrant. In addition to the expected challenges in treating any chronic pain condition, treatment of MS-related pain has the added difficulty of disruption of normal neural pathways that subserve pain transmission and attenuation. This chapter endeavors to describe the classification, epidemiology, evaluation methods, and treatment strategies for this and often confounding pain syndrome.

CLASSIFICATION

The most recent classification described in the medical literature proposed five major categories of pain that effects the patient with MS: nociceptive, neuropathic, psychogenic, idiopathic, and mixed. These categories are generally well described in the literature[1] and are depicted graphically in Fig. 20.1.

Perhaps the biggest distinction in this taxonomy is nociceptive pain, which is pain that arises from actual or threatened damage to nonneural tissue and is due to the activation of nociceptors, versus neuropathic pain, which is caused by a lesion or disease of the somatosensory nervous system. Of note, both neuropathic and nociceptive pain can demonstrate peripheral or central sensitization, which is a process of increased responsiveness of neurons to their normal input and/or recruitment of a response to normally subthreshold inputs. Although this distinction is obvious in some individuals, many patients with MS demonstrate characteristics of both neuropathic and nociceptive pain.[2] Patients with MS can demonstrate nociceptive pain that is prevalent in the non-MS patients, such as degenerative joint disease, as well as nociceptive pain

that is associated directly with the disease process, such as abnormal joint biomechanics secondary to spastic hypertonia. Trigeminal neuralgia, a relatively common neuropathic pain condition, has a higher prevalence in the population with MS. Optic neuritis is a neuropathic pain condition that is almost exclusively associated with MS.

Among the five categories of pain, perhaps the most challenging to define is psychogenic pain. This term refers to both primary psychiatric conditions such as somatoform pains associated with anxiety and depression and the superimposed psychogenic components that often develop in patients with chronic refractory pain. Somatoform pain disorder is defined as a form of mental illness that causes one or more bodily symptoms that causes excessive and disproportionate levels of distress. An example of this disorder would be a middle-aged female with a 10-year history of stable MS with refractory back pain despite relatively benign imaging and extensive trials of oral medication who displays catastrophic behavior and demands inappropriate interventions (such a high doses of opiates).

Idiopathic pain embodies several complex and perhaps poorly understood chronic pain conditions, including fibromyalgia, irritable bowel syndrome, interstitial cystitis, and persistent idiopathic facial pain. Of note, these disorders are not exclusive to MS but may have a higher prevalence in this patient population. These syndromes may share a common genetic predisposition.[3]

The two most common mixed pain syndromes in patients with MS are headache and low back pain. For both of these conditions, there is evidence to suggest that MS-related factors can increase the occurrence of these entities.

Pain can be a consequence of or related to MS treatment. The β-interferons and glatiramer acetate are given as subcutaneous injections and have been associated with local acute pain. Systemic pain syndromes, particularly myalgias, have been associated with interferons. A potential increase in the frequency of preexisting headaches can occur after starting treatment with

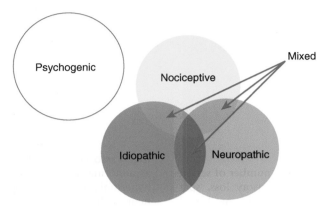

FIG. 20.1 Classification of multiple sclerosis pain types.

interferons.[4] Dalfampridine, an agent that is used to improve walking capacity in patients with MS, has been reported to potentially activate trigeminal neuralgia.[5]

EPIDEMIOLOGY

Given the potential ambiguity of chronic MS-related pain described earlier, attempts at epidemiology can be problematic. Potential confounders include oversampling (because patients may have more than one pain syndrome), adequate pain description, criteria used for chronicity/severity, and appropriate inclusion/exclusion criteria. Based on relatively broad definitions, the prevalence of chronic pain in the population with MS has ranged from 29% to 86%. If one applies a more stringent approach to epidemiology (diagnoses of definite MS, prospective study design, and strict assessment measures), the prevalence range narrows considerably, from 57% to 65%. It is not uncommon for pain to present at the time of initial MS diagnosis, with a reported prevalence from 11% to 21%.[6–8] Roughly 20% of patients report increased pain during an exacerbation.[9] With regard to pain intensity, a general rule of thumb is that about half of patients with MS would self-report their pain as moderate, a quarter would rate their pain as severe, and a quarter would rate their pain as mild. The presence of pain in an individual with MS is associated with decreased emotional and physical functioning.[10] Risk factors reported to be associated with a greater likelihood of pain in patients with MS include older age, longer disease duration,[11] and greater disease severity.[12] Men and women with MS seem to have a comparable risk for pain, although women may have greater severity of pain.[10] The etiology of these observations appears to be multifactorial in nature.

EVALUATION

The approach to MS-related pain should commence in a fashion similar to that of all chronic pain conditions—history, physical examination, and judicious use of diagnostic testing. Information should be obtained regarding the patient's disease onset, course, and progression. Descriptors should be obtained regarding pain history, including time of onset from initial diagnosis, time course, pain location, intensity, quality, alleviating and aggravating factors, past evaluations, treatments (including effectiveness), and pharmacologic assessment. Inquiry into the presence or change in upper motor neuron signs, such as clonus or spasticity, is reasonable. Functional, occupational, and recreational history should be acquired for two reasons. First, these activities may be a contribution factor to the development of pain (e.g., shoulder pain in a wheelchair-dependent individual). Second, the degree of pain interference with these activities allows the clinician to judge the functional impact of the patient's pain condition. Some degree of psychological assessment is warranted with exploration into possible depression, anxiety, personality disorders, substance use, and cognitive impairment. In selected cases, a more formal psychological assessment, including psychometric testing, by either a psychologist or psychiatrist may be appropriate. Lastly, the patient should be queried into what diagnostic tests have been undertaken previously. Newly occurring pain is a potential warning sign that should be thoroughly diagnosed and not "automatically" be attributed to MS. One serious example is spinal cord compression in patients with MS that results from various causes such as vertebral deterioration, tumor, or other anatomic causes.[13,14]

It is also reasonable to attempt assessment of the multidimensional nature of pain in terms of interference with daily activities. Of note, the Initiative on Methods, Measurement, and Pain Assessment in Clinical Trials (IMMPACT) group recommended that measures of pain severity, physical functioning, and emotional functioning be included in all clinical trials of chronic pain interventions.[15] The impact of pain on physical functioning may be obtained through a number by pain interference scales such as the Graded Chronic Pain Disability scale and the Brief Pain Inventory. These scales have demonstrated reasonable reliability and validity in the populations with MS.[16,17]

Many patients with chronic pain disorders and MS have comorbid psychological disorders, including depression, anxiety, anger, psychosis, eating disorders, substance dependence, cognitive impairment, and personality disorders. At a minimum, treating physicians should discuss the existence and severity of these behavioral problems with the patient. Cotreatment with mental health professionals is often warranted for more in-depth neuropsychological assessments. Examples of standardized psychological assessments used in this population include the Beck Depression Inventory and Hospital Anxiety and Depression Scale.[18-20]

The physical examination of the individual with MS-associated pain should focus on the neurologic and musculoskeletal systems. Assessment should include reflex testing, assessment sensory abnormalities (allodynia, hyperalgesia, hyperpathia), motor control (tremor, ataxia), and muscle overactivity (spasms, spasticity, clonus). One particular maneuver is worthy of note: the Lhermitte phenomenon, which is an electrical sensation that runs down the back and into the limbs elicited by bending the head forward. Although this is often considered a classic finding in MS, it can be caused by a number of conditions. Focal examination of a particular pain area would then proceed in a manner similar to that utilized for all pain complaints. Items to be included are inspection, palpation, active and passive range of motion, and provocative maneuvers. Observation of wheelchair propulsion, posture, and gait may be appropriate in selected patients. Appropriate comfort and fit of assistive devices (cane, walker, crutch) and orthotic devices should be undertaken if this equipment appears to be contributing to the pain syndrome. A survey of mood, behavior, personality, and cognition is certainly reasonable given their potential impact on chronic pain treatment.

Although the use of neuroimaging is paramount in the diagnosis and management of MS, the use of imaging modalities for the detection of potential pain generators is less clear. The literature suggests that imaging is often undertaken in the presence of headache and facial pain. Brainstem lesions on MRI appear to be associated with a higher frequency of headache. Given the possible unreliability of abdominal/pelvic examinations in an insensate patient, imaging may also be warranted if visceral pain is suspected. In addition to the traditional MRI and CT imaging modalities, specialized techniques may be warranted for potential pain generator relative to neurogenic bowel and bladder. Examples in this arena might include colonoscopy, cystoscopy, urodynamics testing, etc. Triple phase bone scanning could be appropriate for the evaluation of unsuspected fractures or complex regional pain syndrome.[21]

Similarly, judicious use of laboratory testing is a reasonable undertaking. Care must be exerted with regards to interpretation so as not to "over-read" the importance of a particular abnormality. An example of this pitfall would be to attribute asymptomatic urinary bacterial colonization as the sole cause of visceral pain. Potential laboratory tests in this population might include a complete blood count, erythrocyte sedimentation rate, HbA1c, C-reactive protein, and hormonal assessment (including thyroid/testosterone levels, pregnancy testing). Subtherapeutic vitamin B_{12}[22] and vitamin D[23] have been implicated in neuronal dysfunction and represented potentially reversible abnormalities.

MANAGEMENT
Nonpharmacologic
A generalized exercise program in the form of global strength training, cardiovascular training, or recreational physical activities has the potential to be beneficial for a number of MS-related conditions (e.g., spasticity, muscle atrophy, bone health), but its effect on global pain in this population has not been very satisfactory. Animal studies have suggested that antinociceptive behaviors can be reduced with weeks of exercise training.[24,25] Extrapolation from these experiments to the human condition has not been straightforward. Some human trials have suggested that a long-term exercise program can attenuate global pain complaints[26] but these effects may not persist if regular exercise is discontinued.[27] More targeted exercise programs for specific pain complaints have a much higher likelihood of success. Van der Linden et al. suggested that Pilates was a safe and feasible form of exercise for wheelchair-bound individuals with MS, which resulted in decreased back and shoulder pain.[28] Doulatabad and colleagues suggested the positive effects of yoga on MS-related pain during a randomized clinical trial.[29]

In addition to generalized and specified exercise programs, referral to physical or occupational therapy may be appropriate for the patient with MS with musculoskeletal pain in an effort to address biomechanical abnormalities that can be associated with mobility aids. Modification of orthotics, canes, walkers, crutches, and wheelchairs has the potential to influence detrimental ergonomics. Perhaps the best example of this intervention is adjustment of the rear wheel of a manual wheelchair in an effort to modify the forces about the shoulder that can occur as a result of wheelchair propulsion.[30]

Therapeutic modalities have the potential to be effective in treating MS-related pain. A review of transcutaneous electrical nerve stimulation has suggested that it is a safe and effective treatment of central neuropathic pain.[31] A randomized controlled trial (RCT) of massage therapy suggested enhanced pain reduction compared with a generalized exercise program.[32] Reflexology, which is the application of pressure to the feet and hands with specific thumb, finger, and hand techniques without the use of oil or lotion, failed to demonstrate significant difference compared with nonspecific massage during an RCT. However, both groups exhibited pain relief compared with baseline.[33]

One nonpharmacologic pain intervention that is particularly popular for both the general patient and the population with MS is acupuncture. In 1997 a report from the National Institutes of Health supported the use of acupuncture for certain conditions, including pain.[34] There have been at least 12 studies that have examined the capacity of acupuncture to attenuate MS-related symptoms, including pain. Although the majority of these studies suggest benefit, there is a significant lack of scientific rigor in these investigations.[35]

Pharmacologic

Antiepileptic drugs (AEDs) are considered first-line therapy for central neuropathic pain associated with MS. The most common medications discussed include pregabalin, gabapentin, and lamotrigine. Pregabalin and gabapentin binds to voltage-gated calcium channels. It is hypothesized that this binding that reduces the influx of calcium into the hyperexcited neuron in turn results in a reduction in the release of several neurotransmitters, including glutamate, noradrenaline, serotonin, dopamine, and substance P. Both gabapentinoids have analgesic, anticonvulsant, anxiolytic, and sleep-modulating activities.[36] Lamotrigine is a sodium channel blocker and is thought to exert its pain-modulating activity by enhancing γ-aminobutyric acid and reducing glutamatergic neurotransmission.[37] Less

common AEDs utilized in patients with MS include carbamazepine, oxcarbazepine, topiramate, and phenytoin. The most common adverse events associated with pregabalin and gabapentin are mild or moderate and typically transient. Edema, somnolence, and dizziness are the most commonly reported adverse events, with edema being the most likely reason for discountenance of therapy. Hyponatremia can be seen with oxcarbazepine. AEDs are most commonly utilized in MS-related neuropathic pain, including trigeminal neuralgia, glossopharyngeal neuralgia, and paroxysmal dysesthesias.[38]

The use of antidepressants for neuropathic pain has a long-standing tradition. It would appear that this class of medication is less well tolerated than AEDs. The classic group of medications is the tricyclic antidepressants (TCAs). They can be quite beneficial but can have a significant side-effect profile, including anticholinergic adverse effects such as urinary retention, constipation, dry mouth, cognitive dysfunction, weight gain, cardiac arrhythmia (prolonged QTc), and increased fatigue. These medications may be particularly useful for treating hyperactive detrusor in cases of bladder dysfunction and may reduce sleep disorders.[39] The so-called second-generation TCAs (i.e., secondary amines such as nortriptyline, desipramine, and protriptyline) are preferred because the analgesic efficacy is equivalent and tolerability is better than that of first-generation TCAs (i.e., tertiary amines such as amitriptyline, clomipramine, and doxepin). All TCAs are considered to have a ceiling effect. Thus, once a therapeutic effect is achieved, further increase in dosing should be avoided to minimize adverse effects.[40] When adverse events or effects are encountered with the TCAs, there is a suggestion that additive therapy with AEDs can be beneficial.

One of the more recent additions to the armamentarium of antidepressant use for chronic pain is the dual serotonin and norepinephrine reuptake inhibitors. Medications in this class include duloxetine, milnacipran, levomilnacipran, venlafaxine, and desvenlafaxine. Pain modulation appears to be independent of their antidepressant properties. Duloxetine, the first medication approved for use in the United States within this class, has Food and Drug Administration indication for chronic musculoskeletal pain, fibromyalgia, and diabetic neuropathy. Two trials of this agent with patients with MS have suggested a positive therapeutic effect, although tolerability was somewhat of a concern.[41,42] There are no reports of using any of the other medications for chronic MS-associated pain. One interesting observation is the potential for venlafaxine to be immunomodulatory in preclinical models.[43]

Opioid medications have been suggested as a reasonable option for chronic nociceptive and perhaps neuropathic pain. Perhaps no other decision in medicine causes more anxiety than prescribing opiates for patients with chronic, noncancer pain. Concerns over diversion, misuse, dependence, addiction, monitoring, and cost can make the analysis of utilizing chronic opiate therapy troublesome for even experienced clinicians.[44] In the patient with MS, concerns over the potential exacerbation of neurogenic bowel caused by opioid-related constipation makes this decision even more challenging. There are several new strategies for the management of opioid-related constipation, including peripheral opioid receptor antagonists and prokinetic agents.[45] A review of the use of opioids in neuropathic pain suggested clinical efficacy of this medication class for long-term use. It is relevant to note that this review has a large preponderance of periphery-based neuropathic pain (diabetic neuropathy or postherpetic neuropathy), but some subjects with MS were included.[46] There are several developments within the opioid class medications that may be of specific interest to clinicians treating MS-related pain. Tapentadol is a centrally acting analgesic with dual mechanism of action—agonist activity at the μ-opioid receptor and inhibition of norepinephrine reuptake. A potential therapeutic advantage of this agent is its utility in neuropathic pain. This benefit has been studied with both low back pain with a neuropathic pain component and diabetic peripheral neuropathy.[47,48] There are no specific reports on the use of this agent in MS. In addition, this medication may also have therapeutic advantages over other opiates, including a lower incidence of withdrawal symptoms and decreased frequency of gastrointestinal side effects. However, owing to the activity that this agent has with monoamine metabolism, there is a potential to exacerbate or precipitate serotonin syndrome.[49] Another dual-acting product is tramadol, which is a combination of a serotonin and noradrenaline reuptake inhibitor and a μ-opioid agonist. This medication is noteworthy because its mechanism of action is distinct from those of other opioids. Tramadol has been shown to demonstrate benefit in osteoarthritis, fibromyalgia, and neuropathic pain; however, there is insufficient evidence to definitely define tramadol as more effective than other opioids.[50] There is also some evidence to suggest that opiate use can be detrimental for patients with MS. This hypothesis is supported by the observation that low-dose naltrexone therapy can improve many symptoms of MS, including fatigue, cognition, mood, and pain.[51] The theory behind the mechanism of action of low-dose naltrexone is that

this agent transiently inhibits opioid receptors at low doses, causes the body to increase the production of endorphins, and upregulates the immune system.[52] As with any patient who receives opiates, a screening must be performed to elucidate which patient may be at risk for abuse or diversion. There are several survey instruments available to clinicians that can assist in the decision making relative to chronic opiate therapy. These include the Screener and Opioid Assessment for Patients with Pain-Revised (SOAPP-R), the Opioid Risk Tool (ORT), and the DIRE score (Diagnosis, Intractability, Risk and Efficacy) score. The validity, reliability, sensitivity, and predicative value of these tools are considered fair to good.[53] Additional measures that should be utilized if a clinician is going to engage chronic opiate therapy includes narcotic agreement, query of state prescription drug databases, and in-office drug testing (such as urine, saliva, serum, or hair sampling). Thus the decision to utilize opiates in the patient with MS must undergo a careful risk-benefit analysis.

The relationship between pain and spasticity is complex. Reduction of spasticity may reduce the pain associated with biomechanical pain. Modulation of spasticity may not be effective in reducing neuropathic pain.[54] There are several oral medications that can accomplish spasticity reduction, including baclofen, tizanidine, diazepam, and dantrolene. Of particular interest, tizanidine has a dual mechanism of action, an α2 adrenergic agonism at the spinal level and an influence on descending noradrenergic pathways. The latter mechanism may be of particular interest in the management of MS-related pain.[55] Similarly, botulinum toxins have the potential to reduce muscle overactivity in a focally directed manner.[56] Over and above their antispasticity activities, botulinum toxins have the capacity to exert a therapeutic effect on neuropathic pain.[57] However, there are no formal studies examining the effects of botulinum toxin on MS-related pain independent of their spasticity reduction properties.

Medicinal marijuana and synthetic cannabinoids represent intriguing pharmacologic choices for the management of MS-associated pain. Cannabis contains 60 or more cannabinoids, the most abundant of which are δ-9-tetrahydrocannabinol (THC) and cannabidiol (CBD). At the time of submission of this chapter, roughly half of US states had legalized some form of medicinal marijuana, although it is illegal under federal law. Many states have qualifying conditions for medicinal marijuana use. One of the most common qualifying condition is pain as well as muscle spasms. Some states also use damage to the nervous tissue of the spinal cord a qualifying condition. Availability is a concern in many locations given this legal ambiguity. Several clinical trials have examined the use of cannabinoids for the population with MS. Using a crossover design, it was noted that dronabinol (a synthetic THC product) reduced pain and improved certain quality of life measures but was associated with a high frequency of side effects.[58] In a parallel group trial, a mixture of THC and CBD reduced pain, improved sleep quality, and was reasonably well tolerated in a group of patients with MS with central pain.[59] The use of a THC/CBD oromucosal spray (Sativex) suggested efficacy in open-label[60] and enriched enrollment trials[61] but had somewhat equivocal results during an RCT when used in combination with patients' existing treatment regimen.[62] Nabilone (a synthetic THC analogue) showed promise as additive therapy to gabapentin during an RCT in 15 patients with MS.[62] Side effects may have compromised the blinding in some of these trials, which would make interpretation of the results problematic.

Interventional

Perhaps the most common neuropathic pain syndrome that appears to be the most amenable to interventional procedures is trigeminal neuralgia. Approaches include thermocoagulation in Meckel cave, percutaneous retrogasserian glycerol rhizotomy, radiosurgery with the Gamma Knife, and microvascular decompression. These procedures are typically reserved for recalcitrant cases and appear to the capacity for dramatic pain relief. Recurrence is possible. The most common adverse event is persistent facial numbness.[39]

Spinal cord stimulation (SCS) is defined as posterior epidural stimulation of the dorsal columns. The proposed mechanisms of action of this therapy involve the gate theory of pain, enhancement of parasympathetic activity, inhibition of sympathetic activity, upregulation of descending inhibitory pathways, and downregulation of ascending pain pathways. Owing to concerns over MRI compatibility of SCS devices and the need for routine surveillance MRI to assess disease burden in MS, this intervention has not been utilized very often. Provenzano et al. reported on the successful reduction of neuropathic pain in a patient with MS with the use of an MRI-compatible SCS system.[63]

Intrathecal drug delivery provides direct administration of therapeutic agents to the subarachnoid space where they have enhanced access to receptor sites. Intrathecal baclofen is a well-established technique for the reduction of spasticity associated with MS.[64,65] To the extent that spasticity is related to musculoskeletal pain, this technique has the capacity to attenuate pain in this population. However, the use of intrathecal baclofen as a pure pain-modulating agent is limited.[66] The utility of more traditional intrathecal analgesic agents has not been overwhelmingly successful. Combination therapy with baclofen and clonidine,[67] morphine and clonidine,[68] baclofen and morphine,[69] baclofen and ziconotide,[70] and hydromorphone and ziconotide[71] have resulted in varying degrees of success. Intrathecal gabapentin failed to demonstrate a therapeutic effect in a population with generalized pain.[72]

Peripheral field stimulation is a form of neuromodulation that involves placement of an electrical stimulator that targets small nerve fibers in the subcutaneous tissue, beneath the skin. This technique has been utilized for the management of trigeminal neuralgia and other facial pain in patients with MS.[51] Deep brain stimulation has also been suggested as a potential therapeutic modality for facial pain in this population.[51] The MRI compatibility of these devices has similar concerns to those of the SCS devices described earlier.

SUMMARY

MS-related pain is clearly a challenging pain syndrome. Each element of this review (classification, epidemiology, evaluation, and management) has demonstrated limitations. Patients with MS present unique difficulties to the managing clinician. An individualized approach to evaluation and management is appropriate in this patient population. Treatment decisions should include consideration of nonpharmacologic, pharmacologic, and interventional techniques that weigh the risks and benefits of each method. Further investigation by both the basic scientists and clinicians is warranted in an effort to further delineate the nature of this problem and create more effective treatment strategies.

REFERENCES

1. Boyd D, Butler M, Carr D, et al. *IASP Pain Terminology. An Update on the IASP Taskforce on Taxonomy. Part III: Pain Terms, a Current List with Definitions and Notes on Usage.* IASP Taxonomy; 2011:2011.
2. Jensen TS, Baron R, Haanpaa M, et al. A new definition of neuropathic pain. *Pain.* 2011;152(10):2204–2205.
3. Nickel JC, Tripp DA, Pontari M, et al. Interstitial cystitis/painful bladder syndrome and associated medical conditions with an emphasis on irritable bowel syndrome, fibromyalgia and chronic fatigue syndrome. *J Urol.* 2010;184(4):1358–1363.
4. Girouard N, Theoret G. Management strategies for improving the tolerability of interferons in the treatment of multiple sclerosis. *Can J Neurosci Nurs.* 2008;30(4):18–25.

5. Birnbaum G, Iverson J. Dalfampridine may activate latent trigeminal neuralgia in patients with multiple sclerosis. *Neurology*. 2014;83(18):1610–1612.
6. Indaco A, Iachetta C, Nappi C, Socci L, Carrieri PB. Chronic and acute pain syndromes in patients with multiple sclerosis. *Acta Neurol (Napoli)*. 1994;16(3):97–102.
7. Osterberg A, Boivie J, Thuomas KA. Central pain in multiple sclerosis–prevalence and clinical characteristics. *Eur J Pain*. 2005;9(5):531–542.
8. Stenager E, Knudsen L, Jensen K. Acute and chronic pain syndromes in multiple sclerosis. A 5-year follow-up study. *Ital J Neurol Sci*. 1995;16(9):629–632.
9. Pollmann W, Feneberg W, Erasmus LP. Pain in multiple sclerosis–a still underestimated problem. The 1 year prevalence of pain syndromes, significance and quality of care of multiple sclerosis inpatients. *Nervenarzt*. 2004;75(2):135–140.
10. Hadjimichael O, Kerns RD, Rizzo MA, Cutter G, Vollmer T. Persistent pain and uncomfortable sensations in persons with multiple sclerosis. *Pain*. 2007;127(1–2):35–41.
11. Clifford DB, Trotter JL. Pain in multiple sclerosis. *Arch Neurol*. 1984;41(12):1270–1272.
12. Ehde DM, Gibbons LE, Chwastiak L, Bombardier CH, Sullivan MD, Kraft GH. Chronic pain in a large community sample of persons with multiple sclerosis. *Mult Scler*. 2003;9(6):605–611.
13. Burgerman R, Rigamonti D, Randle JM, Fishman P, Panitch HS, Johnson KP. The association of cervical spondylosis and multiple sclerosis. *Surg Neurol*. 1992;38(4):265–270.
14. Ronthal M. On the coincidence of cervical spondylosis and multiple sclerosis. *Clin Neurol Neurosurg*. 2006;108(3):275–277.
15. Dworkin RH, Turk DC, Peirce-Sandner S, et al. Research design considerations for confirmatory chronic pain clinical trials: IMMPACT recommendations. *Pain*. 2010;149(2):177–193.
16. Ehde DM, Nitsch KP, Smiley JP. Measurement characteristics and clinical utility of the brief pain inventory-short form for individuals with multiple sclerosis. *Rehabil Psychol*. 2015;60(4):365–366.
17. Osborne TL, Raichle KA, Jensen MP, Ehde DM, Kraft G. The reliability and validity of pain interference measures in persons with multiple sclerosis. *J Pain Symptom Manage*. 2006;32(3):217–229.
18. Hanna J, Santo JB, Blair M, Smolewska K, Warriner E, Morrow SA. Comparing depression screening tools in persons with multiple sclerosis (MS). *Rehabil Psychol*. 2017;62(1):20–24.
19. Litster B, Fiest KM, Patten SB, et al. Screening tools for anxiety in people with multiple sclerosis: a systematic review. *Int J MS Care*. 2016;18(6):273–281.
20. Solaro C, Trabucco E, Signori A, et al. Depressive symptoms correlate with disability and disease course in multiple sclerosis patients: an Italian multi-center study using the beck depression inventory. *PLoS One*. 2016;11(9):e0160261.
21. Le Chapelain L, Perrouin-Verbe B, Fattal C. SOFMER French Society for Physical Medicine and Rehabilitation. Chronic neuropathic pain in spinal cord injury patients: what relevant additional clinical exams should be performed? *Ann Phys Rehabil Med*. 2009;52(2):103–110.
22. Petchkrua W, Little JW, Burns SP, Stiens SA, James JJ. Vitamin B12 deficiency in spinal cord injury: a retrospective study. *J Spinal Cord Med*. 2003;26(2):116–121.
23. Hummel K, Craven BC, Giangregorio L. Serum 25(OH)D, PTH and correlates of suboptimal 25(OH)D levels in persons with chronic spinal cord injury. *Spinal Cord*. 2012;50(11):812–816.
24. Hutchinson KJ, Gomez-Pinilla F, Crowe MJ, Ying Z, Basso DM. Three exercise paradigms differentially improve sensory recovery after spinal cord contusion in rats. *Brain*. 2004;127(Pt 6):1403–1414.
25. Kuphal KE, Fibuch EE, Taylor BK. Extended swimming exercise reduces inflammatory and peripheral neuropathic pain in rodents. *J Pain*. 2007;8(12):989–997.
26. Hicks AL, Martin KA, Ditor DS, et al. Long-term exercise training in persons with spinal cord injury: effects on strength, arm ergometry performance and psychological well-being. *Spinal Cord*. 2003;41(1):34–43.
27. Ditor DS, Latimer AE, Ginis KA, Arbour KP, McCartney N, Hicks AL. Maintenance of exercise participation in individuals with spinal cord injury: effects on quality of life, stress and pain. *Spinal Cord*. 2003;41(8):446–450.
28. van der Linden ML, Bulley C, Geneen LJ, Hooper JE, Cowan P, Mercer TH. Pilates for people with multiple sclerosis who use a wheelchair: feasibility, efficacy and participant experiences. *Disabil Rehabil*. 2014;36(11):932–939.
29. Doulatabad SN, Nooreyan K, Doulatabad AN, Noubandegani ZM. The effects of pranayama, hatha and raja yoga on physical pain and the quality of life of women with multiple sclerosis. *Afr J Tradit Complement Altern Med*. 2012;10(1):49–52.
30. Katalinic OM, Harvey LA, Herbert RD. Effectiveness of stretch for the treatment and prevention of contractures in people with neurological conditions: a systematic review. *Phys Ther*. 2011;91(1):11–24.
31. Sawant A, Dadurka K, Overend T, Kremenchutzky M. Systematic review of efficacy of TENS for management of central pain in people with multiple sclerosis. *Mult Scler Relat Disord*. 2015;4(3):219–227.
32. Negahban H, Rezaie S, Goharpey S. Massage therapy and exercise therapy in patients with multiple sclerosis: a randomized controlled pilot study. *Clin Rehabil*. 2013;27(12):1126–1136.
33. Hughes CM, Smyth S, Lowe-Strong AS. Reflexology for the treatment of pain in people with multiple sclerosis: a double-blind randomised sham-controlled clinical trial. *Mult Scler*. 2009;15(11):1329–1338.
34. NIH Consensus Conference. Acupuncture. *JAMA*. 1998;280(17):1518–1524.
35. Karpatkin HI, Napolione D, Siminovich-Blok B. Acupuncture and multiple sclerosis: a review of the evidence. *Evid Based Complement Alternat Med*. 2014;2014:972935.

36. Gajraj NM. Pregabalin: its pharmacology and use in pain management. *Anesth Analg.* 2007;105(6):1805–1815.

37. Johannessen Landmark C. Antiepileptic drugs in non-epilepsy disorders: relations between mechanisms of action and clinical efficacy. *CNS Drugs.* 2008;22(1):27–47.

38. Pollmann W, Feneberg W. Current management of pain associated with multiple sclerosis. *CNS Drugs.* 2008;22(4):291–324.

39. Pollmann W, Feneberg W, Steinbrecher A, Haupts MR, Henze T. Therapy of pain syndromes in multiple sclerosis – an overview with evidence-based recommendations. *Fortschr Neurol Psychiatr.* 2005;73(5):268–285.

40. Mico JA, Ardid D, Berrocoso E, Eschalier A. Antidepressants and pain. *Trends Pharmacol Sci.* 2006;27(7):348–354.

41. Brown TR, Slee A. A randomized placebo-controlled trial of duloxetine for central pain in multiple sclerosis. *Int J MS Care.* 2015;17(2):83–89.

42. Vollmer TL, Robinson MJ, Risser RC, Malcolm SK. A randomized, double-blind, placebo-controlled trial of duloxetine for the treatment of pain in patients with multiple sclerosis. *Pain Pract.* 2014;14(8):732–744.

43. Vollmar P, Nessler S, Kalluri SR, Hartung HP, Hemmer B. The antidepressant venlafaxine ameliorates murine experimental autoimmune encephalomyelitis by suppression of pro-inflammatory cytokines. *Int J Neuropsychopharmacol.* 2009;12(4):525–536.

44. Hallinan R, Osborn M, Cohen M, Dobbin M, Wodak A. Increasing the benefits and reducing the harms of prescription opioid analgesics. *Drug Alcohol Rev.* 2011;30(3):315–323.

45. Walters JB, Montagnini M. Current concepts in the management of opioid-induced constipation. *J Opioid Manag.* 2010;6(6):435–444.

46. Eisenberg E, McNicol E, Carr DB. Opioids for neuropathic pain. *Cochrane Database Syst Rev.* 2006;3(3):CD006146.

47. Steigerwald I, Muller M, Davies A, et al. Effectiveness and safety of tapentadol prolonged release for severe, chronic low back pain with or without a neuropathic pain component: results of an open-label, phase 3b study. *Curr Med Res Opin.* 2012;28.

48. Schwartz S, Etropolski M, Shapiro DY, et al. Safety and efficacy of tapentadol ER in patients with painful diabetic peripheral neuropathy: results of a randomized-withdrawal, placebo-controlled trial. *Curr Med Res Opin.* 2011;27(1):151–162.

49. Riemsma R, Forbes C, Harker J, et al. Systematic review of tapentadol in chronic severe pain. *Curr Med Res Opin.* 2011;27(10):1907–1930.

50. Leppert W. Tramadol as an analgesic for mild to moderate cancer pain. *Pharmacol Rep.* 2009;61(6):978–992.

51. Klein J, Sandi-Gahun S, Schackert G, Juratli TA. Peripheral nerve field stimulation for trigeminal neuralgia, trigeminal neuropathic pain, and persistent idiopathic facial pain. *Cephalalgia.* 2016;36(5):445–453.

52. Agrawal YP. Low dose naltrexone therapy in multiple sclerosis. *Ðed Hypotheses.* 2005;64(4):721–4.

53. Jones T, Moore T, Levy JL, et al. A comparison of various risk screening methods in predicting discharge from opioid treatment. *Clin J Pain.* 2012;28(2):93–100.

54. Ward AB, Kadies M. The management of pain in spasticity. *Disabil Rehabil.* 2002;24(8):443–453.

55. Kamen L, Henney 3rd HR, Runyan JD. A practical overview of tizanidine use for spasticity secondary to multiple sclerosis, stroke, and spinal cord injury. *Curr Med Res Opin.* 2008;24(2):425–439.

56. Dressler D, Bhidayasiri R, Bohlega S, et al. Botulinum toxin therapy for treatment of spasticity in multiple sclerosis: review and recommendations of the IAB-Interdisciplinary Working Group for Movement Disorders task force. *J Neurol.* 2017;264(1):112–120.

57. Intiso D, Basciani M, Santamato A, Intiso M, Di Rienzo F. Botulinum toxin type A for the treatment of neuropathic pain in neuro-rehabilitation. *Toxins (Basel).* 2015;7(7):2454–2480.

58. Svendsen KB, Jensen TS, Bach FW. Does the cannabinoid dronabinol reduce central pain in multiple sclerosis? Randomised double blind placebo controlled crossover trial. *BMJ.* 2004;329(7460):253.

59. Rog DJ, Nurmikko TJ, Friede T, Young CA. Randomized, controlled trial of cannabis-based medicine in central pain in multiple sclerosis. *Neurology.* 2005;65(6):812–819.

60. Rog DJ, Nurmikko TJ, Young CA. Oromucosal delta9-tetrahydrocannabinol/cannabidiol for neuropathic pain associated with multiple sclerosis: an uncontrolled, open-label, 2-year extension trial. *Clin Ther.* 2007;29(9):2068–2079.

61. Notcutt W, Langford R, Davies P, Ratcliffe S, Potts R. A placebo-controlled, parallel-group, randomized withdrawal study of subjects with symptoms of spasticity due to multiple sclerosis who are receiving long-term Sativex(R) (nabiximols). *Mult Scler.* 2012;18(2):219–228.

62. Turcotte D, Doupe M, Torabi M, et al. Nabilone as an adjunctive to gabapentin for multiple sclerosis-induced neuropathic pain: a randomized controlled trial. *Pain Med.* 2015;16(1):149–159.

63. Provenzano DA, Williams JR, Jarzabek G, DeRiggi LA, Scott TF. Treatment of neuropathic pain and functional limitations associated with multiple sclerosis using an MRI-compatible spinal cord stimulator: a case report with two year follow-up and literature review. *Neuromodulation.* 2016;19(4):406–413.

64. Erwin A, Gudesblatt M, Bethoux F, et al. Intrathecal baclofen in multiple sclerosis: too little, too late? *Mult Scler.* 2011;17(5):623–629.

65. Rekand T, Gronning M. Treatment of spasticity related to multiple sclerosis with intrathecal baclofen: a long-term follow-up. *J Rehabil Med.* 2011;43(6):511–514.

66. Saulino M. The use of intrathecal baclofen in pain management. *Pain Manag.* 2012;2(6):603–608.

67. Middleton JW, Siddall PJ, Walker S, Molloy AR, Rutkowski SB. Intrathecal clonidine and baclofen in the management of spasticity and neuropathic pain following spinal cord injury: a case study. *Arch Phys Med Rehabil.* 1996;77(8):824–826.

68. Siddall PJ, Molloy AR, Walker S, Mather LE, Rutkowski SB, Cousins MJ. The efficacy of intrathecal morphine and clonidine in the treatment of pain after spinal cord injury. *Anesth Analg.* 2000;91(6):1493–1498.

69. Saulino M. Simultaneous treatment of intractable pain and spasticity: observations of combined intrathecal baclofen-morphine therapy over a 10-year clinical experience. *Eur J Phys Rehabil Med.* 2011;48(1):39–45.

70. Saulino M, Burton AW, Danyo DA, Frost S, Glanzer J, Solanki DR. Intrathecal ziconotide and baclofen provide pain relief in seven patients with neuropathic pain and spasticity: case reports. *Eur J Phys Rehabil Med.* 2009;45.

71. Saulino M. Successful reduction of neuropathic pain associated with spinal cord injury via of a combination of intrathecal hydromorphone and ziconotide: a case report. *Spinal Cord.* 2007;45(11):749–752.

72. Rauck R, Coffey RJ, Schultz DM, et al. Intrathecal gabapentin to treat chronic intractable noncancer pain. *Anesthesiology.* 2013;119(3):675–686.

CHAPTER 21

Trigeminal Neuralgias

NICOLE M. SPARE, DO • SANTIAGO M. MAZUERA-MEJIA, MD • JEFFREY A. GEHRET, DO

INTRODUCTION

Cranial neuralgias and trigeminal autonomic cephalalgias are potentially disabling neurologic disorders. Trigeminal neuralgia (TN) is also called *tic douloureux (Tic)*. Trigeminal neuropathies are defined as "head and/or facial pain in the distribution of one or more branches of the trigeminal nerve caused by another disorder and indicative of neural damage. The pain is highly variable in quality and intensity according to the cause."[1]

The International Classification of Headache Disorders (ICHD) defines headache as "pain located above the orbitomeatal line."[1] Primary headache, such as migraine and tension-type headache, is a disorder unto itself; no underlying disease process is present. Secondary headache is a manifestation of an underlying disease process. A variety of headaches are frequently associated with facial pain. The ICHD-3 β, the most updated edition, defines facial pain as "pain below the orbitomeatal line, above the neck and anterior to the pinna."

Trigeminal autonomic cephalalgias (TACs) characteristically feature unilateral pain and "share the clinical features of headache, which is usually lateralized, and often prominent cranial parasympathetic autonomic features, which again are lateralized and ipsilateral to the headache."[1] The majority of patients with painful cranial neuralgias present with unilateral facial pain, headache, or both.[2] However, for many headache and facial pain disorders, pain patterns can cross these so-called boundaries. Classification of these disorders often overlaps significantly, leading to misdiagnosis or a prolonged treatment regimen involving trial and error of various pharmacologic and nonpharmacologic therapies. It has been questioned if these overlapping disorders are distinct entities or a continuum of the same disorder.[3,4]

EPIDEMIOLOGY AND DISEASE BURDEN

Epidemiologic evidence shows the prevalence of TN to be approximately 4–28.9/100,000 persons worldwide.[5-7] Onset is usually after age 50 years and increases with advancing age. Women are affected 1.7 times more than men.[7] A large retrospective cohort study demonstrated an increased risk of having comorbid depression or anxiety disorders in patients with TN.[8] Activities of daily living, work productivity, and quality of sleep all may be affected.

Epidemiologic data show a strong association of TN in multiple sclerosis (a 20-fold increased risk of developing TN compared with the general population),[7] as well as in cases of hypertension and stroke.[6,7,9]

Another epidemiologic evaluation was completed to evaluate the diagnostic approaches for patients presenting to a tertiary neurology outpatient clinic with a complaint of side-locked headache and facial pain.[2] Strictly unilateral headaches accounted for 19.2% of total headaches.[2] Patients who present with secondary headaches and cranial neuralgias are more prevalent as age increases.[2] Classical TN and persistent idiopathic facial pain (PIFP) were the most common painful cranial neuropathies.[2]

DIAGNOSTIC CRITERIA

The ICHD is a detailed hierarchical classification of all headache-related disorders and facial pain published by the International Headache Society. The ICHD third β edition (ICHD 3-β) helps to further clarify the terminology used to classify these challenging neuropathic pain syndromes. This schematic classification is divided into three parts containing 14 sections. The first part identifies the primary headache disorders, including the TACs. The second part describes headaches attributed to an underlying (secondary) condition. The third part characterizes painful cranial neuropathies, other facial pains, and other headaches. Section 13 in the ICHD 3-β is further subdivided into other painful cranial neuropathies.

During the development of proper diagnostic criteria, several debates on terminology were created. The ICHD 3-β adds that "trigeminal and glossopharyngeal neuralgias present a problem of terminology. When pain is found to result from compression of the nerve by a vascular loop at operation, the neuralgia should strictly be regarded as secondary. Since many patients do not come to operation, it remains uncertain as to whether they have primary or secondary neuralgias. For this reason, the term classical (see Box 21.1) rather than primary has been applied to those patients with a typical history even though a vascular source of compression may be discovered during its course. The term secondary can then be reserved for those patients in whom a neuroma or similar lesion is demonstrated."[1] The ICHD 3-β no longer lists secondary or symptomatic TN as separate diagnostic categories.[10]

Several grading systems are available, which makes it difficult to classify patients with TN in practice or research. It also hampers the design of clinical guidelines. The International Association for the Study of Pain (IASP)[11] defines TN as "sudden, usually unilateral, severe, brief, stabbing, recurrent episodes of pain in the distribution of one or more branches of the trigeminal nerve."[12] Treede et al. suggested that the following definition of neuropathic pain be revised as "pain arising as a direct consequence of a lesion or disease affecting the somatosensory system."[13,14] Cruccu et al. stated that "formally classifying trigeminal neuralgia as neuropathic pain based on the grading system of the IASP is complicated by the requirement of objective signs confirming an underlying lesion or disease of the somatosensory system."[10] Cruccu et al. reported that with endorsements from the Neuropathic Pain Special Interest Group of the IASP and the Scientific Panel of Pain of the European Academy of Neurology, a new diagnostic grading system for TN was proposed, which is in alignment with diagnostic certainty and was first introduced for neuropathic pain (see Fig. 21.1).[10] The remainder of this chapter utilizes the ICHD 3-β diagnostic criteria for discussion.

NEUROANATOMIC BASIS AND PATHOGENESIS

Sensory axons at the distal aspect of the Gasserian ganglion form the three major divisions (V_1, V_2, and V_3).

BOX 21.1
Trigeminal Neuralgia Criteria From the ICHD 3-β—Part 1

13.1.1 Classical trigeminal neuralgia
Previously used term:
   Tic douloureux
Description:
   Trigeminal neuralgia developing without apparent cause other than neurovascular compression
Diagnostic criteria:
A. At least three attacks of unilateral facial pain fulfilling criteria B and C
B. Occurring in one or more divisions of the trigeminal nerve, with no radiation beyond the trigeminal distribution
C. Pain has at least three of the following four characteristics:
   1. recurring in paroxysmal attacks lasting from a fraction of a second to 2 min
   2. severe intensity
   3. electric shock–like, shooting, stabbing, or sharp in quality
   4. precipitated by innocuous stimuli to the affected side of the face[10]
D. No clinically evident neurologic deficit[1]
E. Not better accounted for by another ICHD-3 diagnosis.
Notes:
1. Some attacks may be, or appear to be, spontaneous, but there must be at least three that are precipitated in this way to meet this criterion.
2. Hypoesthesia or hypoalgesia in the affected trigeminal region always indicates axonal damage. When either is present, there is trigeminal neuropathy and extensive diagnostic workup is necessary to exclude symptomatic cases. There are some patients with hyperalgesia in the painful region, which should not necessarily lead to a diagnosis of trigeminal neuropathy because it may reflect the patient's increased attention to the painful side.

ICHD, International Classification of Headache Disorders.
© International Headache Society 2013; with permission.

Motor axons travel in the mandibular division (V_3). A single neurite, consisting of cell bodies from the trigeminal ganglion, bifurcates and then projects out into the periphery and into the medullary dorsal horn, ultimately forming the major relay center for head and facial pain called the trigeminal nucleus caudalis.[15] The descending root, or spinal tract, extends down through the pons, the medulla, and the upper cervical spinal cord as far down as C2–C4.[15,16]

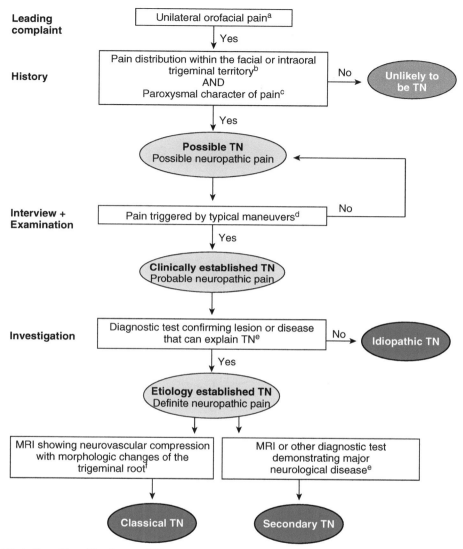

FIG. 21.1 **New Classification and Diagnostic Grading System for Trigeminal Neuralgia (TN).** (From Cruccu G, Finnerup NB, Jensen TS, et al. Trigeminal neuralgia: new classification and diagnostic grading for practice and research. *Neurology.* 2016;87(2):220–228; with permission.)

The nerve fiber peptidergic content plays an integral role in the modulation of pain transmission in the trigeminovascular system.[15] Calcitonin-gene-related peptide, substance P, and neurokinin A are found in meningeal sensory fibers.[15] Sympathetic fibers (containing neuropeptide Y) arise from the ipsilateral superior cervical ganglion, whereas parasympathetic fibers (containing vasoactive intestinal polypeptide) arise from the sphenopalatine and otic ganglia.[15] Vascular

loops can compress sensory roots, thus causing TN.[16] Mechanical, thermal, or chemical stimuli activate sensory fibers and can create central sensitization of meningeal nociceptors (Fig. 21.2).

The classic studies of Ray and Wolff[15] demonstrated that "the brain itself is largely insensitive to pain, but the dura mater, the intracranial segments of the trigeminal, vagus, and glossopharyngeal nerves, and the proximal portions of the large intracranial vessels including

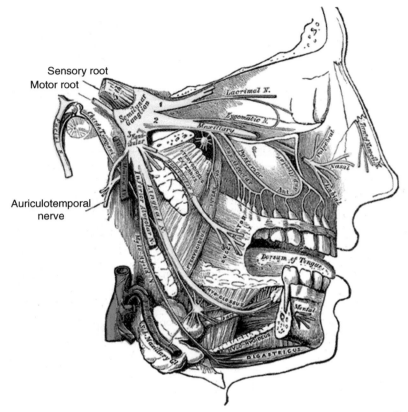

FIG. 21.2 **Anatomy of the Trigeminal Nerve.** (From Gray H. *Anatomy of the Human Body*. Philadelphia: Lea & Febiger; 1918; Bartleby.com, 2000. www.bartleby.com/107/; with permission.)

the basilar, vertebral, and carotid branches, are pain-sensitive."[15] The dura mater consists of a large plexus of unmyelinated fibers, arising from the ophthalmic division of the trigeminal nerve and the upper cervical dorsal roots.[15] Sympathetic and parasympathetic sensory nerve fibers innervate the dura.

There are several hypotheses to describe the relationship of vascular compression and TN.[6,9] Classical TN usually occurs when there is vascular compression of the trigeminal nerve in the cerebellopontine angle. This theoretical model is still not well defined but is accepted in the literature.[5,7] Neuroimaging may reveal a vascular anomaly (most commonly the superior cerebellar artery) or a cerebellopontine angle mass; then a diagnosis of secondary TN is given.[17]

Some believe TN occurs as a result of focal demyelination of the nerve root entry zone due to pulsatile indentation at the impingement site, which often is a result of a tortuous vascular loop (most often the

superior cerebellar artery).[7] The establishment of central sensitization is a plausible mechanism to explain nociception and chronic pain. Other theories suggest a neurobiological mechanism with an underlying predisposing genetic basis.[15]

CLINICAL APPROACH TO DIAGNOSIS

It is important to obtain a detailed clinical history and identify the location of pain—side-locked unilateral, bilateral, side-switching unilateral (before, during, or after attacks), or unilateral spreading to become bilateral. The pain described needs to be localized as central or peripherally based. The duration of the pain attack needs to be well characterized, lasting a fraction of second to minutes to hours or days. The frequency of attacks in TN can be as few as 1 to over 50 per day.[1,10] An attack is an individual episode of pain, whereas remission is defined as a pain-free period in between attacks, with episodes occurring 1–50 times per day.[1,10] One needs to establish if the pain attack consists of headache, facial pain, or both. The quality of the pain as well as associated symptoms, premonitory symptoms (warning signs), radiation pattern, and any medications taken need to be elicited from the patient. Often, pain questionnaires are utilized to obtain more detailed information.

In addition to routine review of past medical history, a thorough neurologic history should include history of orofacial, head, or neck trauma; comorbid psychiatric disorders; quality of sleep; family or personal history of migraine, stroke, multiple sclerosis, or other neurodegenerative disorders; history of skin disorder of the face or scalp; dental disorder or dental procedures; and history of infection or inflammatory disorder of the head and neck. A functional history must be taken.

Physical examination includes inspection of the skin (rash, vesicles etc.) and assessment of range of motion of the cervical spine and temporomandibular joint. Neurologic examination is often normal, but it is important to carefully test cranial nerves, sensation (sometimes a subtle sensory deficit is present, other times allodynia is present), temperature sense, and trigeminal reflexes.

Neuroimaging is utilized to rule out red flags. Gadolinium-enhanced magnetic resonance imaging (MRI) of the brain and fine cuts through the trigeminal nerves should be ordered for patients with acute or newly diagnosed TN. Conventional brain MRI may not always detect symptomatic neurovascular contact.[6] High-resolution "constructive interference in steady state" (CISS) coronal imaging may better visualize neurovascular compression (see Fig. 21.3).[7] The CISS protocol is commonly ordered for detecting intracranial lesions to assist with the diagnosis of TN.[7] A multidisciplinary evidence-based review of the published literature by the American Academy of Neurology and the European Federation of Neurological Societies (EFNS) concluded that standard MRI is currently too insensitive for detecting neurovascular compression of the trigeminal nerve to recommend routine use.[9,12]

Differential Diagnosis for Trigeminal Neuralgia and Other Cranial Neuralgias

A thorough differential diagnosis for TN and other cranial neuralgias with corresponding cranial nerve involvement is depicted in Table 21.1.

The differential diagnosis for chronic orofacial pain includes temporomandibular joint disorders, atypical odontalgias, oral dysesthesias, thalamic pain syndrome, compression of the vagus nerve, or referred pain

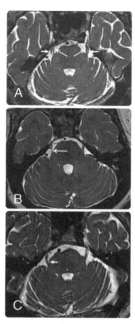

FIG. 21.3 Neurovascular Compression of the Trigeminal Root. Three-dimensional constructive interference in steady-state MRI shows axial sections at the level of trigeminal nerve root entry into the pons. **(A)** Bilateral neurovascular contact without morphologic changes of the root in a patient with left trigeminal neuralgia (TN). Nerve (*long arrows*) and blood vessel (*short arrows*) appear hypointense surrounded by hyperintense cerebrospinal fluid. Contact is seen at the root entry zone as well as mid-cisternal segment. **(B and C)** Morphologic changes exceeding mere neurovascular contact of the trigeminal nerve root are compatible with the diagnosis of classical TN. **(B)** Root atrophy in a patient with right TN. **(C)** Indentation and dislocation of the root in a patient with right TN (*short arrow*). (From Cruccu G, Finnerup NB, Jensen TS, et al. Trigeminal neuralgia: new classification and diagnostic grading for practice and research. *Neurology*. 2016;87(2):220–228; with permission.)

from a distant metastatic site such as in lung cancer.[14] Posterior fossa tumors and extracranial masses along the course of the trigeminal nerve are commonly associated with TN. Typical pain characteristics of TN are associated with vestibular or trigeminal schwannomas, meningiomas, invasive squamous cell carcinoma of the face, Chiari malformation, saccular aneurysm or arteriovenous malformation compressing the trigeminal nerve root, epidermoid cysts, or other skull base tumor.[7,9] Bilateral TN pain in younger patients may indicate a possible diagnosis of multiple sclerosis.[7] Demyelination plaques, intrinsic brain lesions in the

TABLE 21.1
Differential Diagnosis for Cranial Neuralgias

Cranial Neuralgia	Associated Cranial Nerve Involved
Optic neuritis	Optic nerve (CN II)
Recurrent painful ophthalmoplegic neuropathy	Oculomotor (CN III)
Headache attributed to ischemic ocular motor nerve palsy	Oculomotor (CN III), trochlear (CN IV), abducens nerve (CN VI)
Tolosa-Hunt syndrome	Oculomotor (CN III), trochlear (CN IV), abducens nerve (CN VI)
Trigeminal neuralgia	Trigeminal nerve (CN V)
Classical trigeminal neuralgia, purely paroxysmal	
Classical trigeminal neuralgia with concomitant persistent facial pain	
Painful trigeminal neuropathy	Trigeminal nerve (CN V)
Attributed to acute herpes zoster	
Postherpetic trigeminal neuropathy	
Painful posttraumatic trigeminal neuropathy	
Attributed to multiple sclerosis plaque	
Attributed to space-occupying lesion	
Attributed to other disorder	
Paratrigeminal oculosympathetic (Raeder's) syndrome	Trigeminal nerve (CN V)
Burning mouth syndrome	Trigeminal nerve (CN V)
Trigeminal autonomic cephalalgias	Trigeminal nerve (CN V)
Nervus intermedius neuralgia	Facial nerve (CN VII)
Classical nervus intermedius neuralgia	Complex overlapping innervation of external ear[a]
Attributed to herpes zoster (Ramsay Hunt syndrome)	Facial nerve (CNVII)
Persistent idiopathic facial pain	Poorly localized[b]
Glossopharyngeal neuralgia	Glossopharyngeal nerve (CN IX)
Occipital neuralgia	Greater, lesser, and/or third occipital nerves
Central neuropathic pain	Central nervous system
Attributed to multiple sclerosis	
Central poststroke pain	

[a]Deriving from the trigeminal (auriculotemporal nerve), facial, glossopharyngeal, vagus, and second cervical nerve.
[b]Not following the distribution of a peripheral nerve.
Adapted from Headache Classification Committee of the International Headache Society. The International Classification of Headache Disorders, 3rd edition (beta version). *Cephalalgia*. 2013;33(9):629–808; with permission.

thalamus, or lacunar infarcts along trigeminal brainstem pathways should be considered.[9] Patients with trigeminal neuropathic pain caused by trigeminal sensory neuropathy may also have an underlying connective tissue disorder or diabetic neuropathy.[6]

According to the ICHD-3 β, it is clinically complex to differentiate between TN and the TACs, particularly the short-lasting unilateral neuralgiform headache attacks. Moreover, lesions in the posterior fossa may mimic these disorders.[1]

MANAGEMENT OF THE TRIGEMINAL NEURALGIAS

Clinically, when a patient presents with facial pain, first try oral antiepileptics. If this is unsuccessful or beyond one's scope of clinical judgment, next steps include referral and collaboration with a multidisciplinary team (including physiatrists, neurologists, pain specialists, dentists, oromaxillofacial surgeons, neuroradiologists, and neurosurgeons),[14,17] which has been shown to improve tolerability, safety, efficacy, and overall outcomes in the management of TN.[8] Individualizing the type of therapy with each patient addresses one's goals, current and predicted level of functioning, and additional medical or psychological comorbidities before proceeding with a surgical intervention. The EFNS examined randomized controlled trials and later produced guidelines in 2010 for the pharmacologic treatment of neuropathic pain.[17]

Oral Antiepileptics

The first-line pharmacologic therapy includes oral antiepileptics. The initial response rate is about 70%, whereas the remaining 30% have transient improvement.[5] Carbamazepine is the drug of choice for TN (level A evidence).[7] Low dosing, 100 mg two to three times daily, is usually effective as an initial starting point. There is level B evidence for oxcarbazepine, where the starting dose is 300 mg twice daily, with titration to 600–1200 mg twice daily as tolerated. Level C evidence for baclofen shows a starting dose of 5 mg three times daily, titrating to 10–20 mg three times daily as tolerated.[7] Level C evidence includes lamotrigine, with a starting dose of 25 mg every other day and titration to a typical dose of 50–200 mg twice daily.[7] Phenytoin was the first breakthrough found in the 1940s when treating TN.[6] To date, there is level C evidence for the use of phenytoin. The starting dose is 50 mg three times daily, with titration to 300–400 mg at bedtime in the extended-release form.[7] Ensure monitoring for gingival hyperplasia in the long-term use of phenytoin. Acute treatment of TN includes gabapentin 100–900 mg three times daily.[7] In some patients, antiepileptics are not well tolerated. Unlike in migraine where a preventive trial may last up to 6 months, a therapeutic benefit should be noted within days when treating TN.[6,7,15] One can titrate the dose or move on quickly to another agent if the patient is unable to tolerate therapeutic dosing.

In patients with multiple sclerosis with TN or those with baseline ataxia, dizziness, drowsiness, nystagmus, or blurry vision, closer monitoring is required. Adverse events to be aware of when using antiepileptics include atrioventricular block, hepatotoxicity, bone marrow suppression (aplastic anemia or agranulocytosis), Stevens-Johnson syndrome, toxic epidermal necrolysis, electrolyte abnormalities (hyponatremia, hypocalcemia), pancreatitis, nephrotoxicity, and suicidal thoughts.[6,7]

OnabotulinumtoxinA

OnabotulinumtoxinA is a neurotoxin derived from *Clostridium botulinum*. The mechanism involves inhibition of the release of acetylcholine at the neuromuscular junctions, resulting in reduced muscle contraction, mitigation of peripheral sensitization, and, secondarily, suppression of central sensitization. The US Food and Drug Administration approved the use of onabotulinumtoxinA for the prevention of chronic migraine. Micheli and colleagues[8] successfully used onabotulinumtoxinA to relieve pain and twitching in a patient with TN-related hemifacial spasm. A systematic review and meta-analysis explored the evidence in several published randomized controlled trials (RCTs) regarding the safety and efficacy of using onabotulinumtoxinA for the treatment of TN. The outcome measures reported a favorable proportion of respondents (defined as patients with >50% reduction in the mean pain score from baseline to end point), reduction in the mean paroxysm frequency per day, which was significantly lower in the onabotulinumtoxinA group than in the placebo group, and a lower mean visual analog scale score at the end of follow-up. Adverse events and complications of onabotulinumtoxinA treatment included facial asymmetry, which resolved after 5–7 weeks, and edema/hematoma at injection site, which recovered in 5–6 days.[8] There was variation between studies on the amount of onabotulinumtoxinA injected, which ranged from a minimum of 25 units to a maximum of 100 units.[8] Inconclusive data were presented for how long the therapeutic effect of onabotulinumtoxinA lasts, whereas in chronic migraine it has been shown that the duration of treatment is 3 months. The limitation of the systematic review reported that there are currently a small number of trials that investigate the safety and efficacy of using onabotulinumtoxinA for the treatment of TN. Further double-blinded RCTs are needed to optimize the outcomes, the duration of treatment, and the route of administration.

Surgical Interventions

Surgical interventions are divided into ablative (destructive) and nonablative (nondestructive) procedures.[18,19]

Microvascular decompression (MVD), peripheral nerve stimulation, and motor cortex stimulation are nondestructive procedures. Stereotactic radiosurgery, destructive lesioning (chemical, thermal, or mechanical destruction of the trigeminal nerve), and nucleus caudalis dorsal root entry zone lesioning are considered to be destructive procedures.

In a systematic review and meta-analysis, surgical complications were reviewed.[18] MVD is an open-surgical approach that can be performed in both younger patients and the elderly.[6,18] Death, stroke, and thromboembolism were more likely to occur in the elderly population; the analysis could not conclude whether these were independent associations but commented that these potential complications should be reviewed as risks for this type of surgery. No differences between the age cohorts were found for complications such as cerebellar hematoma, cranial nerve deficit, diplopia, facial numbness, hearing loss, vertigo, cerebrospinal fluid leak, and meningitis.[6,18] Compared with rhizotomy procedures, facial sensation can be preserved with MVD.[6] In a systematic review, the best surgical result in the short term (less than 4 years) is seen with MVD, followed by radiofrequency lesioning.[9] After MVD the recurrence rate is about 10% over 10–20 years, in comparison with palliative destructive procedures, which have a recurrence rate of about 50% after 3–5 years.[9]

Stereotactic Gamma Knife radiosurgery targets the trigeminal nerve root entry zone with a concentrated dose of ionizing radiation at the level of the pons.[7,9] There are higher reports of facial paresthesia and dysesthesia with this technique.[7] Risk-benefit ratios and patient satisfaction are significantly higher with this least invasive intracranial treatment for TN.[6]

Partial sensory rhizotomy and percutaneous radiofrequency thermocoagulation or glycerol rhizotomies are less invasive Gasserian ganglion procedures, with pain relief noted to be 91%–99% and recurrence rates from 10% to 25%.[6,9] Balloon compression mechanically presses the trigeminal nerve against the surrounding bone and dural reflections.[9]

Nucleus caudalis dorsal root entry zone lesioning (NC DREZ) of second-order neurons is a more invasive but very effective procedure.[19] A greater than 50% pain reduction and 75% improvement in quality of life were reported by Chivukula and colleagues at 8-year follow-up.[19] NC DREZ is effective for postherpetic neuralgia, chronic cluster headache, vagal or glossopharyngeal neuralgias, and intractable pain syndromes due to secondary causes (cancer, surgery, or trauma).[19]

Motor cortex stimulation, of third-order neurons, is reserved for medically intractable trigeminal deafferentation pain (central facial pain) and for patients who do not respond to NC DREZ.[7,19] This procedure involves an open craniotomy with implantation of electrodes over the motor cortex, ultimately connected to a subcutaneously placed stimulator.[7]

Neuromodulation

Neuromodulation is a promising therapeutic strategy for the treatment of headache and neuropathic facial pain disorders. More controlled studies have been emerging, although the evidence base is still highly variable.[15] Peripheral nerve neurostimulation includes occipital nerve stimulation (ONS), single-pulse transcranial magnetic stimulation, vagus nerve stimulation (which is both implanted and portable transcutaneous), transcutaneous supraorbital neurostimulation, and sphenopalatine ganglion neurostimulation.[15] Central neurostimulation includes hypothalamus deep brain stimulation.[15] Neurostimulation was studied in patients with TACs. Nine patients with medically intractable short lasting unilateral neuralgiform headache with conjunctival injection and tearing (SUNCT) and three patients with short lasting unilateral neuralgiform headache attack with cranial autonomic symptoms (SUNA) achieved greater than 50% improvement with ONS.[15] When comparing invasive procedures and evaluating potential morbidity (adverse events, lead migration, battery failure) of treatment for patients with intractable pain, neurostimulation should be considered a viable option.[15] The evidence available shows that peripheral and central neurostimulation may be effective for both preventive and acute management of intractable head and facial pain disorders.

Nonpharmacologic Therapies

Chronic pain that is poorly localized, deep, or refractory to treatment can respond to an integrative approach.[14] Poor prognosis is seen with patients who have PIFP.[14] This is often an opportunity to consult an integrative medicine specialist.

Empowering the patient to commit to making healthy lifestyle changes promotes a wellness-based therapy plan. Taking extra time to listen and educate your patient during an office-based encounter allows formation of a deeper relationship to understand expectations and create a greater understanding of your patient's pain experience.

Prescribed therapeutic exercise, osteopathic manipulative therapy, and physical therapy (to improve mobility and range of motion of the temporomandibular joint, cervical spine, and scapulothoracic mechanism) are physical treatment modalities. Cognitive behavioral therapy, assisted relaxation therapy, hypnotherapy, biofeedback, and mindfulness-based stress reduction therapy all address the psychological, emotional, and the psychosocial environment impacts the overall pain experience. Supportive social networks, chronic pain groups, and educational seminars are additional ways in which patients can connect with their peers who also have chronic painful neuralgias and cephalalgias. Diet modification and the use of supplements can reduce inflammation seen in chronic pain states.[14] Additional integrative therapies suggested in a 2010 evidenced-based review include[14] acupuncture, Ayurvedic medicine, naturopathic and homeopathic medicine, and energy therapies (Reiki, therapeutic touch, magnets, and Qi Gong). Addressing spirituality may also help to understand the complexity of the whole-person.

When one encounters a patient who appears to fit the definition of TN (see Box 21.2) but one is not entirely convinced, the differential for Tic versus TAC should be recalled. For example, here is a 40-year-old man with a history of hypertension who presented with a 6 months' history of continuous right facial pain associated with severe electric, paroxysmal shocks in the right eye, forehead, and ear. The initial presentation of his pain was mostly in the morning, with no positional component. His primary care physician adjusted blood pressure medications without improvement of pain. There was progression of attack frequency: every 2 min, lasting 15 s, and development of right-sided autonomic symptoms. Dental and ophthalmologic evaluations were normal. MRI of the brain was only positive for microvascular ischemic changes related to hypertension. The patient failed trials of indomethacin, carbamazepine, lamotrigine, gabapentin, verapamil, topiramate, and memantine, as well as physical therapy. He had an elective admission for intravenous lidocaine, which was effective in controlling his pain, and he was discharged home with a prescription for oral mexiletine. After 6 months of controlled pain, attacks recurred and a second admission was required. During the last admission, an MRI/MRA of the brain CISS sequence revealed close proximity of the right superior cerebellar artery to the medial root entry zone of the right trigeminal nerve. MVD was performed without complications and the patient presented complete resolution of headaches and facial pain.

Some rare cases of *hemicrania continua-tic* have responded to both carbamazepine and indomethacin.[20] TN is sometimes referred to as *cluster-tic* syndrome, which occurs when there is the rare co-occurrence of cluster headache and TN attacks.[21] The proposed mechanism commonly shares the theory of venous compression of the trigeminal nerve.[1,21] Short-lasting unilateral neuralgiform headache attacks are usually triggered without a refractory period.[1] In contrast, patients with TN usually have a refractory period after each attack.

BOX 21.2
Trigeminal Neuralgia Criteria From the ICHD 3-β — Part 2

Comments:
The term classical (rather than primary) trigeminal neuralgia is used because, according to current evidence, 13.1.1 Classical trigeminal neuralgia is caused by neurovascular compression, most frequently by the superior cerebellar artery. Imaging (preferably MRI) should be done to exclude secondary causes and, in the majority of patients, to demonstrate neurovascular compression of the trigeminal nerve.

Many patients with 13.1.1 Classical trigeminal neuralgia have a memorable onset of pain.

13.1.1 Classical trigeminal neuralgia usually appears in the second or third divisions. The pain never crosses to the opposite side, but it may rarely occur bilaterally. Following a painful paroxysm there is usually a refractory period during which pain cannot be triggered. When very severe, the pain often evokes contraction of the muscle of the face on the affected side (tic douloureux). Mild autonomic symptoms such as lacrimation and/or redness of the eye may be present.

The duration of pain attacks can change over time and become more prolonged as well as severe. They can result in psychosocial dysfunction, significantly impairing the quality of life and often leading to weight loss.

13.1.1 Classical trigeminal neuralgia may be preceded by a period of atypical continuous pain termed pretrigeminal neuralgia in the literature.

13.1.1.1 Classical trigeminal neuralgia, purely paroxysmal is usually responsive, at least initially, to pharmacotherapy (especially carbamazepine or oxcarbazepine).

13.1.1.2 Classical trigeminal neuralgia with concomitant persistent facial pain has been referred to as atypical trigeminal neuralgia or, recently, as trigeminal neuralgia type 2. Between paroxysms most patients are asymptomatic. In the subform 13.1.1.2 Classical trigeminal neuralgia with concomitant persistent facial pain, there is prolonged background pain in the affected area.

Central sensitization may account for the persistent facial pain. Neurovascular compression on MRI is less likely to be demonstrated. 13.1.1.2 Classical trigeminal neuralgia with concomitant persistent facial pain responds poorly to conservative treatment and to neurosurgical interventions. It is less likely to be triggered by innocuous stimuli.

ICHD, International Classification of Headache Disorders.
© International Headache Society 2013; with permission.

CONCLUSION

Headache and orofacial pain are often challenging to accurately diagnose and treat. Pharmacologic, medical, surgical, and nonpharmacologic therapies have evolved over time to help alleviate the pain that patients with Tics and TACs experience. A person's physical identity and ability to communicate verbally and nonverbally through facial expression is important. Pain affects physical, cognitive, and psychosocial functioning. Diagnostic precision is needed in both clinical practice and in research to improve outcomes of treatment and quality of life.

In the *New England Journal of Medicine*, Dr. Eric Cassel wrote a significant article in 1982 that later became the book of the same title, *"The Nature of Suffering and the Goals of Medicine."* He profoundly wrote, "Suffering is experienced by persons, not merely by bodies, and has its source in challenges that threaten the intactness of the person as a complex social and psychological entity. Suffering can include physical pain but is by no means limited to it. The relief of suffering and the cure of disease must be seen as twin obligations of a medical profession that is truly dedicated to the care of the sick. Physicians' failure to understand the nature of suffering can result in medical intervention that (though technically adequate) not only fails to relieve suffering but becomes a source of suffering itself."[14]

REFERENCES

1. Headache Classification Committee of the International Headache S. The international classification of headache disorders, 3rd edition (beta version). *Cephalalgia.* 2013;33(9):629–808.
2. Prakash S, Rathore C, Makwana P, Dave A. A cross-sectional clinic-based study in patients with side-locked unilateral headache and facial pain. *Headache.* 2016;56(7):1183–1193.
3. VanderPluym J, Richer L. Tic versus TAC: differentiating the neuralgias (trigeminal neuralgia) from the cephalalgias (SUNCT and SUNA). *Curr Pain Headache Rep.* 2015;19(2):473.
4. Charleston L. Do trigeminal autonomic cephalalgias represent primary diagnoses or points on a continuum? *Curr Pain Headache Rep.* 2015;19(6):22.
5. Sivakanthan S, Van Gompel JJ, Alikhani P, van Loveren H, Chen R, Agazzi S. Surgical management of trigeminal neuralgia: use and cost-effectiveness from an analysis of the Medicare Claims Database. *Neurosurgery.* 2014;75(3):220–226. Discussion 225–226.
6. Cheshire WP. Trigeminal neuralgia: for one nerve a multitude of treatments. *Expert Rev Neurother.* 2007;7(11):1565–1579.
7. Cheshire Jr WP. Cranial neuralgias. *Continuum (Minneap Minn).* 2015;21(4 Headache):1072–1085.
8. Morra ME, Elgebaly A, Elmaraezy A, et al. Therapeutic efficacy and safety of botulinum toxin A therapy in trigeminal neuralgia: a systematic review and meta-analysis of randomized controlled trials. *J Headache Pain.* 2016;17(1):63.
9. Zakrzewska JM, Linskey ME. Trigeminal neuralgia. *BMJ.* 2014;348:g474.
10. Cruccu G, Finnerup NB, Jensen TS, et al. Trigeminal neuralgia: new classification and diagnostic grading for practice and research. *Neurology.* 2016;87(2):220–228.
11. International Association for the Study of Pain: Taxonomy. URL: http://www.iasp-pain.org; https://creativecommons.org/licenses/by-sa/3.0/.
12. Gronseth G, Cruccu G, Alksne J, et al. Practice parameter: the diagnostic evaluation and treatment of trigeminal neuralgia (an evidence-based review): report of the Quality Standards Subcommittee of the American Academy of Neurology and the European Federation of Neurological Societies. *Neurology.* 2008;71(15):1183–1190.
13. Treede R-D, Jensen TS, Campbell JN, et al. Neuropathic pain: redefinition and a grading system for clinical and research purposes. *Neurology.* 2008;70(18):1630–1635.
14. Nguyen CT, Wang MB. Complementary and integrative treatments: atypical facial pain. *Otolaryngol Clin N Am.* 2013;46(3):367–382.
15. Silberstein S, Dodick D. *Migraine* Contemporary Neurology Series. 3rd ed. Oxford University Press; 2016:86–88. 243–257.
16. Campbell W. *DeJong's The Neurologic Examination.* 7th ed. Philadelphia: Wolters Kluwer, Lippincott Williams and Wilkins; 2013:227–245.
17. Attal N, Cruccu G, Baron R, et al. EFNS guidelines on the pharmacological treatment of neuropathic pain: 2010 revision. *Eur J Neurol.* 2010;17(9):e1113–e1188.
18. Phan K, Rao PJ, Dexter M. Microvascular decompression for elderly patients with trigeminal neuralgia. *J Clin Neurosci.* 2016;29:7–14.
19. Rahimpour S, Lad SP. Surgical options for atypical facial pain syndromes. *Neurosurg Clin N Am.* 2016;27(3):365–370.
20. Prakash S, Rathore C. Two cases of hemicrania continua-trigeminal neuralgia syndrome: expanding the spectrum of trigeminal autonomic cephalalgia-tic (TAC-TIC) syndrome. *Headache.* 2016.
21. de Coo I, van Dijk JM, Metzemaekers JD, Haan J. A case report about cluster-tic syndrome due to venous compression of the trigeminal nerve. *Headache.* 2016.

FURTHER READING

1. Voiticovschi-Iosob C, Allena M, De Cillis I, Nappi G, Sjaastad O, Antonaci F. Diagnostic and therapeutic errors in cluster headache: a hospital-based study. *J Headache Pain.* 2014;15:56.
2. Stiles A, Silberstein S. Trigeminal neuralgias and other cranial neuralgias. In: Greeenamyre JT, ed. *MedLink Neurology.* San Diego: MedLink Corporation. Available at: www.medlink.com.
3. Spare N, Larsen E. Headache associated with cervical spine dysfunction. In: Greeenamyre JT, ed. *MedLink Neurology.* San Diego: MedLink Corporation. Available at: www.medlink.com.

CHAPTER 22

Thoracic Outlet Syndrome

RENAE FISHER, MD • JEREMY SIMON, MD

INTRODUCTION

Thoracic outlet syndrome (TOS) has all the components of a challenging disease entity. It is a syndrome that can disable young people, yet there is no gold standard for diagnosis or management. Some consider it overdiagnosed, whereas others consider it underdiagnosed. As a result, there is a wide range in prevalence estimates that vary from 0.03% to 8% of the population.[1] The majority of these patients are women aged 30–50 years.[2] Without a gold standard test, the practitioner must rely heavily on history for diagnosis. Knowledge of the subtypes of TOS and the anatomy surrounding the brachial plexus (Fig. 22.1) are valuable tools in better understanding this disease.

TOS is an intentionally broad term. It was named by Peet in 1956 to unite a group of disorders that resulted from compression of the brachial plexus at different sites (Fig. 22.2).[3] Later Wilbourn subdivided TOS, not as before by anatomic compression site, but by the nerve or vessel compressed. He named the subtypes: arterial TOS (aTOS), venous TOS (vTOS), true neurologic TOS, and disputed neurologic TOS.[4] When it comes to management, however, both the vessel and the site of compression must be considered.

The "thoracic outlet" is a neurovascular canal that tunnels over and under muscular and bony structures from the neck to the axilla (Fig. 22.3). The most common sites of compression or entrapment are the interscalene triangle, the costoclavicular space, and the subpectoral triangle.[5,6] The interscalene triangle is formed by the anterior scalene (anterior), middle scalene (posterior), and medial first rib (inferior). The costoclavicular space is formed by the clavicle (anterior) and first rib (posterior). The subpectoral triangle is formed by the coracoid process (superior), pectoralis minor (anterior), and ribs 2–4 (posterior).[7] Anatomic anomalies, such as fibrous bands and the pre- or postfixed brachial plexus, are being increasingly recognized as potential predisposing factors.[5,8] Similarly, cervical ribs may predispose a patient to TOS.

Pathology at these sites can cause either vascular or neurologic TOS, and each subtype presents differently. About 95% of all cases are neurologic TOS, and up to 99% of these cases are the disputed neurologic subtype.[9] In the 1% of neurologic cases that are called "true," there is a bony abnormality such as a cervical rib found or abnormalities on electrodiagnostic studies. The most common mechanism of injury resulting in TOS is neck hyperextension injuries followed by work-related repetitive strain.[10]

Solid malignancies, especially Pancoast tumors in the lung apex, can present similarly. It is also important to consider circulatory conditions such as vasculitis, acute coronary syndrome, and vasospastic disorders. Complex regional pain syndrome and fibromyalgia must also be considered.[11]

NEUROGENIC THORACIC OUTLET SYNDROME
History

Neurogenic TOS (nTOS) is the most common and reported as about 90% of all TOS cases.[12] As previously mentioned, patients may present with symptoms similar to other commonly seen musculoskeletal disorders. The symptoms may be intermittent and positional or involve the upper (upper TOS) or lower trunk.[13] Because the lower trunk of the brachial plexus is typically involved, complaints often involve numbness and tingling in the fourth and fifth digits of the affected side or sides. Reports of "upper TOS" describe compression of the superior plexus in the scalenes.[13] When the upper trunk is affected, patients report neck, shoulder, and facial pain with paresthesias that follow the fifth and sixth cervical nerve roots and upper trunk.[14] Pain and numbness may be exacerbated with overhead activity and having the arm outstretched. The symptoms of nTOS often include the feeling of arm heaviness and fatigability and also depend on the portion of the brachial plexus compressed. Symptoms are exacerbated by overhead activity or prolonged activity without

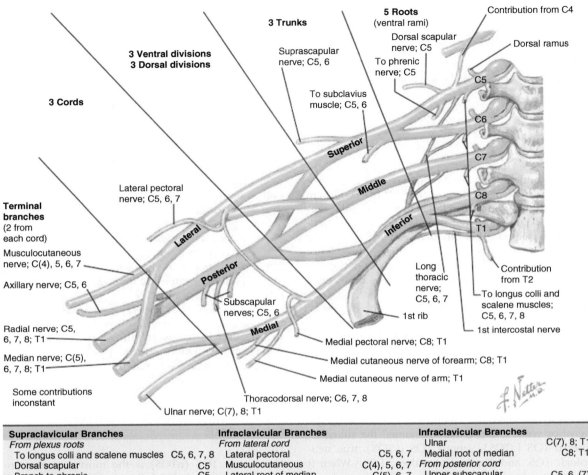

FIG. 22.1 Brachial plexus: schema. (Netter illustration from www.netterimages.com © Elsevier Inc. All rights reserved. Ronthal M. Arm and neck pain. In: *Bradley's Neurology in Clinical Practice*. vol. 31, 324–331.e1 Copyright © 2016, Elsevier Inc. All rights reserved.)

Supraclavicular Branches		Infraclavicular Branches		Infraclavicular Branches	
From plexus roots		*From lateral cord*		Ulnar	C(7), 8; T1
To longus colli and scalene muscles	C5, 6, 7, 8	Lateral pectoral	C5, 6, 7	Medial root of median	C8; T1
Dorsal scapular	C5	Musculocutaneous	C(4), 5, 6, 7	*From posterior cord*	
Branch to phrenic	C5	Lateral root of median	C(5), 6, 7	Upper subscapular	C5, 6, (7)
Long thoracic	C5, 6, 7	*From medial cord*		Lower subscapular	C5, 6
From superior trunk		Medial pectoral	C8; T1	Axillary (circumflex humeral)	C5, 6
Suprascapular	C5, 6	Medial cutaneous nerve of arm	T1	Thoracodorsal	C5, 6
To subclavius muscle	C5, 6	Medial cutaneous nerve of forearm	C8; T1	Radial	C5, 6, 7, 8

arm support.[15] Color changes to the hand are often seen with nTOS from sympathetic fiber activation after nerve compression.[9] In severe cases, muscle weakness and atrophy occurs in the affected nerves' distribution.

The symptoms of nTOS may mimic cervical radiculopathy with neck pain and radiating pain and paresthesias into the shoulder and arm. Numbness in the hand with radiation up the forearm is commonly seen in carpal tunnel syndrome. Ulnar neuropathy at or above the elbow can have a similar distribution of numbness and symptoms in the arm. The so-called double crush syndrome with compression of a cervical nerve root and in the carpal tunnel or cubital tunnel can be mistaken for nTOS.[16]

Physical Examination

Patients may present with altered sensation and/or weakness and wasting of musculature in the affected limb in the distribution of the affected portion of the plexus. There is no gold standard physical examination

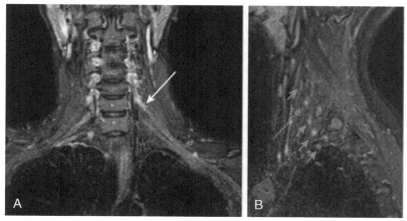

FIG. 22.2 **(A)** In the normal plexus the elements progress in a smooth linear course. **(B)** Nerve-perpendicular views (correlated spatially with the coronal view using radiology software such as eFilm) can be used to sequentially follow nerve caliber and image intensity, while identifying specific elements. In **(A)** the *white arrow* points to an orange cross that the software has placed at the C6 spinal nerve when the corresponding nerve cross-section has been selected at the *red arrow* in **(B)**. Cross-sectional views of the C5, C7, C8, and T1 elements are identified with *small green arrows* in **(B)**. (From Filler AG. Brachial plexus nerve entrapments and thoracic outlet syndromes. In: *Youmans and Winn Neurological Surgery*, vol. 250, 2032–2040.e2 Copyright © 2017 by Elsevier, Inc. All rights reserved.)

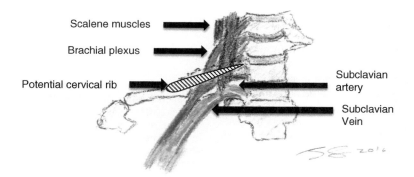

FIG. 22.3 The thoracic outlet.

maneuver for neurogenic TOS.[17,18] Also, the rate of false positives using these maneuvers is high. Patients may have tenderness over the scalene muscles to palpation. Tapping above the clavicle (Tinel sign) may be positive by reproducing the symptoms.

Provocative testing includes the elevated arm stress test ("EAST Maneuver" or Roos test)[19] whereby the patient is instructed to abduct the shoulders and flex the elbows 90 degrees while opening and closing the hands for 3 min. If positive, the patient should have

difficulty as the time progresses in opening and closing the hands or keeping the arms elevated. Rotating the head and placing the ear to the shoulder may cause pain and paresthesias in the opposite upper limb, but this may also be positive in cervical radiculopathy. The modified Upper Limb Tension Test of Elvey[9] (ULTT) involves having the patient abduct both shoulders to 90 degrees without elbow flexion, dorsiflex the wrists, and tilt the head to both sides. If paresthesias or pain occurs in the limb, it is considered positive. Although these tests may be helpful in the diagnosis of TOS, an extremely high rate of false positives may occur. A study from Plewa and Delinger demonstrated a false-positive rate for paresthesias of 15% with the EAST maneuver.[20] A study from Davis et al. showed a false-positive rate of 86.9% for the ULTT.[21]

Diagnostic Criteria and Testing

Imaging and diagnostic support of nTOS is not always clear (Fig. 22.4). Because common conditions such as cervical disc degeneration may be seen on radiography and MRI of the cervical spine, it may be mistaken as the cause of the symptoms. Plain radiographs of the neck may reveal bony anomalies, such as a cervical rib, significantly enlarged C7 transverse process, evidence of a prior fracture/trauma to the clavicle, or calcification of the vasculature in the thoracic outlet, which would point more to vTOS or aTOS (Fig. 22.5). Radiograph views include anteroposterior, lateral, oblique, flexion, and extension to assess for cervical spine pathology that is much more common than TOS.

MRI of the brachial plexus may show inflammatory changes but is often normal.[22] MRI of the cervical spine is often performed to rule out a cervical disc herniation, significant foraminal narrowing, cervical spinal stenosis, or spinal cord compression. The MRI must be interpreted in the clinical context with a careful history and physical examination, as degenerative discs, spondylosis, and disc herniations may occur without clinical symptoms.[23]

Electrodiagnostic testing is often normal in patients with TOS or may show subtle or vague abnormalities. If the lower trunk of the brachial plexus is involved, nerve conduction studies may demonstrate prolonged or absent F-waves in the median and ulnar nerves. In axonopathy, the compound muscle action potentials (CMAPs) may be reduced in the median and ulnar nerves. Classically, the median sensory nerve action potential (SNAP) is preserved as these fibers traverse the upper and middle trunks of the brachial plexus. However, the ulnar SNAP shows a reduction in amplitude as it passes through the lower trunk. The medial antebrachial cutaneous SNAP may be reduced or absent, as well.

Lesions involving the lower plexus are often more sensitive. In a retrospective study of patients with surgically confirmed true nTOS who had electrodiagnostic testing before surgery, Tsao et al. found a reduced median CMAP amplitude in the affected arm with 95% sensitivity.[24]

Differentiating a C8 radiculopathy from nTOS can be challenging but may be aided by electrodiagnostic

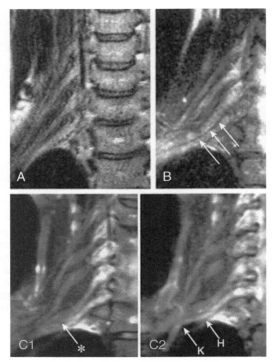

FIG. 22.4 Differentiation of thoracic outlet syndrome (TOS) into categories is often well supported by imaging characteristics. **(A)** In the normal plexus, the cervical spinal nerves and trunks of the brachial plexus follow a straight trajectory with even spacing. **(B)** Scalene syndrome is demonstrated by a gentle deformation of the course of the nerve elements and loss of space between them (*arrows*). In patients with pain only, there is usually no nerve hyperintensity. **(C1)** Distortion of the shape of the C7 element (*asterisk*) associated with a severe TOS case. **(C2)** A more anterior image plane in the same patient showing both a sharp kink (K) in the course of the lower trunk associated with a fibrous band and nerve hyperintensity (H) consistent with lower trunk motor symptoms. (From Filler AG. Applications of MRI and other imaging techniques for studying peripheral nerve and muscle. In: Brown W, Bolton C, Aminoff M, eds. *Neuromuscular Function and Disease: Basic, Clinical, and Electrodiagnostic Aspects*. vol. 2. Philadelphia: WB Saunders; 2002; with permission.)

testing. In C8 or T1 radiculopathies, the ulnar and median SNAPs are maintained. In nTOS, the ulnar SNAP is often reduced.

The needle electromyography (EMG) study may show signs of denervation in the C8-T1 median and ulnar-supplied muscles. This would include the presence of fibrillations and/or positive sharp waves, the presence of polyphasic motor unit potentials (MUPs)

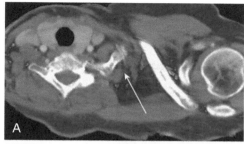

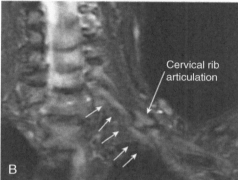

Cervical rib articulation

FIG. 22.5 A bulbous pseudoarticulation between a C7 cervical rib and the first thoracic rib **(A)** caused a growing "mass" that impinged progressively on the plexus **(B)**. This mass is similar to what is described in the first published account of a surgical treatment for a brachial plexus entrapment, which appeared in the *Lancet* in 1861. The *arrow* in **(A)** points to the proximal part of the cervical rib. *Arrows* in **(B)** identify the course of the middle trunk of the brachial plexus as it is impinged upon and distorted by the cervical rib articulation callus. (From Filler AG. Brachial plexus nerve entrapments and thoracic outlet syndromes. In: *Youmans and Winn Neurological Surgery*, vol. 250, 2032–2040.e2 Copyright ©2017 by Elsevier, Inc. All rights reserved.)

upon voluntary activation, and possible reduction in recruitment on voluntary contraction (less available MUPs with a faster firing rate). Reduced recruitment is often the first abnormality seen and generally precedes F-wave and SEP (sensory evoked potentials) abnormalities.[25] No studies have shown the sensitivity and specificity of EMG in the detection of nTOS.

Diagnostic scalene blocks may aid in the diagnosis of nTOS.[26] As with any "diagnostic injection," the possibility of a placebo response is of concern. The block is typically performed by injecting the anterior scalene with an anesthetic, such as lidocaine or bupivacaine, via ultrasound imaging, fluoroscopy, or CT-guidance. Patients should report significant decreased symptoms for the duration of the anesthetic. Using a "pain diary"

where the patient reports the level of pain before injection and then once an hour for several hours helps in documenting the perceived reduction in symptoms. The test is often used in surgical planning and reports of up to 90% success with scalene resection with a positive diagnostic injection are quoted (Fig. 22.6).[26]

Treatment

Conservative management is recommended for all types of TOS before surgical management, except in cases of acute limb ischemia or progressive neurologic deficit.[15] Although there is no gold standard physical therapy treatment program, it has been shown to be effective compared with surgery in regards to decreasing symptoms and returning patients to work.[27,28] The aims of TOS conservative therapy are to decompress the narrowed anatomic spaces, to improve nerve mobility, and to correct muscle imbalances via a targeted stretching and strengthening program. There are differing opinions on how to achieve this; Peet was the first in 1956 to advocate nonsurgical management involving physical therapy, postural education, and moist heat.[3] For many patients, physical therapy is a mainstay of treatment, but supplemental therapies such as acupuncture and massage may also be considered, although evidence is lacking.

The aims of rehabilitation in nTOS are to reduce pain by soft tissue mobilization and muscle conditioning.[5] In regards to patient education, the first lesson is how to control pain at rest while sitting, standing, and sleeping by finding positions of comfort. While the patient is seated, the arms should be placed on pillows or armrests that do not elevate or depress the shoulders. Good posture is encouraged when standing and can be reinforced with the use of front and side mirrors. One method is to ask patients to retract their shoulder blades into a comfortable position and let their head follow.[29] While the patient is standing, weight should be distributed equally over both feet and the back should follow its normal curve. While driving, patients should keep their hands securely but low and relaxed on the wheel. An arm rest should be placed under the affected arm.[29]

Especially in patients with nTOS with entrapment neuropathies, there may be several simultaneous pathologies to address. Rotator cuff tendinopathies, adhesive capsulitis from decreased arm movement, limited range of motion of the neck, and active myofascial trigger points may also compete for the practitioner's attention. According to Walsh, these pathologies should be pinpointed and treated systematically.[5] Ice and/or heat may also be helpful.

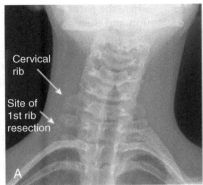
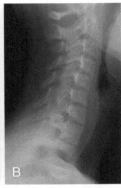

FIG. 22.6 First rib resection with unresected C7 cervical rib. The patient had persistent symptoms after complete first rib resection. A cervical rib is often missed on MRI, so an anteroposterior lordotic chest radiograph **(A)** is an important part of the diagnostic evaluation if there is any reason to suspect a cervical rib. **(B)** Lateral view. (From Filler AG. Brachial plexus nerve entrapments and thoracic outlet syndromes. In: *Youmans and Winn Neurological Surgery*, vol. 250, 2032–2040.e2 Copyright ©2017 by Elsevier, Inc. All rights reserved.)

Once a degree of pain control is achieved, the therapist can then begin the process of mobilizing the soft tissues in the thoracic outlet. Nerve glide exercises are often implemented. With entrapment or compression neuropathies, this gliding movement is impeded. Reasons for reduced nerve mobility include muscle hypertrophy and scar tissue formation. In fact, histology specimens from patients with disputed nTOS showed significantly more scar tissue (36% more) in the scalene muscles compared with the control population.[30]

Botulinum toxin is also utilized in the treatment of nTOS. This is accomplished by injecting the anterior and middle scalenes with an aliquot of the substance, although there is no consensus on dosage. The use of EMG, fluoroscopy, ultrasound imaging, and CT guidance is described.[31,32] The goal is to block the neuromuscular junction of these muscles so they relax and do not cause as much compression. This can also be a tool in establishing the diagnosis and considering surgery if only temporary relief occurs, often up to 3 months because of the half-life of the medication.[32,33]

Surgical Management

Surgery is considered in those who fail conservative therapy and have significant pain and disability because of the condition. The goal of surgical management is to decompress the compromised portion of the brachial plexus. If a cervical rib or prominent C7 transverse process is involved, it is resected often along with the first rib. Decompression of the neural structures through the scalenes is accomplished by removing the anterior and middle scalene muscles. Some practitioners advocate focusing on the scalene resection and not addressing the cervical rib, as they believe this is where most of the compression occurs.[34] Reported surgical success rates for nTOS are up to 70% at 5–10 years from the time of surgery.[15] Complications with these surgeries include infection, brachial plexus injury secondary to retractors, phrenic nerve injury, long thoracic nerve injury, pneumothorax, worsening pain, paresthesias, and seromas.

Measuring and comparing the rate of surgical success is challenging. Because pain is often a major factor in the decision to undergo surgery, reduction in pain greater than 50% is often utilized as a marker of outcome. Comparison of success rates is also complicated by different postoperative follow-up between studies. One study from Altobelli et al. quoted up to 18 months to achieve adequate symptom reduction after nTOS surgery.[35] Quoted success rates range from 46% within 18 months[35] to 70% at 5–10 years after surgery.[15]

VASCULAR THORACIC OUTLET SYNDROME

History

Vascular TOS may involve compression of the subclavian vein or artery and can thus be divided into venous or arterial thoracic outlet syndrome (vTOS or aTOS). vTOS accounts for 2%–3% of all TOS cases. It often occurs in young, active people who engage in strenuous upper extremity activities. After a long period of repetitive external compression of the subclavian or axillary vein at the costoclavicular space, a thrombosis forms. Patients report sudden arm swelling, severe neck and arm pain, stiff cyanotic fingers, and arm heaviness. Fortunately, there is a low rate of pulmonary embolism (10%–20%) compared with lower extremity deep venous thrombosis. If an embolus occurs, it is typically small or unable to travel to the lungs because of the narrowed vein.[36]

aTOS is not only the least common form of TOS but also the most dangerous. It results from subclavian artery stenosis or aneurysm that causes thrombus formation and distal emboli. Pain is usually limited to the hand and spares the shoulder and neck.[9] If not recognized early, patients may present with fingertip ischemia.[14]

Most cases of vTOS and aTOS are secondary to the presence of a cervical rib or a traumatic event at or about the neck and clavicle.[37] aTOS has a higher rate of cervical ribs than nTOS or vTOS. When a thrombus occurs in the subclavian vein, it is also referred to as Paget-Schroetter syndrome. The arterial type is often associated with a large cervical rib that is fused to the T1 rib.[12]

Patients with vascular TOS often complain of pain in the arm, neck, and/or shoulder, which typically worsens with prolonged activity or overhead activity. In more serious cases, a thrombus or arterial embolism can occlude the artery and cause an ischemic limb. Patients may develop edema in the arm from venous occlusion in vTOS and a cold extremity with pallor in aTOS.

Physical Examination

Patients may demonstrate swelling in the base of the neck, shoulder, pectoral region, or upper limb and may mimic lymphedema or deep venous thrombosis from other causes. Dilated veins may be present with vTOS in the upper limb and neck secondary to increased venous pressure from compression of the subclavian vein.[38] Pallor may be present in the hand and digits. Reduced pulses may be present in the radial and/or ulnar arteries. A cervical rib may be palpable, or occasionally there may be a palpable mass in the upper clavicular area.

Provocative and diagnostic maneuvers are used to assist in the diagnosis. The Adson maneuver involves patients taking and holding their breath, looking up and turning their head to the side. If the radial pulse diminishes on palpation or there is a change in blood pressure on the ipsilateral side, it is considered positive.[39] Unfortunately, there is a high rate of false positives with this maneuver and it is neither sensitive nor specific.[20,40,41]

Diagnostic Criteria and Testing

In addition to clinical suspicion, first-line diagnostic testing involves obtaining a blood pressure in the office in both the symptomatic and asymptomatic limbs, as the symptomatic side may have a higher reading. As in nTOS, plain radiographs of the neck may reveal bony anomalies, such as a cervical rib, significantly enlarged C7 transverse process, evidence of a prior break/trauma to the clavicle, or calcification of the vasculature in the thoracic outlet.

An upper extremity Doppler ultrasound imaging can be useful in establishing the diagnosis of vTOS or aTOS. In vTOS, a thrombus may be present and demonstrated in the subclavian vein. In aTOS, vessel abnormalities such as aneurysms may be detectable. In addition, stressing the arm in positions that provoke symptoms may show a change in the arterial blood flow on ultrasound imaging.

The use of upper extremity venography and arteriography can demonstrate the area of compression or blockage. This test is performed selectively, however, as it is invasive. It can be combined to increase the diagnostic value with CT or MRI. After administering the dye, a static traditional image can be taken with either modality. A stress picture can follow such as having the arm in hyperabduction to see if there is a blockage to flow. The structure causing the obstruction is also imaged.

Treatment

Conservative treatment in cases of vTOS and aTOS is considered only if a significant thrombus or occlusion is not present. Therapy may consist of strategies to reduce edema, such as an upper limb wrap or sleeve. Goss et al. advocate the use of anticoagulant medications to avoid thrombus formation in lieu of surgery.[42]

Surgical treatment is considered in cases in which significant obstruction to venous or arterial flow is established, thrombus continues to occur, or morbidity with the condition persists despite efforts of conservative care. If the structures are compressed by a fibrous band, by the presence of a cervical rib or prominent C7 transverse process, or through the scalenes, they are resected. If an aneurysm or significant clot is present, they are resected. Sometimes a bypass may be needed if the distal blood flow is compromised.[12]

CONCLUSIONS

TOS should be considered in the differential diagnosis of upper limb pain. Although rare, it can be a significant source of morbidity and in the vascular cases, life or limb threatening. The presence of a cervical rib on plain films of the cervical spine with the absence of other significant spine pathology may raise suspicion. The presence of upper limb edema and prominent veins may also be a clue to vTOS. As in any other painful condition, careful history and physical examination are essential in making the diagnosis.

REFERENCES

1. Huang JH, Zager EL. Thoracic outlet syndrome. *Neurosurgery.* 2004;55:897–902. Discussion 902–893.
2. Sanders RJ, Hammond SL, Rao NM. Thoracic outlet syndrome: a review. *Neurologist.* 2008;14:365–373.
3. Peet RM, Henriksen JD, Anderson TP, Martin GM. Thoracic-outlet syndrome: evaluation of a therapeutic exercise program. *Proc Staff Meet Mayo Clin.* 1956;31:281–287.
4. Wilbourn AJ. The thoracic outlet syndrome is overdiagnosed. *Arch Neurol.* 1990;47:328–330.
5. Walsh MT. Therapist management of thoracic outlet syndrome. *J Hand Ther.* 1994;7:131–144.
6. Atasoy E. Thoracic outlet syndrome: anatomy. *Hand Clin.* 2004;20:7–14.
7. Hooper TL, Denton J, McGalliard MK, Brismee JM, Sizer Jr PS. Thoracic outlet syndrome: a controversial clinical condition. Part 1: anatomy, and clinical examination/diagnosis. *J Man Manip Ther.* 2010;18:74–83.
8. Aralasmak A, Cevikol C, Karaali K, et al. MRI findings in thoracic outlet syndrome. *Skelet Radiol.* 2012;41:1365–1374.
9. Sanders RJ, Hammond SL, Rao NM. Diagnosis of thoracic outlet syndrome. *J Vasc Surg.* 2007;46:601–604.
10. Sanders RJ, Hammond SL. Management of cervical ribs and anomalous first ribs causing neurogenic thoracic outlet syndrome. *J Vasc Surg.* 2002;36:51–56.
11. Muizelaar JP, Zwienenberg-Lee M. When it is not cervical radiculopathy: thoracic outlet syndrome–a prospective study on diagnosis and treatment. *Clin Neurosurg.* 2005;52:243–249.
12. Hussain MA, Aljabri B, Al-Omran M. Vascular thoracic outlet syndrome. *Semin Thorac Cardiovasc Surg.* 2016;28:151–157.
13. Boezaart AP, Haller A, Laduzenski S, Koyyalamudi VB, Ihnatsenka B, Wright T. Neurogenic thoracic outlet syndrome: a case report and review of the literature. *Int J Shoulder Surg.* 2010;4:27–35.
14. Nichols AW. Diagnosis and management of thoracic outlet syndrome. *Curr Sports Med Rep.* 2009;8:240–249.
15. Mackinnon SE, Novak CB. Thoracic outlet syndrome. *Curr Probl Surg.* 2002;39:1070–1145.
16. Novak CB, Collins ED, Mackinnon SE. Outcome following conservative management of thoracic outlet syndrome. *J Hand Surg Am.* 1995;20:542–548.
17. Roos DB. Thoracic outlet syndrome is underdiagnosed. *Muscle Nerve.* 1999;22:126–129. Discussion 137–128.
18. Wilbourn AJ. Thoracic outlet syndrome is overdiagnosed. *Muscle Nerve.* 1999;22:130–136. Discussion 136–137.
19. Cherington M, Wilbourn AJ. Neurovascular compression in the thoracic outlet syndrome. *Ann Surg.* 1999;230:829–830.
20. Plewa MC, Delinger M. The false-positive rate of thoracic outlet syndrome shoulder maneuvers in healthy subjects. *Acad Emerg Med.* 1998;5:337–342.
21. Davis DS, Anderson IB, Carson MG, Elkins CL, Stuckey LB. Upper limb neural tension and seated slump tests: the false positive rate among healthy young adults without cervical or lumbar symptoms. *J Man Manip Ther.* 2008;16:136–141.
22. Singh VK, Jeyaseelan L, Kyriacou S, Ghosh S, Sinisi M, Fox M. Diagnostic value of magnetic resonance imaging in thoracic outlet syndrome. *J Orthop Surg (Hong Kong).* 2014;22:228–231.
23. Okada E, Matsumoto M, Fujiwara H, Toyama Y. Disc degeneration of cervical spine on MRI in patients with lumbar disc herniation: comparison study with asymptomatic volunteers. *Eur Spine J.* 2011;20:585–591.
24. Tsao BE, Ferrante MA, Wilbourn AJ, Shields RW. Electrodiagnostic features of true neurogenic thoracic outlet syndrome. *Muscle Nerve.* 2014;49:724–727.
25. Passero S, Paradiso C, Giannini F, Cioni R, Burgalassi L, Battistini N. Diagnosis of thoracic outlet syndrome. Relative value of electrophysiological studies. *Acta Neurol Scand.* 1994;90:179–185.
26. Lum YW, Brooke BS, Likes K, et al. Impact of anterior scalene lidocaine blocks on predicting surgical success in older patients with neurogenic thoracic outlet syndrome. *J Vasc Surg.* 2012;55:1370–1375.
27. Landry GJ, Moneta GL, Taylor Jr LM, Edwards JM, Porter JM. Long-term functional outcome of neurogenic thoracic outlet syndrome in surgically and conservatively treated patients. *J Vasc Surg.* 2001;33:312–317. Discussion 317–319.
28. Franklin GM, Fulton-Kehoe D, Bradley C, Smith-Weller T. Outcome of surgery for thoracic outlet syndrome in Washington state workers' compensation. *Neurology.* 2000;54:1252–1257.
29. Anthony MS. *Hand and Upper Extremity Rehabilitation.* 3rd ed. Elsevier; 2006.
30. Sanders RJ, Jackson CG, Banchero N, Pearce WH. Scalene muscle abnormalities in traumatic thoracic outlet syndrome. *Am J Surg.* 1990;159:231–236.
31. Jordan SE, Ahn SS, Freischlag JA, Gelabert HA, Machleder HI. Selective botulinum chemodenervation of the scalene muscles for treatment of neurogenic thoracic outlet syndrome. *Ann Vasc Surg.* 2000;14:365–369.
32. Christo PJ, Christo DK, Carinci AJ, Freischlag JA. Single CT-guided chemodenervation of the anterior scalene muscle with botulinum toxin for neurogenic thoracic outlet syndrome. *Pain Med.* 2010;11:504–511.
33. Jordan SE, Machleder HI. Diagnosis of thoracic outlet syndrome using electrophysiologically guided anterior scalene blocks. *Ann Vasc Surg.* 1998;12:260–264.

34. Sanders RJ, Hammond SL. Supraclavicular first rib resection and total scalenectomy: technique and results. *Hand Clin.* 2004;20:61–70.
35. Altobelli GG, Kudo T, Haas BT, Chandra FA, Moy JL, Ahn SS. Thoracic outlet syndrome: pattern of clinical success after operative decompression. *J Vasc Surg.* 2005;42:122–128.
36. Thompson RW. Comprehensive management of subclavian vein effort thrombosis. *Semin Intervent Radiol.* 2012;29:44–51.
37. Aljabri B, Al-Omran M. Surgical management of vascular thoracic outlet syndrome: a teaching hospital experience. *Ann Vasc Dis.* 2013;6:74–79.
38. Urschel Jr HC, Patel AN. Surgery remains the most effective treatment for Paget-Schroetter syndrome: 50 years' experience. *Ann Thorac Surg.* 2008;86:254–260. Discussion 260.
39. Adson AW. Surgical treatment for symptoms produced by cervical ribs and the scalenus anticus muscle. *Surg Gynecol Obstet.* 1947;85:687–700.
40. Gergoudis R, Barnes RW. Thoracic outlet arterial compression: prevalence in normal persons. *Angiology.* 1980;31:538–541.
41. Malanga GA, Landes P, Nadler SF. Provocative tests in cervical spine examination: historical basis and scientific analyses. *Pain Physician.* 2003;6:199–205.
42. Goss SG, Alcantara SD, Todd GJ, Lantis 2nd JC. Nonoperative management of Paget-Schroetter syndrome: a single-center experience. *J Invasive Cardiol.* 2015;27:423–428.

CHAPTER 23

Neuralgic Amyotrophy

ARI C. GREIS, DO • ZIVA PETRIN, MD • SHIVANI GUPTA, DO • PRIYANCA B. MAGDALIA, DO

INTRODUCTION

Neuralgic amyotrophy, also known as Parsonage and Turner syndrome, is a painful nerve disorder related to a lesion that is severe enough to cause muscle atrophy. It usually presents with acute pain, most commonly affecting the brachial plexus. It is a syndrome that can present with a variety of clinical manifestations. The exact cause is unknown, but autoimmune, genetic, infectious, environmental, and biomechanical processes have been implicated.[1]

INCIDENCE

Neuralgic amyotrophy is a clinical diagnosis. At this time, a definitive diagnosis cannot be made based solely on serologic markers, imaging, or electromyography (EMG), without including the clinical history and physical examination.

Defining a true incidence is therefore difficult, because multiple overlapping clinical definitions and criteria exist when defining the disorder. The clinical picture overlaps with other more common shoulder and neck pathologies and can be overlooked without directed training. The typical syndrome of sudden severe unilateral shoulder pain followed by scapular winging or decreased pinch grip occurs in approximately 70% of cases.[2]

The annual incidence has been described as approximately 2–3/100,000 people in two populations, one in Rochester, Minnesota, and the other in the United Kingdom.[3,4] Following training on how to diagnose neuralgic amyotrophy, the approximate annual incidence increased to 1/1000 people in a population of approximately 14,000 primary care patients in the Netherlands.[2]

However, these incidence studies have been performed primarily in small homogenous populations, and a true worldwide annual incidence is unknown.

The conservative incidence of 2–3/100,000 is comparable with that of Guillain-Barré syndrome (estimated 1–2/100,000)[5] and multiple sclerosis in similar European populations (estimated 1/100,000 to 10/100,000).[6] The condition is more common in men than in women (ratio of 2:1 or 3:2).[4,7]

It is typically asymmetric, involving either exclusively one arm or affecting one side more than the other side. Studies vary and have shown either no statistical preference for sidedness or up to a 2:1 ratio favoring the right arm over the left.[7–9]

Neuralgic amyotrophy has been described in the literature in ages from pediatric patients of less than 3 years old to the elderly, with a median age of 40 years and a normal distribution.[7]

ETIOLOGY

Neuralgic amyotrophy is not a uniform disorder but a syndrome occurring secondary to a variety of precipitating factors and genetic phenotypes (Table 23.1).

The etiology of the disorder can be grossly divided into hereditary, and idiopathic or immune mediated. The hereditary form is more commonly recurrent (up to 74%),[7] whereas the immune-mediated and idiopathic forms primarily occur in a sporadic or epidemic fashion as a one-time event with a minimal recurrence rate. The highest recurrence rate in idiopathic neuralgic amyotrophy reported in the literature was described in a selected series of patients with a 26% recurrence rate.[7]

The condition was first described by Dyke in 1916, in a case report of a peripheral nerve lesion after a patient received antitetanic serum,[10] followed in 1941 by 42 cases of "brachial plexus neuritis" by Wyburn-Mason[11] and 46 cases of "localised neuritis of the shoulder girdle" in 1943 by Spillane.[12] In 1948, Parsonage and Turner reported 136 cases of "neuralgic amyotrophy."[13]

The original case series primarily described adult patients who presented with an acute attack after various precipitating factors such as infections, immunizations, and surgery or trauma. Most commonly, patients suffered a one-time event, with gradual improvement.

TABLE 23.1
Different Subtypes of Neuralgic Amyotrophy

	Hereditary NA	Idiopathic	Hepatitis-E Associated
Median age of onset	20s (Van Alfen 2005)	40s	Middle age (Dartevel)
Sex preference	No	Female:male 2:3	Male
Sidedness	Variable	Unilateral	Bilateral
Involvement outside of brachial plexus	Phrenic, recurrent laryngeal, lumbosacral	Not typical	Phrenic nerve
Recurrence	74%	26%	
Dysmorphic features in patient and family	Yes	No	No

In a minority of cases, patients suffered recurrent attacks on the uninvolved side weeks or months after the initial episode, often after minor precipitating events.[13] Various triggering events have been described in the literature, including infections, immunization, surgery, trauma, exercise, pregnancy, parturition, psychological stress, and burns. Identification of triggering events was reported as 72% in the original series by Parsonage and Turner and 53%[14]–73%[15] in more recent studies. Cases with no pain but otherwise clinical findings of patchy weakness in the upper extremity have been described in 3.7%.[7]

Hereditary Neuralgic Amyotrophy

A hereditary form has been described since 1960.[16] The patients involved have varied expression of dysmorphic features, including hypotelorism, epicanthus, microstomia, dysmorphic ears, cleft uvula and palate, and partial syndactyly of fingers or toes.[17,18] The typical facial dysmorphism has been likened to a Modigliani portrait. Genetic studies of affected families have found mutations in a septin 9 repeat motif, which binds and bundles microtubules, also termed SEPT9. The SEPT9 mutation is located on the 17q25 chromosome and is inherited in an autosomal dominant pattern.[19–22]

The typical patient affected with the familial form presents with an acute episode of neuralgic amyotrophy earlier in life, in the second and third decade, and can have one lifetime episode to multiple recurrent attacks, resulting in significant shoulder weakness. The affected family members show variable expression of dysmorphic features as well as variable presentation of brachial palsies. Most family members have at least one episode. The hereditary form is a systemic disease, and although it more commonly

occurs in the upper extremity, it can affect any peripheral nerve. Besides affecting the lumbosacral plexus, hereditary neuralgic amyotrophy frequently affects the phrenic nerve, recurrent laryngeal nerve, and an episode can present as respiratory distress or dysphagia and hoarseness. Histologic studies have confirmed pathology affecting the lumbosacral plexus.[7,14]

It is unclear whether similar molecular mechanisms and genetic background are involved in immune-mediated and idiopathic neuralgic amyotrophy. A genetic abnormality at 17q25 has been identified in one case of idiopathic neuralgic amyotrophy as occasionally found in some families with hereditary neuralgic amyotrophy. As a single episode of amyotrophy in a patient with hereditary neuralgic amyotrophy is difficult to differentiate from a sporadic case, except on the basis of dysmorphic features or familiar involvement, the importance of this case is unclear. A case of two siblings without dysmorphic features developing neuralgic amyotrophy after Epstein-Barr infection has also been published[23] without clear answer whether the predisposing factor was a genetic predisposition or the infection. However, no cases of SEPT9 mutation have been identified in sporadic cases of neuralgic amyotrophy, further supporting that the hereditary and sporadic forms represent different etiologies of a similar disorder.[24]

Idiopathic Neuralgic Amyotrophy

Since Dyke first described the association between the disorder and tetanus serum administration, multiple immune-mediated triggers for the development of acute neuralgic amyotrophy have been identified, including various infections and vaccinations. Viral infections such hepatitis E, B19,[25] varicella-zoster, and

Epstein-Barr virus[23] have all been implicated in cases of nonhereditary neuralgic amyotrophy.

Van Alfen first described 10 male patients with gross elevations of liver enzymes and severe bilateral brachial plexopathy with phrenic nerve involvement.[7] In 1984 an Italian group described a case of neuralgic amyotrophy associated with non-A non-B hepatitis.[26] Hepatitis E was formally discovered and sequenced in 1990 by Reyes et al., and as such, definitive viral and serologic analysis of the case was not possible in 1984. Although infection with hepatitis E is typically asymptomatic, the virus has also been implicated in other neurologic syndromes such as Guillain-Barré syndrome and meningoencephalitis.[27–30]

In 2009, Fong first described a patient with neuralgic amyotrophy with a confirmed acute hepatitis E infection.[31] Serologic analysis of a cohort of UK and Dutch patients with neuralgic amyotrophy showed that 10% of the patients had anti-hepatitis E virus IgM antibodies, with EMG studies demonstrating bilateral brachial plexus involvement in all patients with positive hepatitis E infection.[32]

Although other infectious agents have been implicated in isolated case reports of neuralgic amyotrophy, there are increasing numbers of cases of confirmed hepatitis E virus infections in association with a subset syndrome of neuralgic amyotrophy. The typical case involves a middle-aged male with bilateral brachial plexus involvement with or without phrenic nerve involvement.[33–35]

At this time, it is still unclear whether the association of neuralgic amyotrophy with infectious agents is a result of direct infection or postinfectious immune-mediated injury to the peripheral nerves. The predilection for nerves of the brachial plexus and phrenic nerve is also unclear. Furthermore, it is still unclear what percentage of sporadic-type neuralgic amyotrophy is associated with an infectious agent, as multiple predilecting events such as trauma, surgery, and psychological stress have all been associated with acute episodes of idiopathic neuralgic amyotrophy and almost half of acute cases do not have an identifiable trigger.

Although an inflammatory-immune mechanism for idiopathic neuralgic amyotrophy is hypothesized, no specific immunologic markers have yet been discovered. Immune complexes such as those found in Guillain-Barré syndrome or acute inflammatory demyelinating polyradiculoneuropathy have not been found in idiopathic neurogenic amyotrophy. Infiltration of the plexus with T cells, mononuclear cells, and B cells has been demonstrated histologically, although it remains unclear whether the inflammatory cells are responding to a pathogen or an autoimmune trigger.[36] Increased antiganglioside antibodies have been found in about one-third of patients with neuralgic amyotrophy. However, they too appear to be nonspecific.[37] Defining the underlying etiology further may help guide targeted treatment in the future.

PRESENTATION

Neuralgic amyotrophy presents with a wide constellation of symptoms, including acute onset of unilateral severe neuropathic shoulder, neck, and/or arm pain. Pain may occur as small isolated episodes that occur for a few weeks and ultimately lead to a major episode that involves severe pain unrelieved by position or analgesics.[7,38,39] The initial stage is continuous intractable shooting and stabbing pain that lasts approximately 4 weeks. Pain symptoms are followed by progressive multifocal neurologic deficits, including paresis and atrophy.[7,40] First signs of paresis may be immediate, with paresis developing in 24 h, or may take up to 2 weeks or longer.[38,41] On average, symptoms first appear in 13.6 days in males and 8 days in females.[7]

Muscles that are normally affected include those innervated by the brachial plexus and most commonly include muscles innervated by the upper and middle trunk of the brachial plexus, including the suprascapular nerve and long thoracic nerve.[7] However, muscles innervated by the cranial nerves, phrenic nerve, and lumbosacral plexus may also be affected.[38] In addition to pain and muscle atrophy, sensory changes may be appreciated but may be patchy in distribution.[38,41] Atrophy is another clinical presentation associated with neuralgic amyotrophy; it develops as early as 2 weeks and may take up to 5 weeks to develop.[7]

DIFFERENTIAL DIAGNOSIS

The differential diagnoses of neuralgic amyotrophy include medical conditions that present with unilateral upper extremity pain, muscle weakness, atrophy, and loss of sensation. The differential diagnosis can be broken down by neurologic, musculoskeletal, and systemic pathology.

Neurologic pathologies that can result in symptoms similar to neuralgic amyotrophy include cervical radiculopathy caused by spinal stenosis and cervical disc herniations,[40] which usually presents with some component of neck pain and follows a single dermatomal pattern. Provocative tests, such as Spurling maneuver (cervical extension with rotation to the ipsilateral side), and imaging, including MRI, can help differentiate whether these compressive etiologies exist. Peripheral neuropathic conditions may also produce similar symptoms, such as mononeuritis multiplex, transverse myelitis, multifocal motor neuropathy, and various motor neuron diseases.[42] Another cause of severe unilateral shoulder pain is herpes zoster and shingles, as well as postherpetic neuralgia.[40]

The differential of unilateral shoulder pain can be expanded to musculoskeletal shoulder joint pathology. This includes, but is not limited to, traumatic injury to the cervical and shoulder girdle musculature, glenohumeral joint osteoarthritis, rotator cuff injuries, adhesive capsulitis, subacromial bursitis, tendinitis, myofascial pain, and complex regional pain syndrome.[8] Neuralgic amyotrophy and adhesive capsulitis may present in a similar fashion including severe unilateral shoulder pain, unrelieved by position, and worse at night. A key difference is that adhesive capsulitis results in restriction of glenohumeral joint range of motion, whereas neuralgic amyotrophy normally does not.[40]

Additional differential diagnosis includes systemic causes of unilateral shoulder pain, including autoimmune, inflammatory, infectious, and vasculitic conditions affecting the brachial plexus.[8,38,40]

DIAGNOSIS

Neuralgic amyotrophy is considered a clinical diagnosis based on its characteristic presentation. In 96% of the cases, a patient presents with a sudden onset of severe neuropathic pain followed by the development of a patchy progressive weakness of the involved extremity that may commence within days to weeks after the onset of pain.[43] In a retrospective study, the diagnosis of neuralgic amyotrophy is often delayed with the mean period of 43.8 weeks and the median being 10.5 weeks.[7] Although no test can definitively confirm or refute its occurrence, further diagnostic studies can be conducted to confirm suspicion or exclude other etiologies.[8,42,43] A thorough history and neurologic and musculoskeletal physical examination is critical in making the diagnosis and to differentiate neuralgic amyotrophy from other neurologic and musculoskeletal diagnoses.

The first test is typically EMG and nerve conduction studies (NCS), which can localize the lesion, confirm the diagnosis, and help determine the extent of the injury. In a consecutive case-series analysis involving 246 patients, 96.3% had abnormal results compatible with neuralgic amyotrophy.[7] A later study evaluated 281 patients with extensive electrodiagnostic studies. The NCS included evaluation of the superficial radial sensory, median sensory, ulnar sensory, median motor, and

ulnar motor and any additional NCS based on clinical presentation. The needle EMG studies included the first dorsal interosseous, extensor indicis, flexor pollicis longus, pronator teres, biceps, triceps, deltoid, paraspinal muscles, and any other clinically involved muscles. The results indicated that the most common nerves involved were pure motor nerves, those with a lack of cutaneous sensory nerve fibers, including the suprascapular, long thoracic, distal motor nerve branches, and anterior interosseous nerve. Although overall the suprascapular nerve had the highest frequency of involvement, the long thoracic nerve was the most injured in patients with mononeuropathy. The second and third group of nerves commonly impacted were, respectively, the predominately motor nerves (axillary and musculocutaneous) and the nerves with a balanced distribution of motor and sensory axonal fibers (radial and median nerves). The least involved group included the cutaneous sensory nerve group, with the lateral antebrachial cutaneous nerve being the most frequently affected.[15] As neuralgic amyotrophy is considered to be primarily an axonopathy, NCS are often normal; however, they may show reduced amplitude, prolonged distal latency, or conduction block. The EMG in the early phases (3–4 weeks after the onset of symptoms) shows evidence of acute denervation, fibrillation potentials and positive sharp waves in muscle fibers, and reduced motor unit recruitment in muscles innervated in a non-myotomal pattern. Later EMG findings, 4–12 months after the onset of symptoms, include evidence of old denervation with early reinnervation, large duration, large-amplitude polyphasic motor units, and decreased recruitment.

An MRI can also be considered as a further extension of the physical examination and helps to exclude disorders with mimicking presentations. Imaging of the cervical spine and shoulder can be used to exclude disc herniation or rotator cuff/shoulder joint pathology as sources of the presenting symptom.[43] Often patients have abnormalities in their cervical spine. Therefore correlation with clinical phenotype is critical to avoid overdiagnosing cervical radiculopathy. MRI also helps to exclude a mass or cyst compressing the suspected nerve, neuritis, or a neural tumor.[38]

MRI T2-weighted images may show evidence of denervated muscles including high signal intensity caused by the increased extracellular water or edema. Imaging immediately after the onset of symptoms may miss these findings as it can take 2–4 weeks after denervation occurs before edematous changes are present.[43] In the subacute to chronic stages, atrophy with and without fatty infiltration may be best seen in T1-weighted images.[44] A study using MRI to identify similar features in 26 patients with neuralgic amyotrophy concluded that it is sensitive for detecting signal abnormalities in the shoulder girdle muscles, most frequently the supraspinatus and infraspinatus.[45] Although the long thoracic nerve is one of the most commonly affected nerves in neuralgic amyotrophy, its small size limits its visibility and can often lead to false-negative MRI results, especially in those patients with a medially winged scapula.[44] In patients with phrenic nerve involvement, a chest radiograph should be ordered to evaluate for a Pancoast lung tumor and also evidence for diaphragmatic palsy.[7]

The use of ultrasonography has been explored as another means of supporting the diagnosis of neuralgic amyotrophy. High-resolution probes greater than 15 Hz allow visualization of nerves less than 1 mm diameter. Evaluation includes scanning of the brachial plexus along with the nerves and muscles thought by clinical examination to be affected. A study in 2016 utilized high-resolution ultrasound imaging to examine six patients with a clinical diagnosis of neuralgic amyotrophy 2 weeks to 6 months from the onset of symptoms. All six patients were found to have focal swelling or fascicular enlargement of peripheral nerves, and those in the later stages had evidence of muscle atrophy. In addition, half of the patients had swelling of the entire visible portion of the long thoracic nerve.[44]

Although nerve biopsies are currently not required for the diagnosis of neuralgic amyotrophy, researchers have studied the peripheral nerve biopsies in patients with neuralgic amyotrophy, which showed multifocal multifascicular inflammatory and constrictive neuritis. Findings included epineural perivascular mononuclear infiltrates associated with active axonal degeneration, a focal decrease in myelinated fibers, and apparent constrictive bands along the course of an affected nerve.[43]

TREATMENT

There is no proven treatment to reduce the neurologic impairment or improve the prognosis of neuralgic amyotrophy.[42] As such, the treatment is focused on improving the quality of life of the patient, including pain control and prevention of further loss of function.

During the initial painful phase, there is anecdotal evidence that corticosteroids shortened the acute phase and helped improve functional recovery.[39] A recommended dose is 60 mg/day of prednisolone for the first week, tapered by 10 mg every day during the next 5 days, ending with 5 mg on day 13, with the median time to start the treatment being 10 days after the onset of symptoms.[7] The limiting factor is that patients are rarely seen so quickly by specialists familiar with neuralgic amyotrophy. One study of 246 neuralgic amyotrophy cases presented data in regards to different modalities for pain control. Both nonsteroidal antiinflammtory drugs (NSAIDs) and a combination of NSAIDs and opioid treatments provided adequate pain control. According to a small study, 31.6% found opioids to provide good control of their pain, whereas 32.2% felt similar relief from an NSAID alone. On the other hand, 60.7% of patients who received both an NSAID and opioid reported adequate pain control.[43] A nonpharmacology option such as rest and immobilization of the affected extremity has also shown to decrease future exacerbations if used during the acute pain phase of the disease process.[43] A study at the Mayo Clinic involving surgical patients with postoperative peripheral neuropathies administered immunotherapy to eight patients, all of whom claimed improvement in neurologic symptoms and function.[40] Typically, 1–2 months after the onset, the acute pain subsides and NSAIDs and/or analgesics may suffice.

After the acute painful attack, lingering neuropathic pain is known to persist. For this, treatment is similar to other neuropathic pain conditions. First-line recommendations for postherpetic neuralgia, including gabapentin, pregabalin, tricyclic antidepressants, lidocaine patch 5%, controlled-release oxycodone, and morphine sulfate, can also be trialed for neuropathic symptoms in neuralgic amyotrophy.[42] If these are ineffective, duloxetine can be considered for persistent neuropathic pain.

As an adjunct to medication, nonpharmacologic options, including physical therapy, osteopathic manipulation, therapeutic modalities, and acupuncture, have been found to play a role in improving the quality of life of patients after the acute painful phase. Positive results are mainly anecdotal. Transcutaneous electrical nerve stimulation and acupuncture may help alleviate pain in prolonged denervated states. Once the acute painful phase has subsided, an aggressive physical therapy approach can be instituted. Any degree of exercise in early reinnervated muscles can overload the muscle, causing more injury. In completely denervated muscles, strengthening exercises are not indicated. Range of motion exercises have been found to be helpful after the hyperalgesic phase, with the goal of preventing loss of function. Desensitization is a modality that can be explored in patients with persistent allodynia. In athletes where overhead activity and high-intensity training are required, working with a therapist on biomechanics and proper form is key to prevent further injury.[40]

Although a conservative approach, including therapy and analgesics, typically brings satisfactory results, in late stages surgical treatments can be considered for secondary complications, including recurrent shoulder dislocations or functional disability from significant weakness. Options explored include neurolysis, nerve grafts, and nerve transfers.[42]

CONCLUSIONS

Neuralgic amyotrophy is a challenging neurologic condition to diagnose and treat. It requires a thorough history and physical examination, imaging studies to rule out other more common causes of a neuropathy, and electrodiagnostic studies to confirm an axonopathy. It usually affects portions of the brachial plexus, most commonly the suprascapular and long thoracic nerves, and can also involve the cervical or lumbosacral plexus, particularly in hereditary neuralgic amyotrophy, where recurrence rates are higher. Multiple immune-mediated triggers have been identified, including the Epstein-Barr, varicella-zoster, and hepatitis E viruses and various immunizations. Treatment is usually conservative, with support for the early use of corticosteroids, and most cases lead to a favorable outcome.

REFERENCES

1. van Alfen N. Clinical and pathophysiological concepts of neuralgic amyotrophy. *Nat Rev Neurol*. 2011;7(6): 315–322.
2. van Alfen N, van Eijk JJ, Ennik T, et al. Incidence of neuralgic amyotrophy (Parsonage Turner syndrome) in a primary care setting–a prospective cohort study. *PLoS One*. 2015;10(5):e0128361.
3. Beghi E, Kurland LT, Mulder DW, Nicolosi A. Brachial plexus neuropathy in the population of Rochester, Minnesota, 1970-1981. *Ann Neurol*. 1985;18(3):320–323.
4. MacDonald BK, Cockerell OC, Sander JW, Shorvon SD. The incidence and lifetime prevalence of neurological disorders in a prospective community-based study in the UK. *Brain*. 2000;123(Pt 4):665–676.
5. Sejvar JJ, Baughman AL, Wise M, Morgan OW. Population incidence of Guillain-Barre syndrome: a systematic review and meta-analysis. *Neuroepidemiology*. 2011;36(2): 123–133.
6. Kingwell E, Marriott JJ, Jette N, et al. Incidence and prevalence of multiple sclerosis in Europe: a systematic review. *BMC Neurol*. 2013;13:128.
7. van Alfen N, van Engelen BG. The clinical spectrum of neuralgic amyotrophy in 246 cases. *Brain*. 2006;129(Pt 2): 438–450.
8. Seror P. Neuralgic amyotrophy. An update. *Joint Bone Spine*. 2016;84(2):153–158.
9. Magee KR, Dejong RN. Paralytic brachial neuritis. Discussion of clinical features with review of 23 cases. *JAMA*. 1960;174:1258–1262.
10. Dyke SC, Lond., L.M.S.S.A. Peripheral nerve lesions after anti-tetanic serum. *Lancet*. 1916;272(466):1.
11. Wyburn-Mason R, Camb, M.B Brachial neuritis occurring in epidemic form. *Lancet*. 1941;238.
12. Spillane JD. Localised neuritis of the shoulder girdle. *Lancet*. 1943;242.
13. Parsonage MJ, Turner JW. Neuralgic amyotrophy; the shoulder-girdle syndrome. *Lancet*. 1948;1(6513): 973–978.
14. van Alfen N, Gabreels-Festen AA, Ter Laak HJ, Arts WF, Gabreels FJ, van Engelen BG. Histology of hereditary neuralgic amyotrophy. *J Neurol Neurosurg Psychiatry*. 2005;76(3):445–447.
15. Ferrante MA, Wilbourn AJ. The lesion distribution among 281 patients with sporadic neuralgic amyotrophy. *Muscle Nerve*. 2017;55(6):858–861.
16. Taylor RA. Heredofamilial mononeuritis multiplex with brachial predilection. *Brain*. 1960;83:113–137.
17. Jacob JC, Andermann F, Robb JP. Heredofamilial neuritis with brachial predilection. *Neurology*. 1961;11:1025–1033.
18. Dunn HG, Daube JR, Gomez MR. Heredofamilial branchial plexus neuropathy (hereditary neuralgic amyotrophy with branchial predilection) in childhood. *Dev Med Child Neurol*. 1978;20(1):28–46.
19. Bai X, Bowen JR, Knox TK, et al. Novel septin 9 repeat motifs altered in neuralgic amyotrophy bind and bundle microtubules. *J Cell Biol*. 2013;203(6):895–905.
20. Collie AM, Landsverk ML, Ruzzo E, et al. Non-recurrent SEPT9 duplications cause hereditary neuralgic amyotrophy. *J Med Genet*. 2010;47(9):601–607.
21. Laccone F, Hannibal MC, Neesen J, Grisold W, Chance PF, Rehder H. Dysmorphic syndrome of hereditary neuralgic amyotrophy associated with a SEPT9 gene mutation–a family study. *Clin Genet*. 2008;74(3):279–283.
22. Kuhlenbaumer G, Hannibal MC, Nelis E, et al. Mutations in SEPT9 cause hereditary neuralgic amyotrophy. *Nat Genet*. 2005;37(10):1044–1046.
23. Tsao BE, Avery R, Shields RW. Neuralgic amyotrophy precipitated by Epstein-Barr virus. *Neurology*. 2004;62(7): 1234–1235.
24. Klein CJ, Wu Y, Cunningham JM, et al. SEPT9 mutations and a conserved 17q25 sequence in sporadic and hereditary brachial plexus neuropathy. *Arch Neurol*. 2009;66(2):238–243.
25. Pellas F, Olivares JP, Zandotti C, Delarque A. Neuralgic amyotrophy after parvovirus B19 infection. *Lancet*. 1993;342(8869):503–504.
26. Del Giudice G, Galli M, Chemotti M, Gasparro M, Franzetti F, Lazzarin A. Brachial paresis complicating acute non-A, non-B hepatitis. *Boll Ist Sieroter Milan*. 1984;63(6):499–504.
27. Kamar N, Marion O, Abravanel F, Izopet J, Dalton HR. Extrahepatic manifestations of hepatitis E virus. *Liver Int*. 2016;36(4):467–472.

28. Bazerbachi F, Haffar S, Garg SK, Lake JR. Extra-hepatic manifestations associated with hepatitis E virus infection: a comprehensive review of the literature. *Gastroenterol Rep.* 2016;4(1):1–15.
29. Dalton HR, Kamar N, van Eijk JJ, et al. Hepatitis E virus and neurological injury. *Nat Rev Neurol.* 2016;12(2):77–85.
30. Dartevel A, Colombe B, Bosseray A, et al. Hepatitis E and neuralgic amyotrophy: five cases and review of literature. *J Clin Virol.* 2015;69:156–164.
31. Fong F, Illahi M. Neuralgic amyotrophy associated with hepatitis E virus. *Clin Neurol Neurosurg.* 2009;111(2):193–195.
32. van Eijk JJ, Madden RG, van der Eijk AA, et al. Neuralgic amyotrophy and hepatitis E virus infection. *Neurology.* 2014;82(6):498–503.
33. Avila JD, Lacomis D, Lam EM. Neuralgic amyotrophy associated with hepatitis E virus infection: first case in the United States. *J Clin Neuromuscul Dis.* 2016;18(2):96–100.
34. Decard BF, Grimm A, Andelova M, et al. Hepatitis-E virus associated neuralgic amyotrophy with sustained plexus brachialis swelling visualized by high-resolution ultrasound. *J Neurol Sci.* 2015;351(1–2):208–210.
35. Silva M, Wicki B, Tsouni P, et al. Hepatitis E virus infection as a direct cause of neuralgic amyotrophy. *Muscle Nerve.* 2016;54(2):325–327.
36. Suarez GA, Giannini C, Bosch EP, et al. Immune brachial plexus neuropathy: suggestive evidence for an inflammatory-immune pathogenesis. *Neurology.* 1996;46(2):559–561.
37. Stich O, Glos D, Brendle M, Dersch R, Rauer S. Cerebrospinal fluid profile and seroprevalence of antiganglioside reactivity in patients with neuralgic amyotrophy. *J Peripher Nerv Syst.* 2016;21(1):27–32.
38. Gupta A, Winalski CS, Sundaram M. Neuralgic amyotrophy (parsonage turner syndrome). *Orthopedics.* 2014;37(2). 75, 130–133.
39. van Alfen N, van Engelen BG, Hughes RA. Treatment for idiopathic and hereditary neuralgic amyotrophy (brachial neuritis). *Cochrane Database Syst Rev.* 2009;(3):CD006976.
40. Feinberg JH, Radecki J. Parsonage-turner syndrome. *HSS J.* 2010;6(2):199–205.
41. England JD, Sumner AJ. Neuralgic amyotrophy: an increasingly diverse entity. *Muscle Nerve.* 1987;10(1):60–68.
42. Smith CC, Bevelaqua AC. Challenging pain syndromes: parsonage-turner syndrome. *Phys Med Rehabil Clin N Am.* 2014;25(2):265–277.
43. Smith DP, Elliott JA, Helzberg JH. Intravenous corticosteroid therapy for bilateral parsonage-turner syndrome: a case report and review of the literature. *Reg Anesth Pain Med.* 2014;39(3):243–247.
44. Lieba-Samal D, Jengojan S, Kasprian G, Wober C, Bodner G. Neuroimaging of classic neuralgic amyotrophy. *Muscle Nerve.* 2016;54(6):1079–1085.
45. Scalf RE, Wenger DE, Frick MA, Mandrekar JN, Adkins MC. MRI findings of 26 patients with Parsonage-Turner syndrome. *AJR Am J Roentgenol.* 2007;189(1):W39–W44.

CHAPTER 24

Piriformis Syndrome: A Review of the Evidence and Proposed New Criteria for Diagnosis

JASON PAN, MD • JOHN VASUDEVAN, MD

INTRODUCTION

Piriformis syndrome is a controversial cause of gluteal pain. Historically, piriformis syndrome has been a diagnosis that may account for as much as 6%–8% of patients seen for a complaint of sciatica (low back/ leg pain in the distribution of the sciatic nerve) in the United States each year.[1-3] The challenge surrounding the diagnosis and treatment of piriformis syndrome is to distinguish it from among the overlapping symptoms seen in other disorders involving the spine, hip, and pelvis. As such, it is generally recognized as a diagnosis of exclusion.

A definitive diagnosis of piriformis syndrome remains difficult because of evolving characterizations of this disease entity over time and the lack of a "gold standard" diagnostic test. A synthesis of the literature leads us to propose the new criteria for diagnosis shown in Box 24.1.

These criteria aim to provide a more clinically applicable approach to piriformis syndrome. Although there is a limited role for therapeutic injections or even surgery, the mainstay of treatment for this condition, once identified using these criteria, is properly directed physical therapy.

The goal of this chapter is to assist the clinician in defining and properly diagnosing this syndrome, to understand the strength of the evidence for proposed treatments, and then to apply an optimal approach to reducing pain and restoring function.

PRESENTATION

Anatomy

The piriformis muscle originates from the anterior sacrum and sacroiliac joint, passes transversely through the greater sciatic foramen via the sciatic notch, and inserts on the greater trochanter (Fig. 24.1). The muscle is innervated by the ventral rami of S1 and S2 (and L5 to a lesser extent), which join to form the nerve to the piriformis.[4] The muscle receives its vascular supply predominantly from a branch off the inferior gluteal artery.[5] When the hip is in extension, the piriformis muscle externally rotates the femur. When the hip is in flexion, the piriformis muscle acts as a weak hip abductor. In greater than 80% of the population, the sciatic nerve traverses beneath the piriformis muscle and exits the pelvis through the greater sciatic foramen. However, several cadaveric studies have demonstrated variable anatomy in a subset of individuals, including 10%–15% of the population with a split sciatic nerve, which travels both through and beneath the piriformis muscle.[3,6] Less common variations include a split nerve traveling through and above the muscle, a complete nerve piercing through the muscle, and a complete nerve traversing above the muscle (Fig. 24.2).[3,6] It is unclear whether or not there is a correlation between these anatomic variants and the development of the syndrome.

Historical Features

Piriformis syndrome presents with a constellation of symptoms that often overlaps with other causes of

---

BOX 24.1
Proposed Piriformis Syndrome Diagnostic Criteria

1. Marked pain in the gluteal region
2. Pain may be focal *or* radiate into the posterior thigh
3. Tenderness to palpation over the sciatic notch
4. Active contraction *or* passive stretching of the piriformis muscle provokes concordant pain
5. There is no alternative explanation for the pain

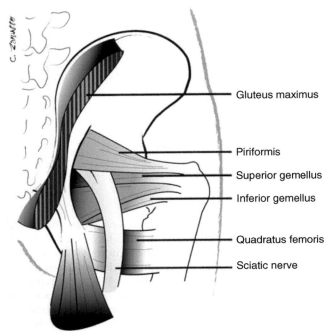

FIG. 24.1 The anatomy of the sciatic nerve, piriformis muscle, and surrounding structures. (From Miller, T. A., et al. The diagnosis and management of piriformis syndrome: myths and facts. Can J Neurol Sci. 2012;39(5): 577–583.)

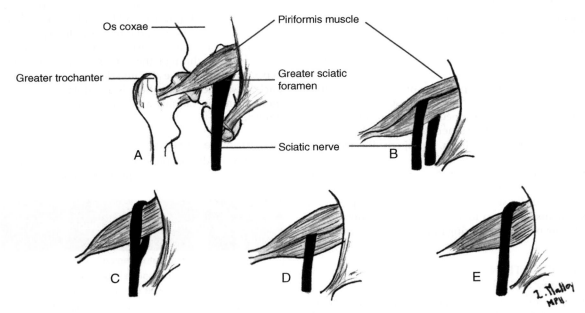

FIG. 24.2 Anatomic variants of the relationship of the sciatic nerve to the piriformis muscle. (From Physio-pedia.com (open-source).)

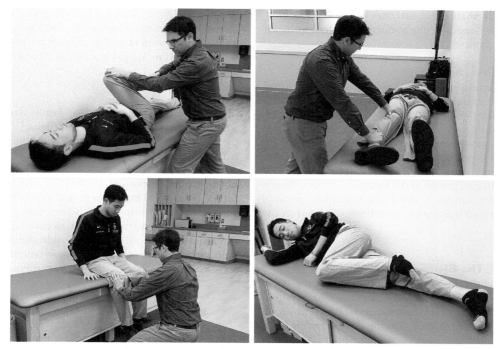

FIG. 24.3 Piriformis examination maneuvers. FAIR maneuver (top left), Freiberg maneuver (top right), Beatty maneuver (bottom left), Beatty maneuver (bottom right).

gluteal pain, such as lumbosacral radiculopathy or sacroiliac joint dysfunction. "Typical" piriformis syndrome often presents as intermittent, sharp/shooting gluteal pain with or without radiation to the posterior thigh. Insidious onset of pain is the most common presentation, with acute pain (e.g., as the result of trauma) being far less common. Classically, the pain may be exacerbated by direct pressure to the region, prolonged sitting, rising from a seated position, stair climbing, and activation or stretching of the piriformis and surrounding musculature. Alleviating factors include changing to a nonpainful position and rest from provocative activity.

Physical Features
Physical examination for piriformis syndrome should evaluate for range of motion, strength, and functional movement patterns that may result in disproportionate strain of the piriformis muscle. The region over the sciatic notch must be palpated to elicit tenderness. A complete evaluation should include focused examination maneuvers that subject the piriformis muscle to active or passive stress. When performing the following tests, they are generally considered "positive" with

reproduction of the patient's concordant gluteal pain. The examination maneuvers are depicted in Fig. 24.3.

The **FAIR test**[7] (flexion, adduction, internal rotation) is performed in the supine or side-lying position. The examiner passively brings the patient's affected side into 90 degrees of hip flexion and 60–90 degrees of knee flexion. The hip is then internally rotated and adducted to place tension on the piriformis muscle.

The **Lasègue maneuver**[8] describes the passive flexion of the hip to 90 degrees and then extending the knee to create neural tension on the sciatic nerve. Note that this is distinct from the straight leg raise test, which involves passively raising the affected limb (with the knee already extended) to reproduce pain in the 30–70 degree range.

The **Freiberg maneuver**[9] involves passive internal rotation of the extended hip joint, placing tension on the piriformis muscle.

The **Beatty maneuver**[10] places the patient in the lateral decubitus position, with the affected side up and the knee resting on the examination surface. The piriformis muscle is then activated as the patient abducts the hip, holding the knee "several inches" off the examination surface.

The Pace maneuver[1] activates the piriformis muscle through resisted active abduction of the hip in the seated position.

Guide to the clinician

Piriformis syndrome presents as insidious-onset gluteal pain that is exacerbated by the activation or stretching of the muscle. Variable anatomic relationships between the piriformis and sciatic nerve have been described and are proposed to predispose a subset of the population to this syndrome. Various diagnostic maneuvers for piriformis syndrome have been described, including the FAIR test, as well as the Lasègue, Freiberg, Beatty, and Pace maneuvers. It should be noted that none of these described maneuvers have been validated in the literature.

DIAGNOSTIC CRITERIA

Throughout the history of piriformis syndrome, there have been multiple proposed definitions of this condition. To date, they remain controversial, with blurred diagnostic criteria. In the following discussion, we highlight two historically important definitions that are often referenced in the literature. In addition, we propose a new set of criteria for piriformis syndrome that emphasizes a myofascial pain component, is more clinically applicable, and better reflects our current understanding of this disease entity.

Robinson

In the early 20th century, the source for sciatic-type pain was disputed. A seminal paper in 1934 by Mixter and Barr described "sciatica" as being caused by intervertebral disc herniation.[11] In that era, other competing theories regarding the etiology of sciatica included the sacroiliac joint, an intrinsic disorder of the sciatic nerve itself, or compression by the piriformis muscle. As early as 1928, the literature had described a relationship between the piriformis muscle, the sciatic nerve, and sciatic-type pain,[12] with detailed analyses of hip and pelvis anatomy using cadavers and radiographs.[9,12,13]

It was not until 1947 that the term "pyriformis [sic] syndrome" was first used by Robinson to describe the particular type of sciatic pain caused by "an abnormal condition of the pyriformis muscle" as opposed to pathology originating in the lumbosacral spine.[14] Robinson initially described the syndrome as having six "cardinal features," including a history of trauma to the sacroiliac/gluteal region, pain in the region of the sacroiliac joint/piriformis muscle radiating down the lower limb causing difficulty with ambulation, symptom exacerbation with bending/lifting, a "sausage-like" mass that is tender to palpation, a positive Lasègue sign, and gluteal atrophy. Although Robinson's labeling of piriformis syndrome was seminal, the clinical field has largely moved on from his description.

Stewart

In 2003, Stewart characterized piriformis syndrome as a sciatic neuropathy with five strict criteria.[15] He defined the syndrome as requiring signs/symptoms of sciatic nerve damage, electrodiagnostic evidence of such damage, normal imaging studies of the back/pelvis/sciatic notch, sciatic compression by the piriformis muscle confirmed by surgical exploration, and relief of symptoms after surgical decompression. Given the exceptionally restrictive requirements of both electrodiagnostic and surgical confirmation, piriformis syndrome is an exceedingly rare phenomenon under Stewart criteria, with only six documented cases meeting all five criteria.[15]

Proposed New Criteria

Millions of people with gluteal pain are diagnosed with "piriformis syndrome" every year,[16] which is in stark contrast to the rarity of true sciatic neuropathy caused by impingement by the piriformis muscle.[15] This discrepancy stems in part from the historical application of "piriformis syndrome" in reference to piriformis-mediated true sciatic neuropathy (e.g., axonal injury), sciatic neural tension at the level of the piriformis, or piriformis-mediated myofascial pain, the last which may be conceptualized as "piriformis myalgia." As such, we propose new, modern criteria for piriformis syndrome (see Box 24.1), which provide a basis for clinically relevant identification and treatment of the spectrum of this syndrome, from the myofascial to neuropathic variants.

Guide to the clinician

The criteria set by Robinson (1947) and Stewart (2003) are generally not used in everyday practice. Our new criteria (Box 24-1) capture the myofascial and neuropathic variants of piriformis syndrome:
1. Marked pain in the gluteal region
2. Pain may be focal or radiate into the posterior thigh
3. Tenderness to palpation over the sciatic notch
4. Active contraction or passive stretching of the piriformis muscle provokes concordant pain
5. There is no alternative explanation for the pain.

COURSE

The symptoms of piriformis syndrome often improve with the avoidance of exacerbating activities and correction of relevant strength and/or flexibility deficits. A majority of cases respond to conservative management, including physical therapy and pharmacologic therapy. Interventional management (e.g., injection therapy) is available but not commonly used. Surgical options are entertained only very rarely for recalcitrant cases.

DIFFERENTIAL DIAGNOSIS
Before arriving at the diagnosis of piriformis syndrome, a wide differential for conditions causing gluteal pain should be considered. Pain in the gluteal region may not only be generated locally, but also be referred from the surrounding structures. Given the extensive differential, it is helpful to categorize the differential diagnosis of gluteal pain by whether or not there is concomitant back pain.

The presence of low back pain suggests pathology involving the lumbosacral spine and its supporting structures. Crucially, pain accompanied by true neurologic deficit (e.g., weakness, sensory disturbance, abnormal reflexes), particularly in a myotomal or dermatomal distribution, should prompt further workup for a neuropathic process (e.g., lumbosacral radiculopathy or neurogenic claudication secondary to spinal stenosis). Bony sources for low back pain include facet arthropathy, spondylolysis, spondylolisthesis, sacroiliac joint dysfunction, and sacral stress fracture. Soft tissue sources for low back pain include lumbar discogenic pain, iliolumbar ligament sprain, muscular strain, and myofascial pain with active trigger points.

In the absence of low back pain, gluteal pain is likely generated by local buttock, hip, or pelvic structures. As with low back pain, the presence of neurologic deficit should prompt evaluation for a neuropathic process (e.g., lumbosacral plexopathy, sciatic neuropathy, or other peripheral mononeuropathy). Neurologic signs and symptoms should not be present in piriformis-mediated myofascial pain.

In considering the broad differential for piriformis syndrome, posterior buttock pain may originate from muscular strain (e.g., gluteal muscles, piriformis, proximal hamstring), ischial bursitis, or ischiofemoral impingement syndrome. Pain at the ischial tuberosity suggests proximal hamstring tendinopathy or ischial bursitis. Ischiofemoral impingement syndrome is a rare impingement phenomenon involving the quadratus femoris muscle as it passes through the ischiofemoral space and may be provoked with the ischiofemoral impingement test (pain with passive extension of the neutral/adducted hip with the patient in the lateral position) and/or the long stride walking test (pain with terminal hip extension during long-stride walking).[17]

Lateral buttock/hip pain may indicate greater trochanteric pain syndrome (GTPS) or iliotibial (IT) band syndrome. GTPS encompasses disorders of the gluteus medius/minimus, trochanteric bursitis, and external snapping hip. Single leg standing and squatting may reveal static or dynamic unleveling of the pelvis, suggesting gluteus medius/minimus dysfunction with or without associated bursitis. IT band syndrome most often presents with pain distally and may also involve discomfort of the anterolateral hip. Examination maneuvers for IT band syndrome include Ober test[18] and Noble compression test.[19] External snapping hip refers to maltracking of the gluteus maximus or IT band complex over the greater trochanter.

Medial hip/buttock pain suggests pathology of the hip joint, gluteus maximus, adductor muscles, or sacrotuberous ligament. Anterior hip/groin pain suggests intraarticular hip pathology, such as osteoarthritis, labral tears, femoroacetabular impingement, femoral stress fracture, or avascular necrosis. In select cases, intraarticular hip pathology can also cause pain in the posterior hip/buttock or through the anterior thigh to knee. Extraarticular sources for anterior pain include hip flexor tendinopathy (e.g., iliopsoas, rectus femoris), osteitis pubis, or athletic pubalgia. Note that the FAIR test is also used in the examination of the hip joint; however, in the case of intraarticular hip pathology, the maneuver typically reproduces anterior/groin pain, as opposed to posterior pain as with piriformis syndrome.

Rare Conditions
When evaluating a patient with gluteal pain and back pain, it is important to consider rare but serious conditions, such as infections (e.g., epidural abscess), cancer (e.g., multiple myeloma), or acute neurologic compromise (e.g., cauda equina syndrome). "Red flag" signs and symptoms include fever, unexplained weight loss, loss of bowel/bladder control, perineal sensory disturbance, and nocturnal pain. Vertebral compression fractures should be considered in patients of advanced age, with poor bone health or recent trauma. In patients with suboptimal bone health, such as those with osteoporosis, a history of chronic corticosteroid use, or suspected female athlete triad, it is important to consider pelvic insufficiency fractures or bone stress injuries as a source for pain. The literature also describes rare piriformis syndrome secondary to space-occupying lesions (e.g., intrapiriformis lipoma[20]).

DIAGNOSTIC TESTING
When the physical examination points toward piriformis syndrome, further diagnostic testing should be

utilized to rule out any alternative explanations for the pain. Imaging modalities, (i.e., CT, MRI, ultrasonography) may evaluate the lumbosacral spine, hip joint, sacroiliac joint, and other nearby structures. It is important to exclude rare but serious disease entities, such as malignancy, infection, vascular malformation, hematomas, and spondyloarthropathies. Electrodiagnostic testing may also be performed to localize a suspected sciatic neuropathy or to exclude radiculopathy or plexopathy.

X-Ray

Radiography is primarily utilized to assess for bony abnormalities that may contribute to back/gluteal pain, such as lumbar spondylolisthesis or hip osteoarthritis. There is no role for X-ray in the direct evaluation of the piriformis muscle or sciatic nerve.

Magnetic Resonance Imaging

Although MRI has been utilized to evaluate for anomalous anatomy of the piriformis and sciatic nerve, there are no set imaging criteria by which piriformis syndrome may be diagnosed. As with plain radiography, MRI is most useful for evaluating for other sources of pain, such as lumbosacral radiculopathy or bone stress injuries, and should be used to rule out other conditions before diagnosing a patient with piriformis syndrome. MRI evaluation of the piriformis syndrome and sciatic nerve may have a role in characterizing variable anatomy, although it is important to note that the presence of anatomic anomalies are not diagnostic of piriformis syndrome. Direct imaging of the sciatic nerve with high-resolution MR neurography may have some predictive value regarding responsiveness to surgical intervention.[21,22] Postinjection side-to-side differences in piriformis muscle volume and thickness have been reported in patients with symptomatic relief of gluteal pain from botulinum toxin injected into the piriformis muscle.[23] However, patients' clinical response to an intervention is most informative and largely supercedes the necessity of postinjection imaging.

Electrodiagnostic Studies (Electromyography/Nerve Conduction Studies)

Electrodiagnostic studies are most useful to evaluate for and rule out other causes of back/gluteal pain, such as lumbosacral radiculopathy, plexopathy, or sciatic neuropathy. However, various approaches to electrodiagnosis of piriformis syndrome have been suggested, including evoked potentials using an epidural recording electrode.[24] Electromyography (EMG) utilizing

invasive[25] and noninvasive[26] spinal nerve root stimulation has also been described in the literature but are not commonly performed.

Fishman's longitudinal study[7] proposed the use of peroneal or tibial H-reflex prolonged latencies in the FAIR position to diagnose piriformis syndrome (sensitivity 88%, specificity 83%) and to predict response to physical therapy. Patients with H-reflex latencies greater than three standard deviations above the latencies of asymptomatic controls were more likely to respond positively to treatment directed toward piriformis syndrome. Successful treatment was defined as at least 50% improvement on the Likert pain scale. The average percent improvement for patients with prolonged H-reflexes was 71%, as compared with 55% improvement in those with a normal H-reflex latency. Despite the large sample size (918 patients, 733 follow-ups), the results of this study are difficult to interpret because of its nonspecific inclusion criteria, lack of exclusion of patients with abnormal imaging findings, nonstandard electrodiagnostic protocol, lack of age-matched control H-reflex values, and variable treatment protocol.

Diagnostic Injection

Image-guided injection of the piriformis muscle with local anesthetic has been described using fluoroscopic and ultrasonographic approaches. These techniques are further described in the Interventional Options section. Upon successful injection into the piriformis muscle, the patient's pain is monitored for the duration of action of the local anesthetic. The patient's pain is more likely to be piriformis mediated if it is no longer present with provocative maneuvers (e.g., FAIR test).

Guide to the clinician

There is no "gold standard" diagnostic test for piriformis syndrome. X-ray, MRI, and EMG/nerve conduction studies may all be utilized in the workup of gluteal pain to evaluate for other conditions, such as lumbosacral radiculopathy or hip osteoarthritis. Image-guided diagnostic injection of the piriformis muscle may be used as a means of ruling in the syndrome when other diagnoses are ruled out, but there is limited supporting evidence for its specificity.

REHABILITATION OPTIONS

Rehabilitation of piriformis syndrome primarily involves stretching and range of motion exercises (adduction, internal rotation). Fishman's longitudinal study described a protocol for physical therapy that places the patient in a lumbosacral corset and positions him/her in the

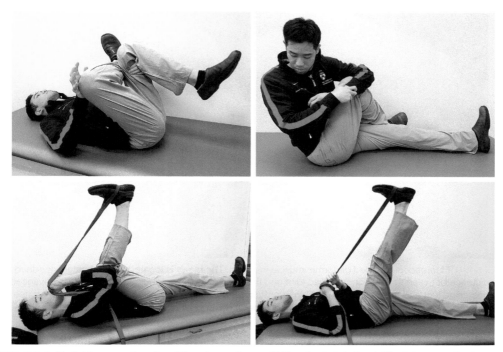

FIG. 24.4 Stretching exercises for piriformis syndrome. Piriformis stretch (top left); gluteus medius/piriformis stretch (top right); proximal hamstring stretch at starting (bottom left) and ending (bottom right) position.

contralateral decubitus and FAIR position.[7] The protocol recommends ultrasound treatment at 2.0–2.5 W/cm² for 10–14 min, heat or cold for 10 min, then manual stretching of the piriformis muscle. Of note, this protocol also includes myofascial release of the lumbar paraspinal muscles and therapeutic exercises per the McKenzie approach. Examples of common stretching exercises for the piriformis and associated gluteal musculature are depicted in Fig. 24.4.

Passive modalities and stretching are followed by progressive strengthening of the hip external rotators, abductors, and extensors to address any asymmetric loading of the piriformis muscle. Kinetic chain abnormalities and weakness of the core musculature (lumbopelvic-hip complex) should be addressed as well. Other possible treatments include foam rolling and massage therapy. Patients should trial these conservative measures before considering more invasive treatment options.

MEDICATION OPTIONS

In the acute phase of injury, nonsteroidal antiinflammatory drugs (NSAIDs) may be used for their analgesic and antiinflammatory properties. Muscle relaxants, with due caution, may be considered when there is evidence of muscle tightness. If the patient presents with neuropathic pain (e.g., burning sensation), neuropathic agents such as gabapentin may provide some relief. Although the abovementioned pharmacologic agents carry no specific evidence with respect to piriformis syndrome, they continue to be administered in the management of this condition with varying degrees of success. Opioids are generally not indicated in the treatment of piriformis syndrome.

INTERVENTIONAL OPTIONS

Image-guided piriformis injections of local anesthetic, steroid, or botulinum toxin have limited evidence for mild to moderate symptom improvement. However, methods described in the literature are inconsistent regarding the precise target for injection (i.e., muscle trigger point, nerve block, peritendinous).

Diagnostic Injection

The clinical use of a diagnostic injection of the piriformis muscle is described in the Diagnostic Testing section. In this section, we detail the fluoroscopic and ultrasonographic approaches.

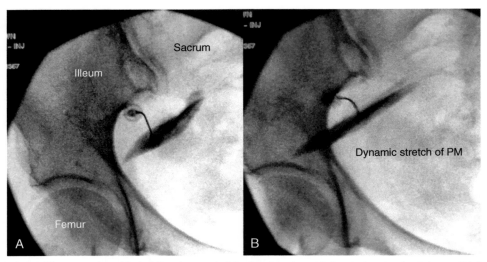

FIG. 24.5 Fluoroscopic-guided piriformis muscle injection. The target is located approximately one-third the distance between the inferior sacroiliac joint and the superolateral acetabulum. The needle is advanced to the posterior ilium and then withdrawn until the contrast pattern above is observed. Panel A demonstrates the desired contrast pattern and key landmarks. Panel B demonstrates a change in the contrast pattern when the muscle is placed in a stretched position. (Image credit: Richard Kinard, MD, used with permission.)

Fluoroscopy

Fluoroscopy may be used in the localization and intramuscular injection of the piriformis muscle. Gonzalez et al. detailed an approach utilizing the anteroposterior view of the pelvis and acetabulum in the prone position.[27] A marker is placed one-third of the distance between the most superolateral aspect of the acetabulum and the inferior aspect of the sacroiliac joint. The needle is advanced to the posterior ilium and then withdrawn 1–2 mm into the piriformis muscle belly. Needle placement may be confirmed with both contrast injection and/or electrical stimulation (Fig. 24.5).[27,28] The overall accuracy of fluoroscopy-guided intramuscular injections (without electrical stimulation) may be as low as 30%, with the most common unintended injection site being the gluteus maximus.[29]

Ultrasound imaging

Ultrasound imaging is the preferred image-guidance technique, as it allows for the direct and dynamic visualization of the piriformis muscle, sciatic nerve, and gluteal vessels. Using the posterior superior iliac spine and posterior inferior iliac spine as bony landmarks, the piriformis muscle may be identified in a longitudinal view when the transducer is just lateral to the sacrum. Before injection, the sciatic nerve should also be identified.[30] The needle trajectory is medial to lateral for a piriformis muscle sheath injection or an intramuscular injection (Fig. 24.6). Under dynamic ultrasound imaging, a sheath injection should demonstrate separation of the sheath from the muscle by the injectate. The use of electrical motor stimulation in addition to ultrasound guidance has also been described as a means of increasing accuracy.[31] In one cadaveric study, with all injections (20 ultrasound guided, 20 fluoroscopy guided) performed by a single experienced investigator, the accuracy of ultrasound-guided piriformis muscle injection was reported as superior (95%) compared with the accuracy of fluoroscopy-guided injection without electrical stimulation (30%).[29] One study that directly compared ultrasound guidance with fluoroscopic guidance with electrical stimulation found no significant difference in clinical outcomes.[32]

Therapeutic Injection
Trigger point

Trigger points are palpable "bands" or "nodules" of muscle tissue that are classically marked by referred pain and tenderness to palpation. Patients may have trigger points in the piriformis muscle itself or the surrounding musculature. If these points are present, they may be directly injected with local anesthetic with or without repeated needle fenestration of the muscle. Ideally, insertion of a needle into the trigger point should produce an involuntary local twitch response.

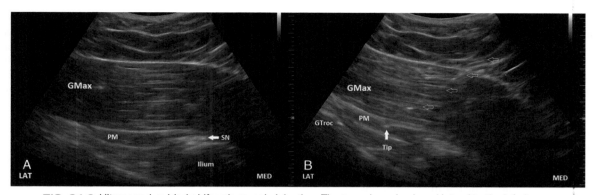

FIG. 24.6 Ultrasound-guided piriformis muscle injection. The transducer is placed lateral to the inferior sacrum, in line with the greater trochanter. The piriformis is observed deep to the gluteus maximus. After the sciatic nerve and gluteal vessels are identified, a needle is advanced in a medial (MED) to lateral (LAT) approach until it passes just through the hyperechoic muscle sheath. Panel A demonstrates key anatomy before injection. *GMax*, gluteus maximus; *PM*, piriformis muscle; *SN*, sciatic nerve. Panel B demonstrates the needle at the target. *GTroc*, greater trochanter; *open arrows*, needle trajectory; *Tip*, needle tip.

Corticosteroid

A limited number of studies describe the injection of corticosteroid medication near the sciatic nerve within the piriformis muscle. In particular, Benzon et al.[33] described a fluoroscopy-guided technique using the lower border of the sacroiliac joint as a point of reference, inserting the needle 0.4–3.0 cm lateral to and 0.5–2.0 cm caudal to this landmark. Electrical nerve stimulation guided the needle to a depth of 7.5–13 cm. Of 19 subjects injected with 40 mg methylprednisolone or 40 mg triamcinolone, 15 reported 75%–100% pain relief lasting 1–3 months (except for one subject who experienced only 3 h of relief). This technique may also be considered if true sciatic neuritis is suspected.

Botulinum toxin

Botulinum toxin injection to the piriformis muscle has been described in a handful of nonrandomized studies. Lang[34] utilized electromyographic guidance to inject 5000–10,000 units of botulinum toxin type B into 20 patients. Over the course of 16 weeks, "fair to excellent efficacy" was reported by 90% of the subjects, although the maximum average numerical improvement for buttock/hip pain was only 1.8 points on the visual analog scale (VAS). Yoon et al.[35] injected 20 subjects with 150 units of botulinum toxin type A under fluoroscopic guidance, reporting at least 50% of pain in 60%–65% of subjects by 8–12 weeks. Of note, nine control subjects were injected with dexamethasone and lidocaine, but this arm of the study was withdrawn after 4 weeks because of lack of improvement.

Guide to the clinician

When considering interventional options, ultrasound guidance is the preferred method over fluoroscopic guidance. Ultrasound imaging allows for the direct and dynamic visualization of relevant structures and may be performed in the office/clinic setting without exposure to ionizing radiation. The accuracy of ultrasound-guided piriformis injection is excellent (95%). Depending on the presentation, the injection target may be a trigger point (using local anesthetic), perisciatic nerve (using steroid), or intramuscular (using botulinum toxin).

SURGICAL OPTIONS

Open and endoscopic approaches to piriformis release with or without neurolysis have been described. The evidence is limited to small studies with carefully selected populations. Generally, open approaches have fallen out of favor, as endoscopic techniques have improved. Of particular interest, Dezawa et al.[36] described a technique for the endoscopic release of the piriformis muscle under local anesthesia. In addition to incising the piriformis muscle at the myotendinous junction, neurolysis of the sciatic nerve was also performed. Performing this surgical intervention under local anesthesia allowed for intraoperative testing for tenderness by direct palpation of the piriformis muscle. However, this study is limited by small sample size (six patients, eight limbs) and lack of follow-up beyond immediate postoperative assessment of symptoms with passive flexion and internal rotation of the hip.

Park et al.[37] reported statistically significant improvement in the mean VAS score from 7.4 to 2.6 after endoscopic sciatic nerve decompression. Release of the nerve was accomplished by radiofrequency cautery of fibrovascular scar bands and splitting the tendinous portion of the piriformis muscle and also the obturator internus and quadriceps femoris muscles. Restrictions included partial weight bearing at postoperative day 1 and full weight bearing at 3 weeks, and no significant adverse events were reported. However, severe sciatic nerve injury has been described as a possible complication of surgical intervention,[38] as well as scar tissue formation leading to the return of symptoms.[39]

PROGNOSIS

The difficulty with treating piriformis syndrome lies in the accurate diagnosis of this disorder. Prognosis is generally favorable, as the symptoms largely improve with conservative measures, such as physical therapy and pharmacologic therapy.

SUMMARY

The spectrum of piriformis syndrome ranges from myofascial to neuropathic variants. In patients presenting with gluteal pain, the differential diagnosis includes various spine, hip, and pelvis conditions. Examination maneuvers that preferentially activate or stretch the piriformis muscle are useful; however, piriformis syndrome is ultimately a diagnosis of exclusion. The workup often includes diagnostic studies (e.g., MRI, EMG) to evaluate for other conditions. There is limited evidence supporting image-guided injections of the piriformis muscle to establish the diagnosis.

Piriformis syndrome generally responds well to conservative measures. Physical therapy is the mainstay of treatment and should focus on stretching the piriformis muscle, core muscle strengthening of lumbopelvic stability, kinetic chain analysis to optimize biomechanics, and ergonomic training.[40,41] Pharmacologic agents may also be used, typically NSAIDs or muscle relaxants. Although it is less common for patients to receive an injection and rare to require surgical intervention, these have been described in the literature.

CONCLUSION

Piriformis syndrome is an entity that encompasses a spectrum of etiologies, from myofascial to neuropathic. Although the evidence for treatment is limited or mixed in the literature, the overall prognosis for this condition is favorable with physical therapy and correction of biomechanical deficits. Therapeutic injections, although uncommon, are safe to consider in assisting with the healing process. Surgical intervention is rarely indicated. Our above-proposed criteria may provide the clinician a basis for clinically relevant diagnosis and evidence-based treatment.

REFERENCES

1. Pace JB, Nagle D. Piriform syndrome. *West J Med.* 1976; 124(6):435–439.
2. Papadopoulos EC, Khan SN. Piriformis syndrome and low back pain: a new classification and review of the literature. *Orthop Clin N Am.* 2004;35(1):65–71.
3. Natsis K, et al. Anatomical variations between the sciatic nerve and the piriformis muscle: a contribution to surgical anatomy in piriformis syndrome. *Surg Radiol Anat.* 2014;36(3):273–280.
4. Kirschner JS, Foye PM, Cole JL. Piriformis syndrome, diagnosis and treatment. *Muscle Nerve.* 2009;40(1):10–18.
5. Gest TR, Schlesinger J. *MedCharts: Anatomy.* New York: ILOC Inc; 1995.
6. Cassidy L, et al. Piriformis syndrome: implications of anatomical variations, diagnostic techniques, and treatment options. *Surg Radiol Anat.* 2012;34(6):479–486.
7. Fishman LM, et al. Piriformis syndrome: diagnosis, treatment, and outcome–a 10-year study. *Arch Phys Med Rehabil.* 2002;83(3):295–301.
8. Borden JN. The Lasègue test. *JAMA.* 1967;201(8):641.
9. Freiberg AH, Vinke TH. Sciatica and the sacro-iliac joint. *J Bone Joint Surg.* 1934;16(1):126–136.
10. Beatty RA. The piriformis muscle syndrome: a simple diagnostic maneuver. *Neurosurgery.* 1994;34(3):512–514. Discussion 514.
11. Mixter WJ, Barr JS. Rupture of the intervertebral disc with involvement of the spinal canal. *N Engl J Med.* 1934;211(5): 210–215.
12. Yeoman W. The relation of arthritis of the sacro-iliac joint to sciatica, with an analysis of 100 cases. *Lancet.* 1928; 212(5492):1119–1123.
13. Beaton LE, Anson BJ. The sciatic nerve and the piriformis muscle: their interrelation a possible cause of coccygodynia. *J Bone Joint Surg.* 1938;20(3):686–688.
14. Robinson DR. Pyriformis syndrome in relation to sciatic pain. *Am J Surg.* 1947;73(3):355–358.
15. Stewart JD. The piriformis syndrome is overdiagnosed. *Muscle Nerve.* 2003;28(5):644–646.
16. Fishman LM. *Piriformis Syndrome: A Pain in the…Back.* The Huffington Post; 2011. Available from: http://www.huffingtonpost.com/loren-fishman-md/piriformis-syndrome-back-pain_b_845270.html.
17. Gomez-Hoyos J, et al. Accuracy of 2 clinical tests for ischiofemoral impingement in patients with posterior hip pain and endoscopically confirmed diagnosis. *Arthroscopy.* 2016;32(7):1279–1284.

18. Puniello MS. Iliotibial band tightness and medial patellar glide in patients with patellofemoral dysfunction. *J Orthop Sports Phys Ther*. 1993;17(3):144–148.

19. Noble CA. Iliotibial band friction syndrome in runners. *Am J Sports Med*. 1980;8(4):232–234.

20. Drampalos E, et al. Intrapiriformis lipoma: an unusual cause of piriformis syndrome. *Eur Spine J*. 2015;24(suppl 4): S551–S554.

21. Filler AG, et al. Sciatica of nondisc origin and piriformis syndrome: diagnosis by magnetic resonance neurography and interventional magnetic resonance imaging with outcome study of resulting treatment. *J Neurosurg Spine*. 2005;2(2): 99–115.

22. Kraus E, et al. Piriformis syndrome with variant sciatic nerve anatomy: a case report. *PM R*. 2016;8(2):176–179.

23. Al-Al-Shaikh M, et al. An MRI evaluation of changes in piriformis muscle morphology induced by botulinum toxin injections in the treatment of piriformis syndrome. *Diagn Interv Imaging*. 2015;96(1):37–43.

24. Nakamura H, et al. Piriformis syndrome diagnosed by cauda equina action potentials: report of two cases. *Spine (Phila Pa 1976)*. 2003;28(2):E37–E40.

25. Chang CW, Lien IN. Spinal nerve stimulation in the diagnosis of lumbosacral radiculopathy. *Am J Phys Med Rehabil*. 1990;69(6):318–322.

26. Chang CW, et al. Measurement of motor nerve conduction velocity of the sciatic nerve in patients with piriformis syndrome: a magnetic stimulation study. *Arch Phys Med Rehabil*. 2006;87(10):1371–1375.

27. Gonzalez P, et al. Confirmation of needle placement within the piriformis muscle of a cadaveric specimen using anatomic landmarks and fluoroscopic guidance. *Pain Physician*. 2008;11(3):327–331.

28. Betts A. Combined fluoroscopic and nerve stimulator technique for injection of the piriformis muscle. *Pain Physician*. 2004;7(2):279–281.

29. Finnoff JT, Hurdle MF, Smith J. Accuracy of ultrasound-guided versus fluoroscopically guided contrast-controlled piriformis injections: a cadaveric study. *J Ultrasound Med*. 2008;27(8):1157–1163.

30. Smith J, et al. Ultrasound-guided piriformis injection: technique description and verification. *Arch Phys Med Rehabil*. 2006;87(12):1664–1667.

31. Huerto AP, Yeo SN, Ho KY. Piriformis muscle injection using ultrasonography and motor stimulation–report of a technique. *Pain Physician*. 2007;10(5):687–690.

32. Fowler IM, et al. A randomized comparison of the efficacy of 2 techniques for piriformis muscle injection: ultrasound-guided versus nerve stimulator with fluoroscopic guidance. *Reg Anesth Pain Med*. 2014;39(2):126–132.

33. Benzon HT, et al. Piriformis syndrome: anatomic considerations, a new injection technique, and a review of the literature. *Anesthesiology*. 2003;98(6):1442–1448.

34. Lang AM. Botulinum toxin type B in piriformis syndrome. *Am J Phys Med Rehabil*. 2004;83(3):198–202.

35. Yoon SJ, et al. Low-dose botulinum toxin type A for the treatment of refractory piriformis syndrome. *Pharmacotherapy*. 2007;27(5):657–665.

36. Dezawa A, Kusano S, Miki H. Arthroscopic release of the piriformis muscle under local anesthesia for piriformis syndrome. *Arthroscopy*. 2003;19(5):554–557.

37. Park MS, et al. Clinical results of endoscopic sciatic nerve decompression for deep gluteal syndrome: mean 2-year follow-up. *BMC Musculoskelet Disord*. 2016;17:218.

38. Justice PE, et al. Piriformis syndrome surgery causing severe sciatic nerve injury. *J Clin Neuromuscul Dis*. 2012;14(1):45–47.

39. Kobbe P, Zelle BA, Gruen GS. Case report: recurrent piriformis syndrome after surgical release. *Clin Orthop Relat Res*. 2008;466(7):1745–1748.

40. Seidenberg P, Bowen JD. *The Hip and Pelvis in Sports Medicine and Primary Care*. Springer; 2010.

41. Willson JD, et al. Core stability and its relationship to lower extremity function and injury. *J Am Acad Orthop Surg*. 2005;13(5):316–325.

Index

Note: Page numbers followed by "f" indicate figures, "t" indicate tables and "b" indicate boxes.

International Association for Study
of Pain (IASP), 31, 37, 37b, 129,
178
International Classification of Disease
(ICD), 12–13
ICD 10, 12–13
International Classification of
Headache Disorders (ICHD), 146,
177
International Classification of
Headaches Beta 3 (ICHD 3-β), 146,
177–178, 182
taxonomy, 147
TN criteria from, 178b, 185b
Interscalene triangle, 187
Interstitial cystitis, 13
Interventional pain management, 65,
93
Intraarticular hip pathology, 209
Intramuscular
botulinum toxin injection, 150
electrical stimulation, 161–162
injection, 212
of methylcobalamin combined
with lidocaine, 101
Intranasal administration, 57
Intrathecal (IT)
baclofen, 140–141, 172
drug delivery, 172
medication, 72–73
medicine, 140–141
pain, 72–73
ziconotide, 140–141
Intravenous (IV), 107
infusion, 69
medications, 140
Intravenous immunoglobulin (IVIG),
84–85
Intravenous regional anesthesia
(IVRA), 68
Ipsilateral arm, 129
Irritability condition, 45–46
IRT. See Infrared thermography (IRT)
Ischial bursitis, 209
Ischial tuberosity, 209
Ischiofemoral impingement syndrome,
209
Isoniazid, 80
Isosorbide dinitrate spray, 84
IT band syndrome. See Iliotibial band
syndrome (IT band syndrome)
IV. See Intravenous (IV)
IVIG. See Intravenous immunoglobulin
(IVIG)
IVRA. See Intravenous regional
anesthesia (IVRA)

K

Ketamine, 58–60, 69, 130
adverse effects, 69
Ketoprofen, 54t
Ketorolac, 54t
Kinesthesia, 10

L

Lacosamide, 82
Lacosamine, 83b
Lamotrigine, 82, 83b, 138–139, 156,
170
LAPS. See Limbically augmented pain
syndrome (LAPS)
Lasègue maneuver, 207
Laser Doppler flowmetry, 66–67
"Latency" characteristic to neuropathic
pain, 46
Lenalidomide, 60
Levetiracetam, 138–139
Levorphanol, 17
Lhermitte phenomenon, 169
Lidocaine, 59, 84, 93, 158, 162
cream or patch, 83b
Limbically augmented pain syndrome
(LAPS), 13
α-Lipoic acid, 83b, 84
Lithium, 139
Long-term potentiation (LTP), 11
LSB. See Lumbar sympathetic chain
(LSB)
Lumbar pain syndromes after TBI,
150–151
Lumbar spondylolisthesis, 210
Lumbar sympathetic chain (LSB),
65–66, 67f
Lumbosacral radiculopathy, 205–207,
210
Lumpectomy, 113
Lyme disease, neurologic
manifestations of, 105–106, 106b
Lyme encephalomyelitis, 105
Lyme neuroborreliosis, 105
Lymphedema, 113–114
Lymphocytic meningitis, 105

M

Magnetic resonance arthrography
(MRA), 160–161
Magnetic resonance imaging (MRI),
41, 159, 181, 210
of brachial plexus, 190
T2-weighted images, 200–201
Mastectomy, 113
McGill Pain, 21
Mechano-heat-insensitive
C-fibers, 32
Mechanoreception, 10
Medicinal marijuana, 171–172
Meloxicam, 54t
Memantine, 59
Meningoencephalitis, 199
MES. See Myalgic encephalomyelitis
(MES)
Metabolic disorders, 79–80
Methacholine, 42
Methadone, 58
Methotrexate, 11–12
N-Methyl-D-aspartate. See N-methyl-D-
aspartic acid (NMDA)

N-Methyl-D-aspartic acid (NMDA),
11, 58
antagonists, 58–59
receptor antagonist, 69
neurotransmitter, 32–33
Methylprednisolone, 54t
Michigan Neuropathy Screening
Instrument (MNSI), 78, 79t
Michigan Neuropathy Symptom
Inventory, 81
Microglia, 11
Microvascular decompression (MVD),
183–184
Microvascular impairment, 80
Migraine Disability Assessment score,
146
Milnacipran, 14–16
Milnaxipran, 83b
Mind-body strategies, 26–27
Mindfulness therapy, 148–149
Minnesota Multiphasic Personality
Inventory, 21
Mirror therapy, 24–25, 157–158
Mirror visual feedback (MVF), 23–25
Miscellaneous medications, 140
MNSI. See Michigan Neuropathy
Screening Instrument (MNSI)
Mobilization, 26–27
Mononeuritis multiplex, 199–200
MOR. See μ Opioid receptor (MOR)
Morphine sulfate, 83b
Morphine3-glucoronide, 11–12
Motivational-affective processing, 3b
Motor cortex stimulation, 150, 184
Motor dysfunction, 37
Motor extinction, 24
Motor imagery plan, 24–25
Motor unit potentials (MUPs),
190–191
MRA. See Magnetic resonance
arthrography (MRA)
MRI. See Magnetic resonance imaging
(MRI)
MS pain. See Multiple sclerosis pain
(MS pain)
Multidimensional systems related to
processing nociceptive stimuli, 3b
Multifocal motor neuropathy, 199–200
Multiple sclerosis pain (MS pain),
167. See also Complex regional pain
syndrome (CRPS); Pain
classification, 167–168, 168f
epidemiology, 168
evaluation, 168–169
management
interventional, 172
nonpharmacologic, 169–170
pharmacologic, 170–172
MUPs. See Motor unit potentials
(MUPs)
Musculoskeletal injuries, 145–146
MVD. See Microvascular
decompression (MVD)